Neighbourhood Structure and Health Promotion

Christiane Stock • Anne Ellaway
Editors

Neighbourhood Structure and Health Promotion

Springer

Editors
Christiane Stock
Unit for Health Promotion Research
University of Southern Denmark
Esbjerg, Denmark

Anne Ellaway
MRC Social & Public Health Sciences Unit
University of Glasgow
Glasgow, UK

ISBN 978-1-4614-6671-0 ISBN 978-1-4614-6672-7 (eBook)
DOI 10.1007/978-1-4614-6672-7
Springer New York Heidelberg Dordrecht London

Library of Congress Control Number: 2013931258

Printed on acid-free paper

Springer is part of Springer Science+Business Media (www.springer.com)

Contents

Contributors

Ursula Berger Department of Medical Informatics, Biostatistics and Epidemiology (IBE), Ludwig-Maximilians-University Munich, München, Germany

Kim Bloomfield Center for Alcohol and Drug Research, School of Business and Social Science, Aarhus University, Copenhagen S, Denmark

Fiona Crawford Glasgow Centre for Population Health, Glasgow, Scotland

Sanne I. de Vries Department of Life Style, Netherlands Organisation for Applied Scientific Research (TNO), Leiden, The Netherlands

Bo Ejstrud Institute of History and Civilization, University of Southern Denmark, Esbjerg, Denmark

Anne Ellaway MRC Social and Public Health Sciences Unit, University of Glasgow, Glasgow, Scotland, UK

Carol Emslie Institute for Applied Health Research, School of Health & Life Sciences, Glasgow Caledonian University, Glasgow, UK

Neil Ferguson Department of Civil Engineering, University of Strathclyde, Glasgow, UK

Katherine L. Frohlich Département de médecine sociale et préventive, Université de Montréal (IRSPUM), Montréal, QC, Canada

Ulrike Grittner Department for Biostatistics and Clinical Epidemiology, Charité-University Medicine, Berlin, Germany

Carlijn Kamphuis Department of Public Health, Erasmus University Medical Centre, Rotterdam, The Netherlands

Karen Lamb MRC Social and Public Health Sciences Unit, University of Glasgow, Glasgow, Scotland, UK

Eva Ladekjær Larsen Unit for Health Promotion Research, University of Southern Denmark, Esbjerg, Denmark

Jolanda Maas Department of Public and Occupational Health, EMGO + Institute, VU Medical Center, Amsterdam, The Netherlands

Mathias Meijer National Institute of Public Health, University of Southern Denmark, København K, Denmark

David Ogilvie UKCRC Centre for Diet and Activity Research (CEDAR), Institute of Public Health, Cambridge, UK

Frank Pierik Department of Urban Environment and Safety, Netherlands Organisation for Applied Scientific Research (TNO), Utrecht, The Netherlands

Oliver Razum Department of Epidemiology and International Public Health, School of Public Health, Bielefeld University, Bielefeld, Germany

Jasper Schipperijn Institute of Sports Science and Clinical Biomechanics, University of Southern Denmark, Odense M, Denmark

Martine Shareck Département de médecine sociale et préventive, Université de Montréal, Montréal, QC, Canada

Reinier P. Sterkenburg Department of Urban Environment and Safety, Netherlands Organisation for Applied Scientific Research (TNO), Delft, The Netherlands

Christiane Stock Unit for Health Promotion Research, Institute of Public Health, University of Southern Denmark, Esbjerg, Denmark

Chalida Svastisalee National Institute of Public Health, University of Southern Denmark, Copenhagen, Denmark

Metropolitan University College, Pustervig 8, 1126 Copenhagen K, Denmark

Pernille Tanggaard Andersen Unit for Health Promotion Research, Institute of Public Health, University of Southern Denmark, Esbjerg, Denmark

Jens Troelsen Institute of Sports Science and Clinical Biomechanics, University of Southern Denmark, Odense M, Denmark

Frank van Lenthe Department of Public Health, Erasmus University Medical Centre, Rotterdam, The Netherlands

Sven Voigtländer Section on Quality of Health Care, Health Economics, Health System Analysis, Bavarian Health and Food Safety Authority, Erlangen, Germany

Department of Epidemiology and International Public Health, School of Public Health, Bielefeld University, Bielefeld, Germany

Chapter 1
Neighbourhood Structure and Health Promotion: An Introduction

Christiane Stock and Anne Ellaway

Introduction to the Theme

A growing body of literature suggests that neighbourhood context may affect the health and health behaviours of adults and young people. It has been hypothesised that socially disadvantaged areas may induce health risks either directly (e.g. air pollution) or more indirectly, through the ability to lead a healthy life. For example, poorer areas may have poorer social and material infrastructure (e.g. fewer local amenities), although this may vary by local and national context and by the neighbourhood resources examined. Beyond neighbourhood features resulting from social deprivation it is also relevant to determine which characteristics of the physical environment promote or discourage healthy lifestyles such as the availability of parks and green spaces, traffic infrastructure, housing characteristics etc. While geographic information systems can be used to provide objective data on the physical environment and neighbourhood structure, individuals' perceptions of their social environment are also important to understand their lifestyle choices. Therefore data on subjective factors, such as peoples' perceptions (e.g. the extent to which it is attractive and safe) of their neighbourhood and the quality of facilities that might encourage them to develop and maintain health-relevant behaviours are also highly relevant.

C. Stock(✉)
Unit for Health Promotion Research, Institute of Public Health,
University of Southern Denmark, Niels Bohrs Vej 9-10, 6700 Esbjerg, Denmark
e-mail: cstock@health.sdu.dk

A. Ellaway
MRC Social and Public Health Sciences Unit, University of Glasgow,
4 Lilybank Gardens, Glasgow G12 8RZ, Scotland, UK
e-mail: anne@sphsu.mrc.ac.uk

C. Stock and A. Ellaway (eds.), *Neighbourhood Structure and Health Promotion*,
DOI 10.1007/978-1-4614-6672-7_1, © Springer Science+Business Media New York 2013

This chapter provides an overview over the content of the book "Neighbourhood Structure and Health Promotion" that is organised into three main parts (1) understanding health as a matter of place, (2) measuring and monitoring neighbourhood structure and (3) neighbourhoods and lifestyle. Taking different perspectives on neighbourhood characteristics and different analytical methods to measure them into account, this book addresses several questions: Which theories and sociological perspectives are relevant to understand how people interact with their neighbourhood? What are innovative, qualitative and quantitative methods for assessing neighbourhood structures and health resources? How does the social and physical structure of neighbourhoods affect a person's ability to maintain a healthy lifestyle? Do neighbourhood influences contribute to social and/or gender inequalities in health? What can we learn from this research to develop health promotion interventions addressing neighbourhoods as well as people?

About this Book

The idea for this book was born during the European Public Health Conference in Amsterdam 2011, where Christiane Stock and Thomas Abel organised a workshop on the topic of neighbourhood structure and health promotion as activity of the health promotion section of the European Public Health Association (EUPHA). Around the workshop, lively discussions about the recent research in Europe arose leading finally to the idea to publish this book. The intention with this book is to addresses theoretical models and pathways through which neighbourhood factors potentially affect health and the ability to lead a healthy life. It also aims to provide information on relevant as well as innovative methods and techniques to study and analyse neighbourhood structure. It specifically summarises present knowledge on the contribution of neighbourhood factors in shaping lifestyle and health-relevant behaviours. The book not only focuses on analysing the relationship between neighbourhood structure and health behaviour of different population groups but also putst an emphasis on the health promotion, policy and intervention implications of this research. We acknowledge that important research on area effects on health has been conducted in the United States, New Zealand or Australia. However, conclusions from this research may not be valid in the European context with different political, economic and social environments as well as different data sources available. The aim was therefore to put a focus on the European setting, and most of the chapters build on examples from European studies. We feel confident that the material presented in this volume will prove a suitable and timely tool for researchers, policy makers, practitioners and teachers who wish to explore and apply this approach in the European context. The book is organised into three parts.

Part 1: Understanding Health as a Matter of Place

This part of the book lays the basis for the relationship between neighbourhood and health by summarising the existing ideas and concepts about the potential influence and its underlying causal pathways. This is done through a number of chapters that provide the reader with theoretical knowledge relevant to study neighbourhood influences on health and health behaviour of residents.

The chapters in this first part of the book are mainly focused on exploring different theoretical approaches to understanding neighbourhood effects on health.

In Chap. 2, Meijer provides an overview of existing research in social epidemiology on area effects, focusing on mortality as an outcome. Drawing on 40 multilevel studies from throughout the world, the results from a meta-analysis show that the relative risk of all-cause mortality is 1.07 among those living in deprived neighbourhoods compared to those living in more affluent areas. Meijer outlines the models and pathways through which neighbourhood factors potentially affect various health outcomes, examining factors such as income inequality, air pollution and the welfare models in different countries and assesses their area-level effects on health. This chapter ends with a proposed theoretical model which suggest that neighbourhoods are connected to mortality through four distinct pathways: health policy and health resources, health behaviour, perceptions of neighbourhood and the physical quality of an area.

This part of the book is laying the basis for the relationship between neighbourhood and health by summarising the existing ideas and concepts about the potential influence and its underlying causal pathways. This is done through a number of chapters that provide the reader with theoretical knowledge relevant to study neighbourhood influences on health and health behaviour of residents.

In Chap. 3, Frohlich draws on social theorists such as Weber and Bourdieu to provide an overview on the distinction between behaviour, lifestyle and collective lifestyles, placing particular emphasis on the role of social constraints and opportunities in shaping individual behaviour. Building on this, Frohlich explores the concepts of environmental and spatial justice and their implication for research, policy and practice. A novel theoretical framework is then outlined which addresses some of these issues.

In Chap. 4, Andersen outlines the ways in which sociological theory can contribute to a deeper understanding on the complexities of individuals' everyday lives in community settings. In doing so, this chapter complements Chap. 3 by drawing on other social theorists such as Schultz (who explored the importance of the norms, assumptions and behaviour of everyday life), Durkheim and Putnam on the concept of social capital and Goffman's notion of social stigma. Anderson then goes on to describe the application of a specific sociological analysis of a health promotion initiative in a deprived neighbourhood in Denmark.

The final chapter in this section is Chap. 5, written by Larsen, and the main purpose of this chapter is to provide a theoretical overview of the interaction between people and place. Drawing on anthropological theory and case studies, the chapter addresses three key issues (1) how social relationships are practised in public places,

(2) how people culturally construct meanings of places and (3) how public places shape human behaviour. The chapter ends by suggesting that the dialectic relationship between people and place are relevant perspectives for understanding how people relate to their neighbourhood and how neighbourhood architecture invites residents to socially interact and how this might be important for creating healthy neighbourhoods.

Part 2: Measuring and Monitoring Neighbourhood Structure

In this part of the book, the chapters are mainly concerned with the various ways in which neighbourhood structure can be measured and analysed.

In Chap. 6, Voigtländer, Berger and Razum examine the challenges facing the study of neighbourhood conditions on health. Issues that present a challenge include the delineation of neighbourhoods, the importance of examining both the sociodemographic composition of the population as well as the amenities in the neighbourhood, the non random distribution of people to places, the differential impact of particular neighbourhood features on particular groups, the importance of studying neighbourhood effects across the life course and finally the effect of changes to the material and social infrastructure of particular places over time. The authors provide an overview of the quantitative and qualitative methods required to address these challenges and apply these methods to a theoretical framework linking social position, neighbourhood environment and health.

In Chap. 7, Ellaway, Ferguson, Lamb and Ogilvie provide a brief overview of the existing literature on the importance of the built environment to obesity and examines how local facilities, such as physical activity amenities, are distributed across different sorts of neighbourhoods. The issue of access to these facilities using different forms of transport (walking, cycling, bus or car) is explored using data from a Scotland-wide study.

In Chap. 8, Schipperijn, Ejstrud and Troelsen introduce geographical information systems (GIS) and their application to research on area effects on health. An overview of the benefits and limitations of GIS for this research theme is provided and an application of GIS to a range of Danish data sets on health is described.

Another new technological development which is increasingly being used in the study of neighbourhoods and health, global positioning systems (GPS) is described by Maas, Sterkenburg, de Vries and Pierik in Chap. 9. While most of the existing research uses relatively general descriptions of neighbourhood characteristics, GPS provides a new approach to study the interaction between a neighbourhood and its residents in the analysis of area of residence on health and health behaviours. The chapter describes the opportunities, as well as the limitations, that the use of GPS devices offers to study this type of interaction. It also outlines the potential of using new methods and gives recommendations for future research.

In Chap. 10, Grittner and Bloomfield explore the use of the statistical technique, multilevel modelling, in the study of neighbourhoods and health. As the authors note, most of the research studying neighbourhood effects on health aims to adjust for individual socio-economic factors in the analysis, and this requires the use of multilevel modelling as data are nested at different levels (e.g. individuals and areas). The authors provide practical guidance on how to apply multilevel modelling to this type of research and how to best present the results of the analysis.

Part 3: Neighbourhood and Lifestyle

In this section, the chapters focus on specific health behaviours such as alcohol use, smoking and obesity-related behaviours such as dietary intake and physical activity and the influence of different neighbourhood spaces in these behaviours.

In Chap. 11, Maas outlines the evidence on the overall health effects of green spaces on health. She discusses the potential pathways through which existing associations can be explained, while putting a special emphasis on the role of physical activity. The chapter finishes by applying findings from existing research in the Netherlands and beyond to the development and implementation of urban health policies and health promotion interventions.

In Chap. 12, Kamphuis and van Lenthe examine the ways in which neighbourhood factors may influence socio-economic differences in physical activity. Through the application of theoretical models such as the Theory of Planned Behaviour, Kamphuis and van Lenthe describe findings from their studies in the Netherlands on participation in sports and walking for recreation and the role of subjective and objective neighbourhood characteristics.

Chapter 13 by Troelsen outlines the role of physical characteristics of the neighbourhood in influencing levels of physical activity and the part played by different approaches to city planning, landscaping, traffic regulation and health policies in different contexts. The chapter describes new approaches to health promotion such as 'nudge' theory and outlines a theoretical model through which physical activity can be encouraged by means of activating space and land use.

In Chap. 14, Shareck and Frohlich review the literature on area effects and social inequities in smoking among young people. They present a health promotion perspective which involves two key principles: the notion that health is produced in everyday life environments (home, work, study and play) and an explicit focus on equity. Shareck and Frohlich end by describing how they have applied this perspective to an ongoing research project on smoking among young people in Montreal.

In Chap. 15, Bloomfield and Stock provide an overview of the existing research on area effects on alcohol and drug use among different population groups and outline the potential and limitations of health promotion and prevention measures aiming at changes in neighbourhood context and resources.

For a number of years, there has been interest in understanding how to successfully promote healthy nutrition in different population groups and whether and how place and income affect nutritional attitudes and behaviour. In Chap. 16, Crawford provides an overview of the existing research on area effects on food choices and nutrition among different population groups and discusses health promotion and prevention measures aiming at changes in neighbourhood context and resources.

Due to the urgency in global health agendas to create community-based and coordinated policies to address obesity in children, in Chap. 17 Swastisalee highlights several primary research study areas aimed at examining built environments surrounding schools and associations with dietary behaviour, active transport, physical activity and obesity. In closing, this chapter addresses the potential contributions of school environments within obesity prevention policy.

In Chap. 18, Ellaway and Emslie review the literature on gender differences in environmental perception. They focus then on two health behaviours (smoking cigarettes and drinking alcohol) in order to explore how relationships between gender, space and smoking and drinking vary across contexts and by scale.

In the concluding chapter of the book, Stock summarises in Chap. 19 the existing knowledge from neighbourhoods and health behaviour studies and discusses how this research can inform policy and health promotion practice. By providing examples from existing programmes aimed at reducing health inequalities between richer and poorer neighbourhoods, Stock suggests the way forward from intervention research to the policy and practice of health promotion.

Limitations

A relevant limitation to mention is that the contributions in this book are mainly from European authors and from Canada. Although we acknowledge that significant contributions to this the field of neighbourhood and health research originates from the USA, New Zealand or Australia, it was the intention of this book to focus on European examples. Although this is a limitation in terms of geographical coverage, such limitation is also necessary because the political and economic context in Europe differs substantially from the USA or other parts of the world.

Even within Europe do political systems and economies show large differences. Some of the Southern European countries are heavily hit by the financial crisis, and some Eastern European countries are still in transition from former socialist economies and governmental structures. This book is unable to cover all the differences in political contexts as it mainly presents examples from the Northern and Western part of Europe (e.g. Scotland, the Netherlands, Denmark and Germany).

This book aimed at not only focusing on analysing the relationship between neighbourhood structure and the health behaviour but also at putting an emphasis on the health promotion, policy and intervention implications of this research. We admit that in most of the chapters the analysis part is still much larger than the intervention and health promotion practice part. This reflects the existing research and knowledge available, which is still sparse in the area of neighbourhood-level interventions.

Conclusions

We hope that this book will be useful for many readers as it covers a very broad range of topics that are relevant to the study of neighbourhoods and health promotion—from the practical application of appropriate techniques to discussing findings which have implications for the development of policy and practice. In particular is our hope that the book will inform further research but even more health promotion practice using environmental and contextual approaches. In line with Lawrence Green's words that "if we want more evidence-based practice, we need more practice-based evidence" (Green 2006), we would like to stimulate multi-sectoral approaches in order to improve the health conditions of neighbourhoods and residential areas and at the same time encourage effectiveness studies and evaluation research around such approaches.

Reference

Green, L. (2006, June). *If we want more evidence-based practice, we need more practice-based evidence: External validity and health promotion research.* 5th Nordic Health Promotion Research Conference, Esbjerg, Denmark

Part I
Understanding Health as a Matter of Place

Chapter 2
Neighbourhood Context and Mortality: An Overview

Mathias Meijer

Introduction

Does where people live affect their health? This question has occupied an increasing number of public health researchers since the 1990s and has resulted in an equally increasing amount of literature. Ever since the first epidemiological neighbourhood studies emerged, the association between neighbourhood characteristics and mortality has received most attention.

The first objective of this chapter is to evaluate the current body of evidence of this association. Several reviews exist on this topic (Ellen et al. 2001; Pickett and Pearl 2001; Riva et al. 2007; Yen et al. 2009; Nandi and Kawachi 2011), but not all were able to isolate neighbourhood effects from individual effects and to account for the hierarchical data structure because they were not restricted to multilevel studies controlling for individual socioeconomic status. In this chapter, focus will be set on reporting from a systematic review with these inclusion criteria and subsequently on presenting results from a meta-analysis estimating the association between area-level socioeconomic status (ALSES) and all-cause mortality. It will also be specified how gender, age, type of welfare state regime and other covariates influence results.

The second objective of the chapter is to identify pathways between neighbourhood characteristics and geographic patterns in mortality. Often the hypothesised pathways from, e.g. the socioeconomic status of areas to mortality are not accounted for in published studies. However, a common understanding has emerged saying that neighbourhoods expose people to sets of social and physical characteristics,

M. Meijer (✉)
National Institute of Public Health, University of Southern Denmark,
Øster Farimagsgade 5A 2., 1353 København K, Denmark
e-mail: matm@si-folkesundhed.dk; matm@niph.dk

C. Stock and A. Ellaway (eds.), *Neighbourhood Structure and Health Promotion*,
DOI 10.1007/978-1-4614-6672-7_2, © Springer Science+Business Media New York 2013

which influence the ability to lead a healthy life and results in variation in morbidity and, ultimately, mortality. Nevertheless, the mechanisms between neighbourhood residence and individual health remain less clear.

Are Characteristics of the Neighbourhood of Residence Associated with Mortality?

Earlier reviews have consistently reported how social and physical neighbourhood features are associated with mortality. The first two reviews appeared in 2001 and concluded that neighbourhood characteristics were modestly associated with individual mortality (Ellen et al. 2001; Pickett and Pearl 2001). Possibly due to the limited number of studies conducted at the time these conclusions were partly drawn from ecological and non-multilevel studies. At this early stage, a number of methodological challenges were identified. Most importantly, it was discussed how neighbourhoods should be defined, how neighbourhood influences should be measured, how confounding factors should be eliminated and the importance of using multilevel modelling. Later reviews benefited from the increasing numbers of multilevel studies. They echoed the prior methodological concerns but concluded that there was consistent evidence for associations between neighbourhood characteristics and individual health (Nandi and Kawachi 2011; Riva et al. 2007; Yen et al. 2009).

In the systematic review reported in this chapter studies were included if they used multilevel modelling and evaluated the association between area characteristics and mortality or cancer incidence while controlling for individual demographic and socioeconomic factors. 40 studies fullfilled these criteria (Meijer et al. 2012b). The study characteristics and main results are presented in Table 2.1.

All-Cause Mortality

A total of 24 of the studies investigated the association between ALSES and all-cause mortality. Significant ALSES effects were found in 16 of these studies (Anderson et al. 1997; Blakely et al. 2006; Curtis et al. 2004; Henriksson et al. 2006; Jaffe et al. 2005a, b; Jerrett et al. 2003, 2005; Malmstrom et al. 2001; Marinacci et al. 2004; Martikainen et al. 2003; Naess et al. 2007; Turrell et al. 2007; Veugelers et al. 2001; Waitzman et al. 1999; Yen and Kaplan 1999) whereas eight studies found no associations (Blakely et al. 2003; Bosma et al. 2001; Dahl et al. 2006; Jones et al. 2000; Kravdal 2007; Lochner et al. 2001; Naess et al. 2005; Roos et al. 2004). Studies reporting an association suggest that living in areas with low ALSES increases all-cause mortality when individual level characteristics (such as

Table 2.1 Overview of the characteristics of the reviewed studies

First author, publication year, country	Outcome variable and study years	Sample size of individuals (age range), sample size of area unit(s)	Individual characteristics (+ age and sex)	Area-level characteristics	Conclusion on area-effect after adjustment for individual characteristics	Area effect estimates
Anderson et al. (1997), USA	All-cause 1979–1989	239,187 (>25), census tracts (*n* not stated)	Race, urbanization, family income	Median census tract income	Higher mortality in low income areas for persons aged >65 years. No effect on 65+ year-olds. Stronger effect on men than women	1.10 (1.07–1.13) All cause mortality in low income areas vs. high income areas
Backlund et al. (2007), USA	All-cause 1979–1990	521,248 (>25), 50 states	Race, Hispanic origin, urbanization, family income, household size, education, employment status, marital status	State income inequality, % of blacks	Higher mortality in areas with high income inequality for persons aged <65. No effect on 65+ year-olds. Higher effect in males. High mortality in areas with high % of blacks adjusted for income inequality except on men aged 65+	1.08 (1.04–1.12) All cause mortality in areas with higher income inequality vs. areas with lower income inequality
Bentley et al. (2008), Australia	Breast-, prostate-, lung and all-cancer mortality 1996–2000	5,995,661 (25–64), 9 states and territories, 59 statistical divisions, 187 statistical subdivisions, 1,315 statistical local areas	Occupation	Index of relative socio-economic disadvantage	Premature cancer mortality was highest in most disadvantaged areas for all-cancer mortality, and for lung cancer mortality	See Turrell et al. (2007)
Blakely et al. (2003), New Zealand	All-cause and mortality from CVD, cancer, injury and suicide 1991–1994	1.4 million (25–64), 14 regional councils, 35 health funding authority sub-regions, 73 territorial authorities	Ethnicity, equivalent household income, rural/urban	Average household income, income inequality	No association	1.00 (0.97–1.02) All cause mortality in low income areas vs. high income areas
Blakely et al. (2006), New Zealand	All-cause, mortality from CVD, cancer, injury and suicide 1996–1999	Not stated, 1,683 census area units	Marital status, ethnicity, equivalent household income, education, car access, employment	Social capital, deprivation index urbanization	Higher mortality in deprived and urban areas. No association between neighborhood social capital and mortality	1.09 (1.08–1.11) All cause mortality in more deprived areas vs. less deprived areas

(continued)

Table 2.1 (continued)

First author, publication year, country	Outcome variable and study years	Sample size of individuals (age range), sample size of area unit(s)	Individual characteristics (+ age and sex)	Area-level characteristics	Conclusion on area-effect after adjustment for individual characteristics	Area effect estimates
Blomgren et al. (2004), Finland	Alcohol related mortality 1990–1996	1.1 million men (25–64), 84 regions	Education, socioeconomic status, marital status, mother tongue	Proportion of manual workers, unemployment, median household income, income inequality, family cohesion, voting turnout, urbanization, % of Swedish-speaking inhabitants	Higher alcohol-related mortality in areas with higher proportion of manual workers. Protective effect of high level of urbanization	1.10 (1.08–1.12) Alcohol related mortality for areas with higher proportion of manual workers vs. areas with lower proportion of manual workers
Borrell et al. (2002), Spain	All injury mortality, death caused by traffic injury, falls, drug overdose, suicide 1991–1998	1.6 million (>19 years), 38 city-defined neighborhoods	Education	% unemployed men, % men aged >21 who had been in preventive jail	Higher % of unemployed men was associated with high overall injury mortality and mortality from falls among men only. Higher % of men in jail was associated with higher mortality from drug overdose	1.05 (1.03–1.07) All injury mortality in neighborhoods with higher rate of unemployed men vs. neighborhoods with lower rate of unemployed men
Bosma et al. (2001), Netherlands	All-cause 1991–1997	8,506 (15–74), 86 administrative neighborhoods	Education, occupation, being unemployed or disabled, having severe financial problems	% with only primary schooling, % unskilled manual workers, % unemployed, % with severe financial problems	Higher mortality in areas with high % of unemployed, disabled and persons with severe financial problems. Area-level education and occupational was modestly associated with mortality	1.06 (0.97–1.15) All cause mortality in areas with higher financial problems level vs. areas with lower financial problems level

Chaix et al. (2006), Sweden	Mortality from ischemic heart disease, lung cancer and chronic obstructive pulmonary disease 1980–1993	*n* not stated (55–75), 370 parishes	Education, income	Population density, median income	Neighborhood income had effect on mortality from ischemic disease. Higher mortality from all outcomes in areas with high population density	1.04 (1.01–1.08) Mortality from ischemic heart disease in areas with lower median income vs. areas with higher median income
Chaix et al. (2007a), Sweden	Ischemic heart disease mortality 1996–2002	341,048 (50–79), not stated	Marital status, education, occupation 25 years before baseline, cumulated income over 20 years	Population density, mean income	Greater mortality in low-income areas. Stronger effects for younger people and urban areas	1.15 (1.08–1.22) Ischemic heart disease mortality in lower mean income areas vs. higher mean income areas
Chaix et al. (2007b), Sweden	Ischemic heart disease mortality 1986–1996	69,815 in 1986, 73,547 in 1996 (50–64), 652 neighborhoods	Marital status, education, occupation, 15-year averaged income	Median income rank	Greater mortality in low income neighborhoods	1.20 (1.16–1.24) Ischemic heart disease mortality in lower income neighbor-hoods vs. higher income neighborhoods
Chaix et al. (2008), Sweden	Acute myocardical infarction mortality 1987–2003	7791 (>45), 1533 neighborhoods	Marital status, diseases diagnosed, self-rated health, education, income, self-reported financial strain, social participation, perceptions of neighborhood social interactions, smoking, physical activity	Neighborhood safety, neighborhood cohesion, neighborhood income, population density, % residents from low-income countries, residential stability, distance to hospital	Low neighborhood income was associated with higher mortality	1.76 (1.28–2.41) AMI mortality in lower income neighborhoods vs. higher income neighborhoods

(continued)

Table 2.1 (continued)

First author, publication year, country	Outcome variable and study years	Sample size of individuals (age range), sample size of area unit(s)	Individual characteristics (+ age and sex)	Area-level characteristics	Conclusion on area-effect after adjustment for individual characteristics	Area effect estimates
Curtis et al. (2004), England and Wales	All-cause 1939, 1971–1991	62,719 (0–16 years in 1939), 192 residential areas	Social class, housing tenure, unemployment, marital status	1939: Depressed areas, population density, % of semi-skilled or unskilled manual workers, over-crowded housing, unemployment rate 1981: Carstairs index, broad regional locations	Lower mortality for inhabitants living in affluent areas in 1939, even after control for SES in 1981	1.15 (1.11–1.19) All cause mortality for lower SES areas vs. higher SES areas
Dahl et al. (2006), Norway	All-cause 1994–1999	2,197,231 (25–66), 88 economic regions	Marital status, income, education, health related welfare benefits	Mean income, income inequality	Region mean income had no effect on mortality. Mortality increased with higher regional income inequality after adjustment for region-level mean income	1.01 (0.99–1.02) All cause mortality for lower mean income areas vs. higher mean income areas

Franzini and Spears (2003), USA	Years lost premature CVD mortality 1991	50,268 (>25), 12,344 census block groups; 3,788 census tracts; 247 counties	Race/ethnicity, age adjusted education	Census block groups: Median house value Census tracts: Education, % blacks, % Hispanics, house ownership Counties: Education, house ownership, median income, poverty rate, unemployment rate, % blacks, % Hispanics, crime index, income inequality	Block-group level: Higher median house value was associated with reduced mortality. Census tract level: Greater % Blacks and % Hispanics was associated with reduced mortality for Blacks and Hispanics. County level: Higher % of homeownership was associated with lower mortality; worse crime index was associated with increased mortality	1.05 (1.01–1.09) Years lost because of premature CVD mortality in blocks with lower median house value vs. blocks with higher median house value
Henriksson et al. (2006), Sweden	All-cause 1990–1998	2,573,708 (40–64), 284 municipalities	Disposable family income, occupation	Income inequality, mean income, % of manual workers, % poor, % living in confined quarters, municipality size	No association	1.03 (0.94–1.13) All-cause mortality in areas with high income inequality vs. areas with low income inequality
Henriksson et al. (2007), Sweden	All-cause 1990–1998	1,578,186 (40–64), municipalities	Occupation, disposable family income	Income inequality, population size in municipalities, % of manual and non-manual workers, mean income	High level of income inequality had a protective effect for high-level non manual workers and an adverse effect for unskilled manual workers	1.05 (0.90–1.23) All cause mortality in areas with high income inequality vs. areas with low income inequality

(continued)

Table 2.1 (continued)

First author, publication year, country	Outcome variable and study years	Sample size of individuals (age range), sample size of area unit(s)	Individual characteristics (+ age and sex)	Area-level characteristics	Conclusion on area-effect after adjustment for individual characteristics	Area effect estimates
Jaffe et al. (2005a), Israel	All-cause, CVD mortality 1983–1992	141,683 (45–89), 882 statistical areas	Marital status, education, country of birth, continent of origin	Religious affiliation, SES index	Mortality increased with lower religious affiliation and lower SES	See Jaffe et al. (2005b)
Jaffe et al. (2005b), Israel	All-cause 1983–1992	131,156 (45–89), 882 statistical areas	Marital status, education, income, origin, number of rooms in the house, household amenities score	SES index	Greater deprivation was associated with greater risk of mortality	1.22 (1.15–1.29) All cause mortality for lower SES areas vs. higher SES areas
Jerrett et al. (2003), USA	All-cause 1982	550,000 (30+), 151 cities	Smoking, education, exposure to dust or fumes at work, BMI, marital status, alcohol consumption	Pollution, population change, race, doctors per hospital bed, education, mean income, poverty rate, income inequality, unemployment rate	Greater mortality in lower SES areas and areas with high levels of air pollution	1.11 (1.03–1.20) All cause mortality for lower income areas vs. higher income areas
Jerrett et al. (2005), USA	All-cause and cause specific mortality 1982–2000	22,905 (not stated), 267 zip code areas	44 variables including lifestyle, demography, occupation, education	Income, income inequality, education, population size, racial composition, unemployment, % having air-condition, air pollution	Higher mortality in areas with more air pollution	1.11 (0.99–1.25) All-cause mortality in areas with higher air pollution vs. areas with lower air pollution adjusted for individual and ecological factors

Jones et al. (2000), UK	All-cause 1981–1997	8,720 (not stated), 396 wards, 207 constituencies, 22 regions	Ownership of dwelling, social class, employment, smoking, exercise, diet, alcohol	Deprivation index	No significant area SES effect on mortality. Residence in deprived areas had protective effect for high SES groups and adverse effect for low SES groups	1.03 (0.98–1.07) All cause mortality for more deprived areas vs. less deprived areas
Kravdal (2007), Norway	All-cause 1980–1999	Whole Norwegian population (50–89), 435 municipalities	Education, income, marital status	% never married, % divorced, average education, average income	Average income had no association. Reduced mortality for men in areas with high % of divorces and in areas with high % of never married. Mixed effects for women. High average education reduced mortality for men below 80	0.99 (0.97–1.02) All cause mortality for lower income areas vs. higher income areas
LeClere et al. (1998), USA	Heart disease mortality 1986–1990	199,211 (>18), 5,921 census tracts	Race/ethnicity, BMI, pre-existing conditions, income, education, marital status, employment status	% female-headed families, % blacks, median family income, % on public benefits, % in deep poverty, % poor families with children headed by women, unemployment	Higher mortality in communities with high % female-headed families	No overall estimate due to missing 95 % CI and standard errors
Lochner et al. (2001), USA	All cause 1991–1995	546,888 (18–74), 48 states	Race/ethnicity, marital status, annual income	State income inequality, state poverty rate	No significant association between area poverty rate and mortality. Greater mortality in areas with greater income inequality also after adjustment for state poverty	1.00 (0.99–1.01) All cause mortality for lower poverty rate areas vs. higher poverty rate areas
Malmstrom et al. (2001), Sweden	All-cause 1988–1996	22,236 (25–74), 8,519 small area markets statistics	Socioeconomic position, housing tenure, marital status, social network	Composite care need index	Significant area effect, higher mortality in least deprived areas	1.03 (1.01–1.05) All cause mortality for higher deprived areas vs. lower deprived areas

(continued)

Table 2.1 (continued)

First author, publication year, country	Outcome variable and study years	Sample size of individuals (age range), sample size of area unit(s)	Individual characteristics (+ age and sex)	Area-level characteristics	Conclusion on area-effect after adjustment for individual characteristics	Area effect estimates
Mari-Dell'Olmo et al. (2007), Spain	HIV mortality 1991–2001	2,250 (>20), 38 neighborhoods	Education, HIV transmission group	Male unemployment	Areas with high male unemployment had high HIV mortality. Strongest effect in most deprived areas	1.35 (1.15–1.58) HIV mortality in more deprived areas vs. less deprived areas
Marinacci et al. (2004), Italy	All cause. Cause specific mortality: diabetes; stomach and lung cancer; CHD; cerebrovascular diseases; respiratory diseases. 1971–1999	799,564 in 1971–1980; 889,432 1981–1991; 821,736 in 1991–1999 (≥15 years), 23 city-defined neighborhoods	Education, place of birth, composite index of housing conditions	Deprivation index	Greater deprivation was associated with higher risk of mortality	1.03 (1.02–1.05) All cause mortality for higher deprived neighborhoods vs. lower deprived neighborhoods
Martikainen et al. (2003), Finland	All-cause. Cause specific mortality: lung cancer; other cancers; disease of circulatory system; accidents/violence; alcohol-related 1990–1995	251,509 (>25), 55 city-defined neighborhoods	Education, occupation-based social class, housing tenure, housing density, living arrangements	% manual workers, % over 60 years, social cohesion	Greater % of manual workers and lower social cohesion associated with higher risk of all-cause mortality	1.06 (1.03–1.08) All cause mortality for areas with higher proportion of manual workers vs. areas with lower proportion of manual workers

Naess et al. (2005), Norway	All-cause 1960–1998	219,518 (30–69), 473 neighborhoods	Education, housing conditions	Education, income	No significant association for education. Greater income was associated with lower mortality but became insignificant after adjustment for individual deprivation throughout the life course	1.35 (0.96–1.89) All-cause mortality for neighborhoods with higher rates with primary education only vs. neighborhoods with lower rates
Naess et al. (2007), Norway	All-cause, Cause specific mortality: CVD, lung and stomach cancer, chronic obstructive pulmonary disease, psychiatric causes of death, violence 1992–1998	105,359 (50–74), 468 neighborhoods	Education, household income, occupational class, ownership of dwelling, type of dwelling, crowding	Air pollution, education, household income, occupational class, ownership of dwelling, type of dwelling, crowding.	Higher socioeconomic position reduced mortality. Deprived neighborhoods were more exposed to air pollution	1.14 (1.11–1.18) All cause mortality for lower income areas vs. higher income areas
Petrelli et al. (2006), Italy	Mortality from coronary events 1997–2002	523,755 (35–74), 23 neighborhoods	Education, employment status, median census tract income	Deprivation index	No significant association	1.05 (0.995–1.11) Mortality from coronary events for areas with lower level of deprivation vs. areas with higher level of deprivation

(continued)

Table 2.1 (continued)

First author, publication year, country	Outcome variable and study years	Sample size of individuals (age range), sample size of area unit(s)	Individual characteristics (+ age and sex)	Area-level characteristics	Conclusion on area-effect after adjustment for individual characteristics	Area effect estimates
Robert et al. (2004), USA	Breast cancer incidence 1988–1995	14,667 (20–79), census tracts and zip-codes (*n* not stated)	Education, mammography use, family history of breast cancer, parity, age at first birth, alcohol intake, BMI, hormone replacement use, oral contraceptive use, menopausal status	Composite index of community SES, urbanicity	Living in high SES areas or urban areas associated with higher risk of breast cancer	0.95 (0.946–0.96) Breast cancer incidence in higher SES areas vs. lower SES areas
Roos et al. (2004), Canada	All-cause 1990–2002	2,116 Nova Scotia 8,032 Manitoba (18–75), census enumeration areas (*n* not stated)	Income, education, smoking, diabetes, BMI, residential mobility	Household income, dwelling value, education, unemployment, % single mother	No significant main area effects. For Manitoba only, lower income individuals had greater mortality risk in more affluent areas than in less affluent areas	1.07 (0.92–1.23) All cause mortality for low income areas vs. high income areas
Sanderson et al. (2006), USA	Prostate cancer incidence 1999–2002	407 cases and 393 controls (65–79), 265 zip code areas	Education, race, age, prostate-specific antigen testing	Composite socioeconomic status	Higher prostate cancer incidence in lower SES areas	1.19 (1.06–1.34) Prostate cancer incidence in lower SES areas vs. higher SES areas
Turrell et al. (2007), Australia	All-cause 1996–2000	5,995,661 (25–64), 9 states and territories, 59 statistical divisions, 187 statistical subdivisions and 1,317 statistical local areas.	Occupation	Index of relative socio-economic disadvantage	Living in disadvantaged areas increased probability of premature death. Premature death varied systematically at each geographical scale	1.12 (1.11–1.13) All cause mortality for more disadvantaged areas vs. less disadvantaged areas

Veugelers et al. (2001), Canada	All-cause 1990–1999	2,116 (18–75), 705 enumeration areas	Education, income, smoking, diabetes, BMI	Household income, dwelling value, education, unemployment rate, % single mothers	No significant main area effects. Within affluent area only, mortality risks were lower among high-income individuals	See Roos et al. (2004)
Waitzman et al. (1999), USA	All-cause 1986–1995	136,956 (35–65), 34 metropolitan areas	Race, education, income	Spatial inequality/ economic segregation, income inequality, median income	Higher economic segregation and income inequality was associated with higher mortality	1.58 (1.41–1.77) All-cause mortality in metropolitan areas with higher income inequality vs. metropolitan areas with lower income inequality
Webster et al. (2008), USA	Breast cancer incidence 1980–1993	811 in 1980, 1,264 in 1990 (all ages), 1990: 141 census blocks, 34 census tract levels, 1980: 167 enumeration-districts	Education, race, BMI, alcohol use, history of breast cancer, menstrual history, reproductive history, history of mammography, oral contraceptive use, exposure to ionizing radiation	% with incomes below US poverty line, SES composite index, urbanization	Higher-SES communities had increased risk of breast cancer. Increased effect of neighborhood when allowing for a latency period	0.90 (0.87–0.92) Breast cancer incidence in lower SES communities vs. higher SES communities
Yen and Kaplan (1999), USA	All-cause 1983–1994	996 (36–96), census tracts (*n* not stated)	Income, education, race/ethnicity, perceived health status, smoking status, BMI, alcohol consumption	Population SES	Mortality risks were higher in low SES neighborhoods	1.58 (1.13–2.24) All-cause mortality in lowest tertile of neighborhood social environment score vs. higher tertiles

Reprinted from Meijer, M., Röhl, J., Bloomfield, K., & Grittner, U. (2012). Do neighbourhoods affect individual mortality? A systematic review and meta-analysis of multilevel studies. *Social Science & Medicine*, *74*(8), 1204–1212 with permission by the publisher

age, sex and socioeconomic position) have been accounted for. However, due to differences in study designs, population size, age distribution, etc., this apparent association is subject to discussion and furthermore lacks information about the size of the association. Some of these issues are dealt with below in the meta-analysis results section.

Income Inequality

Seven studies investigated the effect of income inequality, i.e. the gap between rich and poor inhabitants within a neighbourhood, city or region. Two studies, one from New Zealand (Blakely et al. 2003) and one from Sweden (Henriksson et al. 2006), found that income inequality on the area level was not associated with all-cause mortality. However, four other studies concluded that there was an effect: A US study showed that mortality was higher in cities with higher income inequality (Waitzman et al. 1999). In Norwegian regions, an association was also found and showed that effects were stronger among individuals with lower SES (Dahl et al. 2006). Two US investigations using states as the area unit also found associations (Lochner et al. 2001; Backlund et al. 2007). A study conducted in Swedish municipalities found that a high level of income inequality had a protective effect for high-level non-manual workers and an adverse effect for unskilled manual workers (Henriksson et al. 2007). Overall, the seven studies point to a possible link between high mortality from all causes and high-income inequality on the area level. This is confirmed in a meta-analysis finding an adverse effect of income inequality on health (Kondo et al. 2009).

Air Pollution

Three multilevel studies examining air pollution were retrieved, and they all reported findings of higher all-cause mortality in areas with higher traffic related air pollution (Jerrett et al. 2003, 2005; Naess et al. 2007). In addition to individual SES, two of these studies controlled for individual smoking (Jerrett et al. 2003, 2005) and one controlled for 44 individual confounders in total (Jerrett et al. 2005). One of the studies found significantly higher levels of air pollution in low ALSES neighbourhoods (Naess et al. 2007).

Population Density

One study examined the influence of area characteristics over the life course and concluded that mortality is higher among people who, in early life, lived in areas with high population density (Curtis et al. 2004). In New Zealand, higher mortality was reported for people living in urban areas (Blakely et al. 2006). These effects persisted after controlling for ALSES and mirror a Danish study where high population density was found to be associated with excess all-cause mortality after controlling for SES at both the individual and area level (Meijer et al. 2012a).

Other Area Characteristics

Some studies found that all-cause mortality was higher in areas with low social cohesion (Martikainen et al. 2003), low religious affiliation (Jaffe et al. 2005a) and in areas with high percentage of black people (though this was not the case for mortality among elderly men) (Backlund et al. 2007). One study examined the effect of social capital on mortality but found no associations (Blakely et al. 2006). Excess mortality was reported for women living in areas with high proportions of unmarried persons; however, this effect was not found for men (Kravdal 2007). For individuals younger than 65 years, high mortality was also observed in areas characterised by high proportions of residents over 60 years old (Martikainen et al. 2003).

Cancer Mortality and Incidence

Four studies investigated neighbourhood influences on general cancer mortality. In Finland, a U-shaped effect of social cohesion was found among men under 65 years old but not for older age groups (Martikainen et al. 2003). In New Zealand, the association between cancer mortality and having performed unpaid voluntary work in the neighbourhood was investigated, but no such link was found (Blakely et al. 2006). No associations were found between cancer mortality and income inequality on the area level among men, but for women, lower cancer mortality appeared to be linked with higher inequality, although this effect was based on a few observations (Blakely et al. 2003). The probability of premature cancer mortality was highest for people living in disadvantaged areas in Australia (Bentley et al. 2008).

Three studies reported that lung cancer mortality was associated with low ALSES (Bentley et al. 2008), high population density (Chaix et al. 2006) and with medium to low proportion of manual workers (Martikainen et al. 2003).

According to one study area disadvantage was not significantly associated with prostate or breast cancer mortality (Bentley et al. 2008). Examinations of the association between neighbourhood characteristics and cancer incidence found that high ALSES was associated with increased breast cancer incidence (Robert et al. 2004; Webster et al. 2008) and that residence in areas with low SES was associated with higher prostate cancer incidence (Sanderson et al. 2006).

Cardiovascular Disease

Three Swedish studies have demonstrated solid evidence for a link between low ALSES and increased mortality from ischemic heart disease (Chaix et al. 2006, 2007a, b) and a fourth concluded the same for acute myocardial infarction (Chaix et al. 2008). The analyses showed that, in addition to the effect of ALSES, inhabitants in areas with high population density were at higher risk and that younger age groups in particular were affected by the socioeconomic contextual effect (Chaix et al. 2006, 2007a). Furthermore, mortality from acute myocardial infarction increased with decreasing neighbourhood safety and cohesion (Chaix et al. 2008) after adjustment for SES on both the individual and the area level. Another study investigated the effect of neighbourhood volunteerism on cardiovascular disease (CVD) but found no evidence for an association (Blakely et al. 2006).

Two studies found no association between ALSES and CVD (Blakely et al. 2003; Petrelli et al. 2006) whereas two others did (Marinacci et al. 2004; Martikainen et al. 2003). While not investigating ALSES directly, a study from the USA showed that high median house value, higher percentages of black people and Hispanics, higher percentages of house owners and low crime were all factors associated with lower CVD mortality. Areas in Israel with high percentage of religious inhabitants also had lower CVD morality (Jaffe et al. 2005a), and in the USA, a lower percentage of female-headed families had a protective effect (LeClere et al. 1998).

Respiratory Diseases

Only two studies examined the influence of neighbourhoods on mortality from respiratory diseases. Both found that inhabitants in neighbourhoods with low socioeconomic status had increased mortality (Chaix et al. 2006; Marinacci et al. 2004). However, Chaix et al. found that population density had much greater impact; only among persons aged 65 age at baseline (as oppose to those aged 55 and 75 at baseline) an additional effect of ALSES was found (Chaix et al. 2006). Marinacci et al. showed that the effect of ALSES was stronger among persons younger than 65 years (Marinacci et al. 2004).

Others Causes of Death

Neighbourhood effects on suicide were investigated in two studies but neither found any effects (Blakely et al. 2003, 2006). The same two studies examined neighbourhood influences on mortality from injuries. One of them showed that there were no contextual effects (Blakely et al. 2003) while the other concluded that there was a higher risk among men living in neighbourhoods with low neighbourhood voluntarism (Blakely et al. 2006). Living in areas with high male unemployment was also associated with higher all-injury mortality both for men and women

(Borrell et al. 2002). Low social cohesion and a medium to high proportion of manual workers was linked with high alcohol-related mortality as well as mortality from accidents and violence (Martikainen et al. 2003). Similarly, Blomgren et al. showed that low ALSES was associated with high mortality from alcohol-related causes (Blomgren et al. 2004). Finally, in a Spanish study with a small sample, it was demonstrated that areas with high male unemployment had high HIV mortality and that the effect was strongest in the most deprived areas (Mari-Dell'Olmo et al. 2007).

Results from a Meta-Analysis on ALSES and All-Cause Mortality

Eighteen of the studies retrieved in the systematic review were included in a meta-analysis evaluating the association between ALSES and all-cause mortality (Meijer et al. 2012b). ALSES refers to the average income, education level or socioeconomic position in a given neighbourhood. ALSES estimates from each study were used to calculate an overall estimate and 95 % confidence interval as shown in Fig. 2.1.

Combining all 18 studies revealed that the relative risk (95 % CI) of all-cause mortality was 1.07 (1.04–1.10) for inhabitants living in areas with low SES compared to those living in areas with high SES. This demonstrates that, over and above individual characteristics such as age, sex, education level or income, the socioeconomic status of the area in which people live is associated with all-cause mortality. Figure 2.1 also shows that the relative risk of all-cause mortality was 1.11 (1.08–1.14) for inhabitants in low ALSES areas when the investigated area unit contained fewer than 5,000 persons per area unit. When studies used area units containing more than 7,000 persons per area unit, the effect was smaller and the relative risk for inhabitants in low ALSES areas was only 1.02 (1.00–1.03). The analysis also showed that there was strong heterogeneity between studies. This means that there was significant variation in ALSES effects between studies, which may be caused by differences in study design or study populations. A meta-regression was therefore conducted to investigate if some selected study characteristics could account for the observed heterogeneity.

Results of the meta-regression revealed that the ALSES effect on all-cause mortality was higher for men, for younger age groups and in area units with fewer persons. Furthermore the analysis showed that estimates did not vary between social democratic, conservative or liberal welfare state regimes as defined by Gösta Esping-Andersen (1990). After adjusting for age and sex, the odds ratio of all-cause mortality in lower SES areas compared to high SES areas was 1.05 (1.04–1.06) in studies with more than 7,000 persons per area unit and 1.10 (1.06–1.15) in studies with less than 5,000 persons per area unit. Despite these adjustments, a significant amount of variance between studies was found. There was no evidence of publication bias using the Begg test ($p=0.363$) (Begg and Mazumdar 1994).

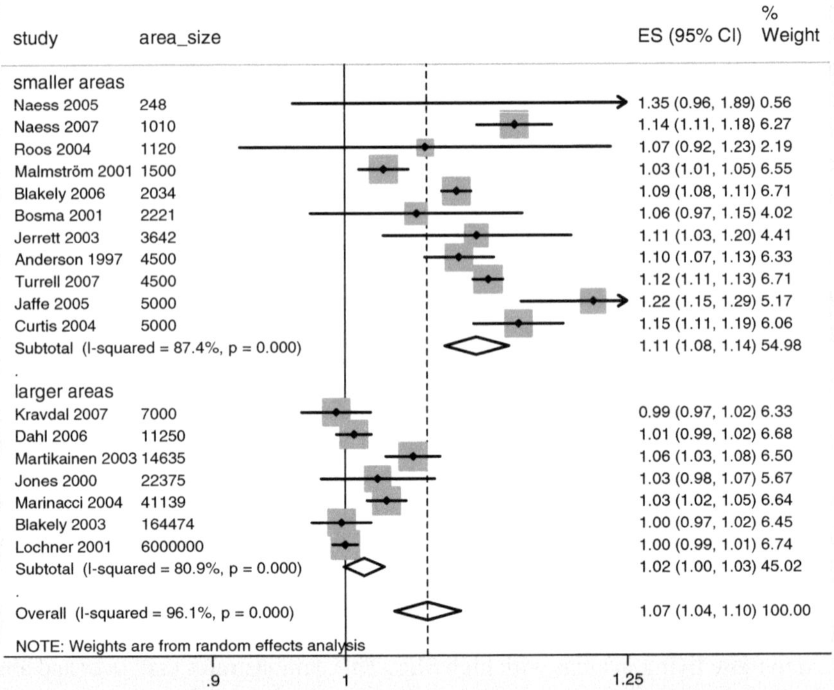

Fig. 2.1 Results of meta-analysis: relative risks for mortality in low-SES areas compared to high-SES areas, with weight of each study and between-study heterogeneity (I^2). Studies are grouped according to number of inhabitants per area unit (<7,000 versus >7,000) (Reprinted from Meijer, M., Röhl, J., Bloomfield, K., & Grittner, U. (2012). Do neighbourhoods affect individual mortality? A systematic review and meta-analysis of multilevel studies. *Social Science & Medicine*, *74*(8), 1204–1212 with permission by the publisher)

Pathways from Neighbourhoods to Health

In the remaining part of the chapter, possible pathways between neighbourhood characteristics and mortality will be discussed. Only few studies actually account for the hypothesised pathways they are investigating. Macintyre et al. have called the impact of the neighbourhoods “a black box, an unspecified ‘miasma’ which somehow, but we do not know how, influences some aspects of health, health-related behaviour or health risks in some population groups” (Macintyre et al. 2002, p. 129). The focus of this chapter is mortality, and indeed, the hypothesised pathways between neighbourhood characteristics and mortality are many and the “storylines” are often long and complicated. An example of a pathway between neighbourhood SES and mortality could be that retailers selling healthy food do not locate their businesses in low-income areas because the customer base there cannot afford their

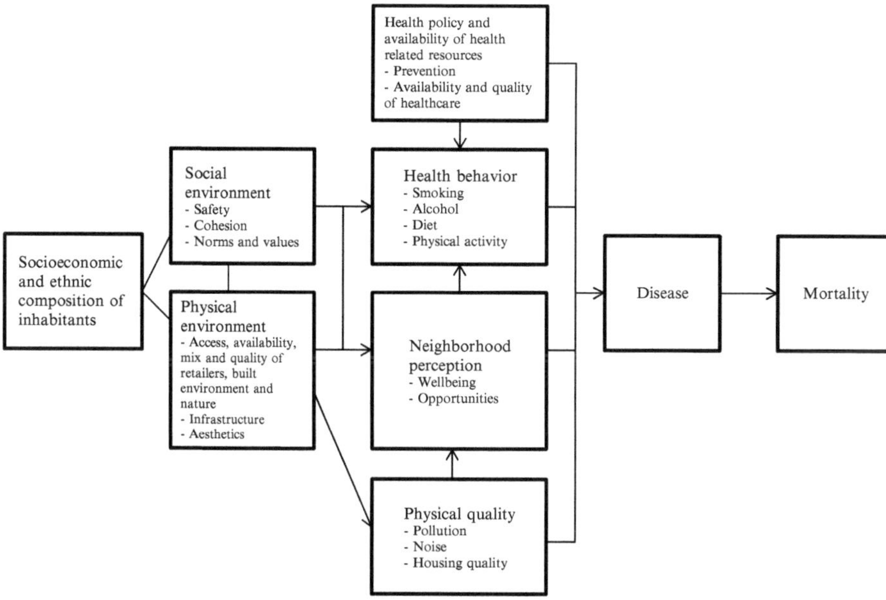

Fig. 2.2 Neighbourhood characteristics and their pathways to inequalities in disease and mortality

products. Inhabitants in these areas therefore have fewer opportunities to purchase healthy food in their local area and may for this reason be more likely to buy unhealthy food, maybe even fast food. As time passes, inhabitants in these areas are at higher risk of becoming obese, which could lead to cardiovascular diseases and ultimately premature death. Not only is the chain of events long but it also stretches over a long period of time.

Previous literature theorising on the link between neighbourhoods and health (Diez Roux and Mair 2010; Macintyre et al. 2002; Stafford et al. 2007; Cummins et al. 2007) overall operate with a model where health outcomes are affected by the social and the physical environment of the neighbourhood. Diez Roux and Mair (2010) describe the social environment as safety/violence, social connections, cohesion, local institutions and norms while the physical environment includes environmental exposures, food and recreational resources, built environment, aesthetic quality/natural spaces, services and quality of housing. Building on this work, a model with four major pathways is presented, which in greater detail specifies how neighbourhood features can affect the individual and translate into spatial patterns in disease and mortality. The model is presented and depicted in Fig. 2.2.

As demonstrated in Fig. 2.2, there is a mutual relationship between socioeconomic status, the social environment and the physical environment. The socioeconomic composition of inhabitants affects both the social environment in terms of social norms and levels of safety/violence, but it also affects the physical environment by, e.g. attracting certain retailers, workplaces and public services. Social and physical neighbourhood features such as shared social values, housing quality, house prices, level of graffiti and access to nature may also regulate where people live.

This chapter suggests that geographic characteristics mainly transmit to individual health and mortality through four overall paths: (1) health policy and distribution of heath-related resources, (2) health behaviour, (3) neighbourhood perception and opportunities and, finally, through (4) physical quality. The first pathway mainly refers to the national and regional levels, the second and third pathways refer to the local neighbourhood level and the fourth pathway stretches from the national level to the street level.

The first pathway, health policy and distribution of health-related resources, refers to how, e.g. health prevention, screening programmes and distribution of doctors, health clinics and hospitals are governed and administered locally. Such geographic differences can cause inequalities in health because some programmes, e.g. smoking cessation programmes or cancer screening programmes, are offered in some areas and not in others or simply because the quality of the programmes differ by area. In Denmark, for instance, mammography was introduced in 1991 in the city of Copenhagen while other counties did not introduce mammography until 2007. Since some studies report of 25–29 pct. reductions in breast cancer mortality in areas with organised mammography screening, this is an example of how local public health policy can affect mortality (Nystrom et al. 1993; Olsen et al. 2005). Targeted health promotion in deprived areas is another. There has also been recent initiatives to examine the effect of local policy on obesity (Michael and Yen 2009) and smoking (Biener et al. 2010; Lipperman-Kreda et al. 2012; Yang et al. 2011) which are both important determinants of health and mortality. Many studies have also investigated how geographical remoteness or distance to hospitals affects mortality (Turrell et al. 2006; Chaix et al. 2008) or how presence of healthcare facilities (e.g. healthcare centres and public hospitals) in neighbourhoods affected CVD incidence (Kawakami et al. 2011).

The second pathway refers to how neighbourhood of residence may affect health behaviours such as alcohol consumption, smoking, diet and physical activity, which are closely linked with disease and mortality. This is by far the best-studied pathway. The link between neighbourhood characteristics and individual health behaviour has been examined in a range of studies (Adams et al. 2009; Duncan et al. 1993; Ecob and Macintyre 2000; Giskes et al. 2006; Karasek et al. 2012; Stafford et al. 2010). Physical features of neighbourhoods can affect individual health behaviour through access to health-promoting and health-damaging goods. Studies have, for instance, shown that consumption of alcohol is higher in neighbourhoods with higher concentrations of outlets (Connor et al. 2010; Kavanagh et al. 2011). Other studies have found that inhabitants have poorer diets if they live in neighbourhoods with higher densities of fast-food restaurants (Moore et al. 2009) or that inhabitants with easier access to supermarkets and other shops selling healthy food products have healthier diets and lower body-mass index (Larson et al. 2009;

Moore et al. 2008). Similarly it has been shown that people smoke more if they live in neighbourhoods with higher densities of stores selling cigarettes (Chuang et al. 2005). Two reviews, however, maintain that the relationship between outlet density and alcohol consumption remains inconclusive (Livingston et al. 2007; Popova et al. 2009).

Another puzzling finding is that it seems to be impossible to automatically equal neighbourhood deprivation with low availability of healthy goods and high availability of unhealthy goods. A study focusing on fast-food outlets in Copenhagen found that deprived neighbourhoods had fewer fast-food outlets than affluent areas (Svastisalee 2011), and a study from Glasgow showed that this also applied to a range of other neighbourhood resources (Macintyre et al. 2008).

The social environment also plays a central role since behaviours can be transmitted between inhabitants due to the normative influence of focused and unfocussed interaction among people in the same neighbourhoods. A qualitative study based on interviews with inhabitants in a deprived Glasgow neighbourhood showed how people were expected to smoke by fellow inhabitants and that teenagers needed strong legitimate reasons, such as asthma, before smoking cessation was accepted by peers. Moreover it was shown how smoking fostered social participation and feelings of belonging (Stead et al. 2001). Neighbourhood social norms towards smoking have also been found to be associated with smoking cessation (Karasek et al. 2012). Lower crime rates may also promote physical activity (van Lenthe et al. 2005; Diez Roux and Mair 2010) and reduced smoking levels among residents (Begg and Mazumdar 1994).

The third pathway refers to individuals' perceptions of their local area. The hypothesis is that safe and socially well-functioning neighbourhoods that offer housing, job opportunities and physical surroundings which meet residents' needs will support the well-being of people. Through positive perceptions of the neighbourhood, inhabitants will feel more comfortable and psychological problems and stress related to the neighbourhood will be reduced and result in healthier lifestyles, reduced morbidity and longer life expectancy. Typical measures of the social environment include social cohesion, social capital, levels of safety and violence, etc. The association between such measures and mortality has been examined in many studies (Blakely et al. 2006; Blomgren et al. 2004; Chaix et al. 2008; Martikainen et al. 2003).

Physical neighborhood features affecting people's perception of their local area could be access to and connectivity between public offices, institutions, banks, libraries, infrastructure, public transport, job opportunities, quality of the built environment, aesthetics, etc. However, as noted by Macintyre et al., the relevance of easy access to local facilities varies from persons to person; to some, it is important to have all facilities within walking distance while others prefer to live in remote and quiet areas (Macintyre et al. 2008). Living in neighbourhoods which increase stress and reduce general well-being is usually linked with psychological problems such as anxiety, depression or other mental health disorders. In two studies, it is shown that neighbourhood perceptions and satisfaction are associated with mental health (Leslie and Cerin 2008; Rocha et al. 2012).

As discussed above, there is not always a connection between ALSES and neighbourhood facilities; a comprehensive study from Glasgow showed that access to many resources was just as good in poor neighbourhoods as it was in wealthier neighbourhoods but that there was a difference in the type of resources found in affluent and deprived areas (Macintyre et al. 2008).

The fourth pathway is named physical quality and covers air pollution, ground pollution, radiation, traffic noise, water quality as well as lack of heating, sanitation and physical deterioration of housing, etc. Humans are either exposed to pollutants when breathing, drinking the water or, in the case of radiation and low housing quality, simply by being present in the area. This pathway covers much of classical environmental epidemiology. As shown above, there was substantial evidence for the influence of air pollution on lung cancer mortality and all-cause mortality (Jerrett et al. 2003, 2005; Naess et al. 2007). Studies with modelled geocoded air pollution levels showed that air pollution significantly differs between neighbouring streets and even between houses on the same street (Robsahm and Tretli 2005). This also applies to traffic noise and radiation and suggests that environmental exposures are sensitive to the geographic scale being used.

Interconnections Between Pathways

As illustrated in Fig. 2.2, the first three pathways following the social and physical characteristics of neighbourhoods are interconnected. The first pathway *health policy and distribution of health-related resources* is connected to the second pathway *health behaviour* when local health policy changes people' health behaviour by, e.g. introducing screening programmes or targeted health interventions. The third pathway, *perception of neighbourhoods*, is also connected to *health behaviour* since studies have shown that negative neighbourhood perception increases smoking (Stead et al. 2001). Similarly neighbourhood disorder, which has fundamental impact on neighbourhood perception, has been associated with reduced sports participation and obesity (Stafford et al. 2007).

Conclusion

This chapter has shown how neighbourhood characteristics are associated with all-cause mortality, cause-specific mortality and cancer incidence. The dominant area-level measures used in most studies belonged to the socioeconomic composition of inhabitants and showed that residence in areas with low-average SES generally was associated with higher mortality regardless of individual socioeconomic background. Studies using indicators of the social environment generally came to inconclusive results across outcomes, although these results should be treated with caution since theoretical considerations, operationalisations and types of measurement differed substantially between studies.

In the meta-regression, it was demonstrated that the odds ratio (95 %CI) for all-cause mortality in low-SES areas was 1.05 (1.04–1.06) in studies with more than 7,000 persons per area unit and 1.10 (1.06–1.15) in studies investigating area units with maximum 5,000 persons after having controlled for a number of study characteristics. The results also showed that the type of welfare state regime in which studies were conducted did not have a significant effect on the overall estimate.

Four pathways between neighbourhood characteristics and mortality were suggested: through (1) health policy and distribution of health-related resources, (2) health behaviour, (3) neighbourhood perception and through (4) physical quality. Since the association between ALSES and mortality has been established, there is now a need for evaluations trying to disentangle the connecting and linking mechanisms between these endpoints.

References

Adams, R. J., Howard, N., Tucker, G., Appleton, S., Taylor, A. W., Chittleborough, C., et al. (2009). Effects of area deprivation on health risks and outcomes: A multilevel, cross-sectional, Australian population study. *International Journal of Public Health, 54*(3), 183–192.

Anderson, R. T., Sorlie, P., Backlund, E., Johnson, N., & Kaplan, G. A. (1997). Mortality effects of community socioeconomic status. *Epidemiology, 8*(1), 42–47.

Backlund, E., Rowe, G., Lynch, J., Wolfson, M. C., Kaplan, G. A., & Sorlie, P. D. (2007). Income inequality and mortality: A multilevel prospective study of 521 248 individuals in 50 US states. *International Journal of Epidemiology, 36*(3), 590–596.

Begg, C. B., & Mazumdar, M. (1994). Operating characteristics of a rank correlation test for publication bias. *Biometrics, 50*(4), 1088–1101.

Bentley, R., Kavanagh, A. M., Subramanian, S., & Turrell, G. (2008). Area disadvantage, individual socio-economic position, and premature cancer mortality in Australia 1998 to 2000: A multilevel analysis. *Cancer Causes & Control, 19*(2), 183–193.

Biener, L., Hamilton, W. L., Siegel, M., & Sullivan, E. M. (2010). Individual, social-normative, and policy predictors of smoking cessation: A multilevel longitudinal analysis. *American Journal of Public Health, 100*(3), 547–554.

Blakely, T., Atkinson, J., Ivory, V., Collings, S., Wilton, J., & Howden-Chapman, P. (2006). No association of neighbourhood volunteerism with mortality in New Zealand: A national multilevel cohort study. *International Journal of Epidemiology, 35*(4), 981–989.

Blakely, T., Atkinson, J., & O'Dea, D. (2003). No association of income inequality with adult mortality within New Zealand: A multi-level study of 1.4 million 25–64 year olds. *Journal of Epidemiology and Community Health, 57*(4), 279–284.

Blomgren, J., Martikainen, P., Makela, P., & Valkonen, T. (2004). The effects of regional characteristics on alcohol-related mortality-a register-based multilevel analysis of 1.1 million men. *Social Science & Medicine, 58*(12), 2523–2535.

Borrell, C., Rodriguez, M., Ferrando, J., Brugal, M. T., Pasarin, M. I., Martinez, V., et al. (2002). Role of individual and contextual effects in injury mortality: New evidence from small area analysis. *Injury Prevention, 8*(4), 297–302.

Bosma, H., van de Mheen, H. D., Borsboom, G. J., & Mackenbach, J. P. (2001). Neighborhood socioeconomic status and all-cause mortality. *American Journal of Epidemiology, 153*(4), 363–371.

Chaix, B., Lindstrom, M., Merlo, J., & Rosvall, M. (2008). Neighbourhood social interactions and risk of acute myocardial infarction. *Journal of Epidemiology and Community Health, 62*(61), 62–68.

Chaix, B., Rosvall, M., Lynch, J., & Merlo, J. (2006). Disentangling contextual effects on cause-specific mortality in a longitudinal 23-year follow-up study: Impact of population density or socioeconomic environment? *International Journal of Epidemiology, 35*(3), 633–643.

Chaix, B., Rosvall, M., & Merlo, J. (2007a). Assessment of the magnitude of geographical variations and socioeconomic contextual effects on ischaemic heart disease mortality: A multilevel survival analysis of a large Swedish cohort. *Journal of Epidemiology and Community Health, 61*(4), 349–355.

Chaix, B., Rosvall, M., & Merlo, J. (2007b). Recent increase of neighborhood socioeconomic effects on ischemic heart disease mortality: A multilevel survival analysis of two large Swedish cohorts. *American Journal of Epidemiology, 165*(1), 22–26.

Chuang, Y. C., Cubbin, C., Ahn, D., & Winkleby, M. A. (2005). Effects of neighbourhood socio-economic status and convenience store concentration on individual level smoking. *Journal of Epidemiology and Community Health, 59*(7), 568–573.

Connor, J. L., Kypri, K., Bell, M. L., & Cousins, K. (2010). Alcohol outlet density, levels of drinking and alcohol-related harm in New Zealand: A national study. *Journal of Epidemiology and Community Health, 65*(10), 841–846.

Cummins, S., Curtis, S., Diez-Roux, A. V., & Macintyre, S. (2007). Understanding and representing 'place' in health research: A relational approach. *Social Science & Medicine, 65*(9), 1825–1838.

Curtis, S., Southall, H., Congdon, P., & Dodgeon, B. (2004). Area effects on health variation over the life-course: Analysis of the longitudinal study sample in England using new data on area of residence in childhood. *Social Science & Medicine, 58*(1), 57–74.

Dahl, E., Ivar Elstad, J., Hofoss, D., & Martin-Mollard, M. (2006). For whom is income inequality most harmful? A multi-level analysis of income inequality and mortality in Norway. *Social Science & Medicine, 63*(10), 2562–2574.

Diez Roux, A. V., & Mair, C. (2010). Neighborhoods and health. *Annals of the New York Academy of Sciences, 1186*, 125–145.

Duncan, C., Jones, K., & Moon, G. (1993). Do places matter? A multi-level analysis of regional variations in health-related behaviour in Britain. *Social Science & Medicine, 37*(6), 725–733.

Ecob, R., & Macintyre, S. (2000). Small area variations in health related behaviours; do these depend on the behaviour itself, its measurement, or on personal characteristics? *Health & Place, 6*(4), 261–274.

Ellen, I. G., Mijanovich, T., & Dillman, K.-N. (2001). Neighborhood effects on health: Exploring the links and assessing the evidence. *Journal of Urban Affairs, 23*(3–4), 391–408.

Esping-Andersen, G. (1990). *The three worlds of welfare capitalism*. London: Polity.

Franzini, L., & Spears, W. (2003). Contributions of social context to inequalities in years of life lost to heart disease in Texas, USA. *Social Science & Medicine, 57*(10), 1847–1861.

Giskes, K., van Lenthe, F. J., Turrell, G., Brug, J., & Mackenbach, J. P. (2006). Smokers living in deprived areas are less likely to quit: A longitudinal follow-up. *Tobacco Control, 15*(6), 485–488.

Henriksson, G., Allebeck, P., Weitoft, G. R., & Thelle, D. (2006). Income distribution and mortality: Implications from a comparison of individual-level analysis and multilevel analysis with Swedish data. *Scandinavian Journal of Public Health, 34*(3), 287–294.

Henriksson, G., Allebeck, P., Weitoft, G. R., & Thelle, D. (2007). Are manual workers at higher risk of death than non-manual employees when living in Swedish municipalities with higher income inequality? *European Journal of Public Health, 17*(12), 139–144.

Jaffe, D. H., Eisenbach, Z., Neumark, Y. D., & Manor, O. (2005a). Does living in a religiously affiliated neighborhood lower mortality? *Annals of Epidemiology, 15*(10), 804–810.

Jaffe, D. H., Eisenbach, Z., Neumark, Y. D., & Manor, O. (2005b). Individual, household and neighborhood socioeconomic status and mortality: A study of absolute and relative deprivation. *Social Science & Medicine, 60*(5), 989–997.

Jerrett, M., Burnett, R. T., Ma, R., Arden Pope, I. C., Krewski, D., Newbold, K. B., et al. (2005). Spatial analysis of air pollution and mortality in Los Angeles. *Epidemiology, 16*(16), 727–736.

Jerrett, M., Burnett, R. T., Willis, A., Krewski, D., Goldberg, M. S., DeLuca, P., et al. (2003). Spatial analysis of the air pollution-mortality relationship in the context of ecologic confounders. *Journal of Toxicology and Environmental Health. Part A, 66*(16–19), 1735–1777.

Jones, K., Gould, M. I., & Duncan, C. (2000). Death and deprivation: An exploratory analysis of deaths in the health and lifestyle survey. *Social Science & Medicine, 50*(7–8), 1059–1079.

Karasek, D., Ahern, J., & Galea, S. (2012). Social norms, collective efficacy, and smoking cessation in urban neighborhoods. *American Journal of Public Health, 102*(2), 343–351.

Kavanagh, A. M., Kelly, M., Krnjacki, L., Thornton, L., Jolley, D., Subramanian, S., et al. (2011). Access to alcohol outlets and harmful alcohol consumption: A multilevel study in Melbourne, Australia. *Addiction, 106*(10), 1772–1779.

Kawakami, N., Li, X., & Sundquist, K. (2011). Health-promoting and health-damaging neighbourhood resources and coronary heart disease: A follow-up study of 2 165 000 people. *Journal of Epidemiology and Community Health, 65*(10), 866–872.

Kondo, N., Sembajwe, G., Kawachi, I., van Dam, R. M., Subramanian, S. V., & Yamagata, Z. (2009). Income inequality, mortality, and self rated health: Meta-analysis of multilevel studies. *BMJ, 339*, b4471.

Kravdal, O. (2007). A fixed-effects multilevel analysis of how community family structure affects individual mortality in Norway. *Demography, 44*(3), 519–537.

Larson, N. I., Story, M. T., & Nelson, M. C. (2009). Neighborhood environments: Disparities in access to healthy foods in the US. *American Journal of Preventive Medicine, 36*(1), 74–81.

LeClere, F. B., Rogers, R. G., & Peters, K. (1998). Neighborhood social context and racial differences in women's heart disease mortality. *Journal of Health and Social Behavior, 39*(2), 91–107.

Leslie, E., & Cerin, E. (2008). Are perceptions of the local environment related to neighbourhood satisfaction and mental health in adults? *Preventive Medicine, 47*(3), 273–278.

Lipperman-Kreda, S., Grube, J. W., & Friend, K. B. (2012). Local tobacco policy and tobacco outlet density: Associations with youth smoking. *Journal of Adolescent Health, 50*(6), 547–552.

Livingston, M., Chikritzhs, T., & Room, R. (2007). Changing the density of alcohol outlets to reduce alcohol-related problems. *Drug and Alcohol Review, 26*(5), 557–566.

Lochner, K., Pamuk, E., Makuc, D., Kennedy, B. P., & Kawachi, I. (2001). State-level income inequality and individual mortality risk: A prospective, multilevel study. *American Journal of Public Health, 91*(3), 385–391.

Macintyre, S., Ellaway, A., & Cummins, S. (2002). Place effects on health: How can we conceptualise, operationalise and measure them? *Social Science & Medicine, 55*(1), 125–139.

Macintyre, S., Macdonald, L., & Ellaway, A. (2008). Do poorer people have poorer access to local resources and facilities? The distribution of local resources by area deprivation in Glasgow, Scotland. *Social Science & Medicine, 67*(6), 900–914.

Malmstrom, M., Johansson, S., & Sundquist, J. (2001). A hierarchical analysis of long-term illness and mortality in socially deprived areas. *Social Science & Medicine, 53*, 265–275.

Mari-Dell'Olmo, M., Rodriguez-Sanz, M., Garcia-Olalla, P., Pasarin, M., Brugal, M., Cayla, J. A., et al. (2007). Individual and community-level effects in the socioeconomic inequalities of AIDS-related mortality in an urban area of southern Europe. *Journal of Epidemiology and Community Health, 61*(3), 232–240.

Marinacci, C., Spadea, T., Biggeri, A., Demaria, M., Caiazzo, A., & Costa, G. (2004). The role of individual and contextual socioeconomic circumstances on mortality: Analysis of time variations in a city of north west Italy. *Journal of Epidemiology and Community Health, 58*(3), 199–207.

Martikainen, P., Kauppinen, T. M., & Valkonen, T. (2003). Effects of the characteristics of neighbourhoods and the characteristics of people on cause specific mortality: A register based follow up study of 252,000 men. *Journal of Epidemiology and Community Health, 57*(3), 210–217.

Meijer, M., Kejs, A., Stock, C., Bloomfield, K., Ejstrud, B., & Schlattmann, P. (2012). Population density, socioeconomic environment and all-cause mortality: A multilevel survival analysis of 2.7 million individuals in Denmark. *Health & Place, 18*(2), 391–399.

Meijer, M., Röhl, J., Bloomfield, K., & Grittner, U. (2012). Do neighborhoods affect individual mortality? A systematic review and meta-analysis of multilevel studies. *Social Science & Medicine, 74*(8), 1204–1212.

Michael, Y. L., & Yen, I. H. (2009). Invited commentary: Built environment and obesity among older adults – can neighborhood-level policy interventions make a difference? *American Journal of Epidemiology, 169*(4), 409–412. discussion 413–414.

Moore, L. V., Diez Roux, A. V., Nettleton, J. A., & Jacobs, D. R., Jr. (2008). Associations of the local food environment with diet quality–a comparison of assessments based on surveys and geographic information systems: The multi-ethnic study of atherosclerosis. *American Journal of Epidemiology, 167*(8), 917–924.

Moore, L. V., Diez Roux, A. V., Nettleton, J. A., Jacobs, D. R., & Franco, M. (2009). Fast-food consumption, diet quality, and neighborhood exposure to fast food: The multi-ethnic study of atherosclerosis. *American Journal of Epidemiology, 170*(1), 29–36.

Naess, O., Piro, F. N., Nafstad, P., Smith, G. D., & Leyland, A. H. (2007). Air pollution, social deprivation, and mortality: A multilevel cohort study. *Epidemiology, 18*(6), 686–694.

Naess, O., Leyland, A. H., Smith, G. D., & Claussen, B. (2005). Contextual effect on mortality of neighbourhood level education explained by earlier life deprivation. *Journal of Epidemiology and Community Health, 59*(12), 1058–1059.

Nandi, A., & Kawachi, I. (2011). Neighborhood effects on mortality. In R. G. Rogers & E. M. Crimmins (Eds.), *Handbook of adult mortality* (pp. 413–439). London: Springer.

Nystrom, L., Rutqvist, L. E., Wall, S., Lindgren, A., Lindqvist, M., Ryden, S., et al. (1993). Breast cancer screening with mammography: Overview of Swedish randomised trials. *Lancet, 341*(8851), 973–978.

Olsen, A. H., Njor, S. H., Vejborg, I., Schwartz, W., Dalgaard, P., Jensen, M. B., et al. (2005). Breast cancer mortality in Copenhagen after introduction of mammography screening: Cohort study. *BMJ, 330*(7485), 220.

Petrelli, A., Gnavi, R., Marinacci, C., & Costa, G. (2006). Socioeconomic inequalities in coronary heart disease in Italy: A multilevel population-based study. *Social Science & Medicine, 63*(2), 446–456.

Pickett, K. E., & Pearl, M. (2001). Multilevel analyses of neighbourhood socioeconomic context and health outcomes: A critical review. *Journal of Epidemiology and Community Health, 55*(2), 111–122.

Popova, S., Giesbrecht, N., Bekmuradov, D., & Patra, J. (2009). Hours and days of sale and density of alcohol outlets: Impacts on alcohol consumption and damage: A systematic review. *Alcohol and Alcoholism, 44*(5), 500–516.

Riva, M., Gauvin, L., & Barnett, T. A. (2007). Toward the next generation of research into small area effects on health: A synthesis of multilevel investigations published since July 1998. *Journal of Epidemiology and Community Health, 61*(10), 853–861.

Robert, S. A., Strombom, I., Trentham-Dietz, A., Hampton, J. M., McElroy, J. A., Newcomb, P. A., et al. (2004). Socioeconomic risk factors for breast cancer: Distinguishing individual- and community-level effects. *Epidemiology, 15*(4), 442–450.

Robsahm, T. E., & Tretli, S. (2005). Weak associations between sociodemographic factors and breast cancer: Possible effects of early detection. *European Journal of Cancer Prevention, 14*(1), 7–12.

Rocha, K., Perez, K., Rodriguez-Sanz, M., Obiols, J. E., & Borrell, C. (2012). Perception of environmental problems and common mental disorders (CMD). *Social Psychiatry and Psychiatric Epidemiology, 47*(10), 1675–1684. doi:10.1007/s00127-012-0474-0.

Roos, L. L., Magoon, J., Gupta, S., Chateau, D., & Veugelers, P. J. (2004). Socioeconomic determinants of mortality in two Canadian provinces: Multilevel modelling and neighborhood context. *Social Science & Medicine, 59*(7), 1435–1447.

Sanderson, M., Coker, A. L., Perez, A., Du, X. L., Peltz, G., & Fadden, M. K. (2006). A multilevel analysis of socioeconomic status and prostate cancer risk. *Annals of Epidemiology, 16*(12), 901–907.

Stafford, M., Brunner, E. J., Head, J., & Ross, N. A. (2010). Deprivation and the development of obesity a multilevel, longitudinal study in England. *American Journal of Preventive Medicine, 39*(2), 130–139.

Stafford, M., Cummins, S., Ellaway, A., Sacker, A., Wiggins, R. D., & Macintyre, S. (2007). Pathways to obesity: Identifying local, modifiable determinants of physical activity and diet. *Social Science & Medicine, 65*(9), 1882–1897.

Stead, M., MacAskill, S., MacKintosh, A. M., Reece, J., & Eadie, D. (2001). "It's as if you're locked in": Qualitative explanations for area effects on smoking in disadvantaged communities. *Health & Place, 7*(4), 333–343.

Svastisalee, C. M. (2011). *Physical activity, fruit and vegetable intake and the built environment: Ecological and epidemiological studies among youth.* PhD thesis, University of Southern Denmark, Copenhagen.

Turrell, G., Kavanagh, A., Draper, G., & Subramanian, S. (2007). Do places affect the probability of death in Australia? A multilevel study of area-level disadvantage, individual-level socioeconomic position and all-cause mortality, 1998–2000. *Journal of Epidemiology and Community Health, 61*(1), 13–19.

Turrell, G., Kavanagh, A., & Subramanian, S. V. (2006). Area variation in mortality in Tasmania (Australia): The contributions of socioeconomic disadvantage, social capital and geographic remoteness. *Health & Place, 12*(3), 291–305.

van Lenthe, F. J., Brug, J., & Mackenbach, J. P. (2005). Neighbourhood inequalities in physical inactivity: The role of neighbourhood attractiveness, proximity to local facilities and safety in the Netherlands. *Social Science & Medicine, 60*(4), 763–775.

Veugelers, P. J., Yip, A. M., & Kephart, G. (2001). Proximate and contextual socioeconomic determinants of mortality: Multilevel approaches in a setting with universal health care coverage. *American Journal of Epidemiology, 154*(8), 725–732.

Waitzman, N. J., Smith, K. R., & Stroup, A. (1999). The direct and indirect effects of metropolitan area inequality on mortality. A hierarchical analysis. *Annals of the New York Academy of Sciences, 896*, 347–349.

Webster, T. F., Hoffman, K., Weinberg, J., Vieira, V., & Aschengrau, A. (2008). Community- and individual-level socioeconomic status and breast cancer risk: Multilevel modeling on Cape Cod, Massachusetts. *Environmental Health Perspectives, 116*(8), 1125–1129.

Yang, T., Xu, X., Rockett, I. R., Guo, W., & Zhou, H. (2011). Effects of household, workplace, and public place smoking restrictions on smoking cessation. *Health & Place, 17*(4), 954–960.

Yen, I. H., & Kaplan, G. A. (1999). Neighborhood social environment and risk of death: Multilevel evidence from the Alameda County Study. *American Journal of Epidemiology, 149*(10), 898–907.

Yen, I. H., Michael, Y. L., & Perdue, L. (2009). Neighborhood environment in studies of health of older adults: A systematic review. *American Journal of Preventive Medicine, 37*(5), 455–463.

Chapter 3
Area Effects on Behaviour and Lifestyle: The Spatiality of Injustice

Katherine L. Frohlich

Introduction

In 1993 David Mechanic, American medical sociologist, wrote the following in an article published in the journal *Social Science and Medicine*:

> …there is little appreciation of the extent to which life imperatives and social opportunities and constraints either enhance or inhibit harmful personal behaviours. Relative to personal behaviour change, such alternatives as the improvement of living conditions, the development of new technologies, regulatory incentives and environmental modifications receive little emphasis. (Mechanic 1993, p. 97)

In this chapter we will elaborate on what Mechanic called social opportunities and constraints in the context of area-effect studies on behaviour. To do so we begin by making the distinction between the concepts of behaviour, lifestyle and collective lifestyles. We discuss a critical element to collective lifestyles, in distinction from behaviour or lifestyle alone, the role of structural constraints and opportunities in shaping people's actions. From there we entertain the idea that the massive urbanisation of the last few decades brings to the fore not only the role of these constraints and opportunities but also their inequitable distribution at the neighbourhood level. We then move on to describe some of the most commonly used theories in health promotion and social epidemiology to explain the relationship between area effects and health-related behaviours, most of them emphasising structural constraints and opportunities, but to varying degrees. The effects of the inequitable distribution of opportunities and constraints on behaviour across space will then be considered. In so doing, we will draw on a well-developed discussion from within social geography regarding spatial injustice. Here, we will describe the concepts of environmental

K.L. Frohlich (✉)
Département de médecine sociale et préventive, Université de Montréal (IRSPUM),
C.P. 6128, succ. Centre-ville, Montréal, QC H3C 3J7, Canada
e-mail: katherine.frohlich@umontreal.ca

C. Stock and A. Ellaway (eds.), *Neighbourhood Structure and Health Promotion*,
DOI 10.1007/978-1-4614-6672-7_3, © Springer Science+Business Media New York 2013

and spatial justice and their potential implications for practice and research in a health promotion concerned with area effects and collective lifestyles. The chapter ends with a description of a novel theoretical approach that addresses many of the concerns and issues raised here, the Interdisciplinary Study of Inequalities in Smoking (ISIS) framework, developed by researchers in Montreal, Canada.

Behaviour, Lifestyle and Collective Lifestyles

With the reduction of infectious diseases as the main causes of morbidity and mortality in the early twentieth century, increasing epidemiological attention was focused on identifying the determinants of chronic diseases associated with an ageing population and modern living conditions (Hansen and Easthope 2007). Among the main contributors to these chronic diseases were cancer, cardiovascular disease and diabetes. By the mid-1970s, epidemiological evidence gathered on the determinants of these diseases pointed increasingly towards health-related behaviours such as smoking, physical activity and diet as some of their main causes.

This etiologic research was followed by the development of public health interventions that focused attention on health risk behaviours. More specifically, these interventions targeted the segment of the population with the highest level of risk exposure determined by their health-related behaviours such as the MRFIT, COMMIT and other programmes (MRFIT 1981, 1982; COMMIT 1995). The assumption was that the high prevalence of chronic diseases was the result of unhealthy behaviours or lifestyle, both of which were viewed to be chosen and under an individual's control. Consequently, particular emphasis in these interventions was placed on personal responsibility and individuals' ability to make personal change towards better health and health behaviours, largely through increased education. This approach was championed by the Lalonde Report of 1974 in which Lalonde insisted on the importance of intervening on populations 'at risk', populations composed of individuals all showing elevated risk for some specific disease based on their behavioural profile. This focus, Lalonde argued, would lead to the greatest public health impact (Lalonde 1974).

The Lalonde approach was challenged early on from within health promotion with the Ottawa Charter (WHO 1986). The charter placed new emphasis on the importance of the 'structure' of lifestyle, that is, the social conditions for individuals' daily life conduct (Kickbusch 1986; Rütten 1995; Frohlich et al. 2001; WHO 2008). The reintroduction of structure into the discussion of lifestyle draws, in part, from the original attributes of lifestyle as delineated by Max Weber (1978), the first social theorist to discuss the term. Weber viewed lifestyle to be comprised of two concepts: life choices and life chances. Life choices were understood as the decisions people make. These choices, differently from those of Lalonde, health education and some epidemiology, were viewed to be embedded in life chances, the opportunities that people encounter due to their social situation. Life chances were therefore understood to either enable or constrain choices, with both choices and chances interacting to shape outcomes. What Weber highlighted, in distinction from mid-twentieth-century thoughts on lifestyle, was that both chances and choices are socially determined, and thus choices are not just under an *individual's* control. Weber also emphasised the collective nature of lifestyle by associating it with status groups and not solely with individuals. He viewed choices made by individuals to be shaped by their position within the social hierarchy, with people from different social classes tending to share certain behaviours and practices.

Since Weber, French sociologist Pierre Bourdieu has further developed this notion of lifestyle by arguing that 'choices' are an expression of *habitus* that itself is a dynamic, evolving inculcation of structuring structures (or 'chances', to use Weber's term) (Bourdieu 1980). The *habitus*, according to Bourdieu, is produced by the objective conditions of existence combined with positions in the social structure, and it generates practices and tastes that together result in a lifestyle. While there is an element of choice with regard to one's lifestyle, people are seen to be predisposed by their *habitus* towards a certain choice of lifestyle. Bourdieu therefore viewed it as being entirely misleading to separate, analytically, 'choices' and 'chances'.

This chapter builds on the premise that research and practice concerned with area effects on behaviour should take inspiration from the idea that behaviours are not just determined by choices but also by the structural opportunities and constraints of people's environments (their chances). Since Bourdieu, and from within health promotion and medical sociology, the term 'collective lifestyles' has been developed to describe this important interplay between social structural constraints and opportunities and people's ability to act, their agency (Cockerham et al. 1997; Cockerham 2005; Frohlich et al. 2001, 2012; Abel and Frohlich 2012).

The collective lifestyles framework develops further the issue of choices and chances by adopting current sociological language. Within the framework we speak of social practices (Giddens 1984; Bourdieu 1980) (or behaviours) and the social structure (or social conditions). Social practices are routinised and socialised behaviours common to groups. Social structure is defined as the way in which society is organised, involving norms, resources, policy and institutional practices. Similarly to choices, social practices are understood as emerging from the structure, and thus the relationship between structure and practices is always explicit. In this way, an individual behaviour, or social practice, is never divorced from its position within the social structure. Further, this relationship is not unidirectional; the structure is seen to shape people's social practices, but in turn, people's social practices are understood to influence the structure, by both reproducing and transforming it. So, social practices are embedded within the social structure but have a critical role in transforming it. A third component to the collective lifestyle framework, in contrast to past perspectives, is a focus on the constraints on agency and what the implications of the constraints are for true empowerment to take place. People's position within the social structure clearly shapes their agency (i.e. their ability to act). Approaches that focus on changing health behaviours give attention to agency, but what is often missing is a well-developed analysis of the structural constraints to individual agency, that is, a direct link established between structure and agency (Frohlich et al. 2012).

The consideration of collective lifestyles, as opposed to behaviours alone, has three important implications for health promotion and the study of area effects. First, it suggests that when studying area effects on behaviour, we must move beyond an individually based focus to one that considers both the structural barriers and opportunities in areas for people to act in particular ways. Second, these barriers and opportunities may affect groups differentially based on their position within the social structure; it is a socially shaped, group phenomena. These group effects are often termed ecological, in reference to group-level exposures. In better understanding these ecological effects, we might be better able to intervene on a population level rather than on one individual at a time. Lastly, a focus on collective lifestyles introduces a social justice agenda; if these barriers and opportunities for healthy behaviour are inequitably distributed throughout areas, and we view the social structure to be mutable, health promotion should be addressing this issue as one of injustice.

Urban Areas and Collective Lifestyles

A growing focus for health promotion's concern with inequities in collective lifestyles is urban areas. Urbanisation is likely the single most important demographic shift worldwide during the past and in the new century, and it represents a sentinel change from how most of the world's population has lived for the past several 1,000 years (Galea and Vlahov 2005). Cities such as Los Angeles, New York, London and Hong Kong now have income disparities that rank among the highest in the world. It is of little surprise, therefore, that new justice movements are arising in these highly urban areas of the world (Soja 2010), including movements such as Occupy Wall Street (a movement arising from general feelings of indignation with regard to the financial crisis in the first decade of the 2000s). Although resources are made available to urban residents through private, public and volunteer conduits, socio-economic inequities in cities are linked to differential access to these resources. As a result, people at different ends of the socio-economic spectrum may have inequitable opportunities to benefit from the resources available in cities, leading to differential distributions of collective lifestyles.

One area of urban studies of particular importance to social inequities in health is that of neighbourhoods. Most commonly these studies focus on spatial groupings of individuals and typically consider the impact of one's community of residence within an urban area either on an individual's health or on the health of the population living in the neighbourhood (at the aggregate level). As early as 1942, sociologists Shaw and McKay from the Chicago School demonstrated that Chicago neighbourhoods characterised by poverty, residential instability and dilapidated housing were found to suffer disproportionately higher rates of infant mortality, delinquency, crime, low birth weight, tuberculosis, physical abuse and other factors detrimental to health. They observed that high rates of adverse outcomes tended to persist in the same communities over time despite the movement of different population groups from them. Based on these empirical findings, they deduced that neighbourhoods possess relatively enduring features that transcend the idiosyncratic characteristics of their inhabitants (Sampson 2003).

Until the last 15 years or so, little interest was shown in health promotion with regard to the relationship between area characteristics and inequitable collective lifestyles. Increasing evidence, however, demonstrates that health-related behaviours, or health practices, tend to be substantially poorer in areas characterised by high levels of social and economic disadvantage, relative to areas characterised by social and economic advantage (Drewnowski 2009; Pearce et al. 2010; Pabayo et al. 2011). Because where people live is the basis for health practices, experiences of engaging in them are to a certain extent constrained or encouraged by several aspects of these areas: the physical environment, the cultural expectations about appropriate behaviour and the social experiences possible there (Fitzpatrick and LaGory 2011). Physical and social qualities of place therefore make some collective lifestyles more possible than others and some preferences and expectations more plausible than others. Indeed, while it is argued, on the one hand, that for each health practice there is a unique pathway between area effects and its inequitable distribution, others argue that many area-level characteristics have salience across multiple 'problem' health practices (Pearce et al. 2011).

Current Approaches and Theories Used to Study the Link Between Area Effects and Health-Related Behaviours

The scholarly literature on urban area effects and health-related behaviours offers a plethora of concepts, theories and approaches with which researchers are attempting to understand cause and effect relationships. We choose to focus on a certain number of these ideas, selecting the most current and those we consider to have had the most impact on the field up until now. Of note, nearly all studies referenced here were concerned with behaviours as outcomes, not collective lifestyles per se. We will come back to collective lifestyles in later sections of this chapter.

One of the most important of the approaches from within health promotion is the settings approach, developed through the desire to move beyond an individual-based behavioural approach to health to one that focuses on the creation of supportive environments to help people make healthier choices. From social epidemiology, medical sociology and geography more specifically, numerous hypotheses have been put forward as to how areas, or neighbourhoods in particular, may be shaping the inequitable distribution of health-related behaviours. Among the most common current theories are those of the social and physical environments, opportunity structures, social capital and social disorder. We will examine each of these briefly, describing their strengths and limitations with regard to their explanatory power concerning social inequities in health behaviours.

The Settings Approach

Inspired in part by the work of Aaron Antonovsky on salutogenesis (Antonovsky 1996), as well as the ecological approach (McLeroy et al. 1988; Richard et al. 1996), the settings approach is concerned with the interplay of the physical, organisational and social contexts in which people live, work and play as the objects of inquiry and intervention. The focus is not just the people contained in or defined by that setting (Poland et al. 2009), an approach that commonly results from epidemiological studies of area effects. Through its focus on the interplay between different levels of determinants of health, the settings approach offers an interesting opportunity to influence inequities in health. Indeed, the recent WHO Commission on the Social Determinants of Health has affirmed that the settings approach could be an essential ingredient for reducing health inequities by connecting healthy people with healthy places (WHO 2008).

In theory the settings approach could serve to connect people's health with area effects. In practice, however, this approach has been difficult to operationalise in accordance with its purported objectives. For instance, while the Healthy Cities movement, one of the most important movements to operationalise the settings approach, has been successful in raising awareness about the role of cities in shaping health outcomes (Galea and Vlahov 2005), the movement as a whole has been slow to move beyond treating settings (workplaces, schools, neighbourhoods) as containers or venues for delivering health promotion programming, otherwise known as health promotion *in* settings. Instead, however, the settings approach was intended to directly address the aspects of settings that influence health outcomes and behaviours (*health-promoting* settings) (Masuda et al. 2010). The tendency in practice towards health promotion *in* settings has to date set limitations in our ability to analyse and intervene on the structures and opportunities of areas using this approach.

The Social Environment

Many social epidemiological researchers conceive of the neighbourhood urban environment in terms of two categories: social and physical environments. Exposure to neighbourhood social and physical environments has been linked to health behaviours such as smoking (Duncan et al. 1996, 1999; Frohlich et al. 2002; Chow et al. 2009), diet (Chow et al. 2009) and physical activity (ibid, Tolbert Kimbro et al. 2011). The social environment of urban areas has been described as the collective norms and values shared by members of social groups along with the interpersonal relationships and interactions shared among urban residents and communities (Galea 2007). It has also been defined to include '....occupational structure, labour markets, social and economic processes, wealth, social, human and health services, power relations, government, race relations, social inequalities, cultural practices, the arts, religious institutions and practices, and beliefs about place and community' (Galea and Vlahov 2005, p. 347). Somewhat often the social environment tends to be conflated with the social processes arising from the social environment, with researchers suggesting that social environment can be either collective efficacy, social cohesion or more material aspects of the social environment such as those detailed above by Galea and Vlahov (2005).

Other researchers in this area describe the abundant plausible mechanisms through which the social environment is believed to potentially influence behaviour: (1) shaping norms, (2) enforcing patterns of social control (which can be salutogenic or deleterious to health), (3) providing or not providing opportunities to engage in certain behaviours and (4) reducing or producing stress which might lead to certain behaviours as coping mechanisms (Berkman and Kawachi 2000). The point of this description is not to be comprehensive in our definition of the social environment but rather to demonstrate the lack of agreement and fuzziness in the current definitions of the social environment. While rather fundamental to our understanding of area effects on behaviour, the broad range of phenomena subsumed under the loose umbrella of the social environment leads to conceptual, and later empirical, confusion. We will later argue for a more solid definition both of what a social environment is comprised of and how it can affect health behaviours differentially.

The Physical Environment

The urban physical environment refers to the natural and built environments. The former includes trees, bodies of water and geological and climactic conditions of the particular area of the city one is concerned with. The built environment, on the other hand, is often discussed as including housing, roads and footpaths, transport networks, shops, markets, parks and other public amenities. The physical environment, similarly to the social environment, can be pathogenic or salutogenic for the residents exposed to it. Several studies from the United Kingdom and other European countries have indeed found that poverty levels are positively associated with poorer-quality physical environments (Higgs and Langford 2009; Walker et al. 2005). Examples of the deleterious influence of these inequities include inequitable access across neighbourhoods to green or open spaces, playgrounds and good quality grocery stores and their relationship to the engagement in physical activity and levels of obesity (Lang and Caraher 1998; Rose and Richards 2007). Further hypothesised health benefits of access to physical aspects of the environment, such as green spaces, include the psychosocial mechanisms that may lower levels of stress and blood pressure.

Opportunity Structures

Despite the tendency for some researchers to focus on either the social *or* the physical environment in their empirical explorations of neighbourhood effects on health behaviours, it is generally accepted that there are important interactions between these two environments (Galea 2007). Furthermore, a heavy reliance on evidence narrowly defined as a small subset of variables in the physical environment in some studies obscures a larger picture of the full range of environmental impact on people's health (Masuda et al. 2010). One of the more celebrated explanations of the inequitable distribution of health and health behaviours in neighbourhoods that brings together both social and physical environments is that of Macintyre, Ellaway and colleagues (Macintyre et al. 1993, 2002; Macintyre and Ellaway 2003). Macintyre and Ellaway have melded the importance of the physical and social environments in the work they have conducted in Glasgow, Scotland, since 1987. Through their framework of opportunity structures, or socially constructed and socially patterned features of the physical and social environment, they surmise that, along with collective social functioning and practices, possibilities for people to live more or less healthy lives become socially distributed (Macintyre et al. 2002).

Macintyre and Ellaway's conceptual framework proposes five features of neighbourhoods they view as being health promoting or damaging. Similar to other researchers, they propose that the first feature is physical. Here, they include the quality of air and water, latitude and climate. They propose that this aspect of a local area is likely to be shared by all residents within a locality. In a somewhat similar vein to the settings approach, the second feature of their model is conceptualised as the availability of health environments at home, work and play. They argue that areas vary in their provision of resources through these environments, and this inequity may affect those less well off more than their more fortunate counterparts. Third, they posit that services provided, publicly or privately, to support people in their daily lives can also inequitably affect people's health and health behaviours. Here they include services such as education, transport, street cleaning and lighting, policing, health and welfare services. The fourth feature includes sociocultural features of neighbourhoods, including the political, economic, ethnic and religious history of a community. Lastly, they argue that residents' perceptions of their neighbourhood, the neighbourhood's reputation, may influence the infrastructure of a neighbourhood as well as the morale and self-esteem of its residents.

While useful as a general guide for understanding how area effects influence health outcomes and behaviours, Macintyre and Ellaway have themselves criticised their framework for being somewhat limited in that it does not specify exactly what we need to study, within each category, in order to fully understand how social and physical environments inequitably influence health. And indeed, the same critique can be launched towards all of the aforementioned studies on the social or physical environments; the focus rests on correlates of health behaviours rather than explanations of how these behaviours come about, particularly inequitably.

Social Capital

Another common theory used to explain the relationship between neighbourhoods and health behaviours is social capital. Researchers who borrow from social capital theory generally believe that neighbourhood effects on health are due to social processes that involve collective aspects of neighbourhood life such as social cohesion, support networks and informal social control (Sampson 2003). Competing theories of social capital are those of Putnam (1993) and Coleman (1990), the former defining social capital as social networks, shared norms and mutual trust with the latter defining social capital as a resource stemming from the structure of social relationships which facilitate the achievement of specific goals (Sampson 2003).

In social epidemiology the application within the last 10 years of social capital to our understanding of area effects and inequitable health outcomes has focused largely on Putnam's definition of social capital, most notably tested and discussed by Kawachi and Kennedy (1997a, b). These social epidemiologists argue that the core meaning of social capital is tied to the broader notion of social cohesion, referring to the absence of social conflict coupled with the presence of strong social bonds and mutual trust between residents of an area. This attribute of local areas, they claim, is differentially distributed according to various social determinants and results in the inequitable distribution of health behaviours and health outcomes.

While most of Kawachi and Kennedy's early work on social capital was performed at the state level, their interest in the relationship between social capital and broad area effects set the stage for an enormous amount of research to follow that narrowed in on the pertinence of studying social capital in relationship to health behaviours and neighbourhoods. In the area of tobacco, for instance, Siahpush et al. (2006) found that individual smoking was associated with residence in communities where people are less likely to trust their neighbours. Similarly, work in England and Finland has found that low levels of social cohesion promote higher levels of smoking (Karvonen et al. 2008; Poortinga 2006). From Scandinavia, Martine Lindstrom and colleagues have attempted to unpack the relationship between community-level social capital and smoking (Lindstrom 2003, 2010; Lindstrom et al. 2003). They link smoking to the notion of 'miniaturisation of community', a process involving more narrowly based forms of social participation and, subsequently, lower levels of trust. Lindstrom has tested the relationship between a number of different aspects of social capital and smoking, consistently finding that lower levels of social capital are associated with higher levels of smoking and decreased cessation rates.

Social Disorder

Lastly, we turn to the theory of social disorder. Deborah Cohen and colleagues have been examining these issues for several years (Cohen et al. 2000, 2003). Their research has borrowed from what political scientist James Q. Wilson refers to as 'broken windows' (Wilson and Kelling 1989). James Q. Wilson's 'broken windows' theory suggests that disorder in the physical environment can be associated with crime. The theory suggests that a neighbourhood's physical condition sends out messages about the kinds of behaviour that are permitted. A neglected and disorderly physical environment signals to residents that behaviours that are usually prohibited are tolerated.

Cohen et al. (2000, 2003) have extended Wilson's theory to examine health-related outcomes such as gonorrhoea rates. The research team created a 'broken windows index' to examine the possible association of neighbourhood deterioration and high-risk sexual behaviour and gonorrhoea rates in 55 New Orleans neighbourhoods. The index is a scale representing conditions in the neighbourhood, and it accounts for such problems as rubbish, abandoned cars, graffiti and homes and schools in poor repair. Researchers mapped all cases of gonorrhoea between 1994 and 1996 and calculated the rate of disease by neighbourhood 'block group'. Using data from the 1990 US Census and 1995 updates, they determined the relationship between gonorrhoea rates, neighbourhood deterioration and poverty and other demographic characteristics. The broken windows index was found to be a significant predictor of gonorrhoea rates. Poor neighbourhoods with high broken windows scores had significantly higher gonorrhoea rates than did poor neighbourhoods with low broken windows scores. Indeed, the level of neighbourhood deterioration as measured by the broken windows index was a better predictor of neighbourhood gonorrhoea rates than were demographic characteristics as measured by a poverty index.

Moving Beyond Current Theories

In many of the above-described frameworks and/or theories, an overarching theme is the desire to understand the correlates of various societal, political and institutional phenomena with income-deprived groups and their occupation of spaces of multiple environmental deprivation. Researchers concerned with physical and social environments, however, tend to lack explanatory power, as they focus almost exclusively on these correlates of inequities. Theories of social capital and disorder attempt to explain mechanisms but are able to only partially explain how areas lead to inequitable outcomes in behaviours. We propose that what is needed is a framework that explains both what neighbourhoods are and how resources in these neighbourhoods come to be inequitably distributed. To this end, our ISIS framework is offered as the focus of the last section of this chapter.

Environmental and Spatial (In)justice

Despite this growing area of work in neighbourhoods and health, the spatial dimension had tended to be treated as a kind of fixed background, a physically formed environment that has some influence on our lives (and health) but that remains external to the social world as well as to efforts to make the world more socially just (Soja 2010). However, for certain segments of the population, it seems that being in an unhealthy place is not a matter of timing or accident but rather a function of the social structure (Macintyre 2007; Fitzpatrick and Lagory 2011), a structure that is amenable to change if the political will is present. It is also now recognised in both health promotion and environmental justice literatures that marginalised populations face a double burden: being socially marginalised and being subject to the inequities resulting from being located in poor social and physical environments (Masuda et al. 2010). 'Given that the majority of the world's population now lives in cities, contextualising spatial (in)justice becomes to a significant degree a matter of locating it in the specific conditions of urban life and in the collective struggles to achieve more equitable access of all residents to the social resources and advantages that the city provides' (Soja 2010, p. 32). Since cities are artificially constructed environments, i.e. 'intentional', 'built' environments, they should as easily be engineered to promote more desirable health outcomes (Fitzpatrick and Lagory 2011).

One area of research and advocacy that has developed to confront these issues is the environmental justice movement. Environmental justice has been defined as the disproportionate exposure to and burden of harmful environmental conditions experienced by people of lower socio-economic position (Taylor et al. 2006). The environmental justice movement, which has become global in scope and includes collaborations among researchers, non-governmental organisations, public health professionals, legal advocates and community leaders, involves a theoretical positioning linking environmental research to debates around human rights and social equity (Masuda et al. 2010). In this sense, environmental justice offers a remarkably important framework for thinking about the inequitable distribution of collective lifestyles across areas.

Importantly for health promotion, the focus of environmental justice has moved from its original focus on the distributional outcomes of hazardous facilities found in low-income communities (Taylor et al. 2006) to a deeper an. multilevel structural analysis of the socio-economic and political processes involved in the production of environmental health injustices. Within this framework cities and neighbourhoods can be considered resource spaces where the goods and services capable of protecting and enhancing the health of their residents can be more or less equitably distributed (Fitzpatrick and LaGory 2011). Urban spaces are home to various social groups, sorted and sifted according to political and economic resources (what we earlier called life chances). Those with the greatest resources generally reside in areas containing the most health-promoting resources, while those with the least personal resources find their access restricted to less desirable areas with the fewest health-promoting resources. Exposure to risk, constraints and opportunities are thus associated with life chances. As a logical conclusion, these same groups with the least exposure to health-promoting resources have collective lifestyle choices that are constrained by reduced life chances. And indeed as we have seen, studies continue to show that the most socially disadvantaged neighbourhoods lack the resources necessary to promote good health and healthy collective lifestyles. For instance, high-poverty ghettos have a difficult time keeping or attracting the supermarket chains that offer healthy foods. Environmental justice has also been used to demonstrate inequities in physical activity and obesity (Drewnowski 2009). Additionally, the absence of health-promoting places such as parks or chain grocery stores is complemented only by the prevalence of liquor stores, pawn shops and drug dealers (Fitzpatrick and LaGory 2011). In a study from Canada, it was found that children from low socio-economic backgrounds are more likely to use active transport to and from school (which is a good thing) but are more likely to do so in unsafe environments (in terms of rates of vehicle-pedestrian collisions and neighbourhood decay) (Pabayo et al. 2012).

In sum, environmental justice can challenge the historical reproduction of neighbourhoods which relegate socio-economically disadvantaged groups to the margins, depriving them of access to health-promoting amenities enjoyed by others and limiting their chances to be healthy. Working with frameworks such as those of environmental justice, with their distinct equity and mechanism focus, health promotion and area-effects research could be instrumental in identifying the uneven power relations embedded in institutional policies and practices that reproduce and legitimate social and spatial inequities in health and collective lifestyles.

The Interdisciplinary Study of Inequalities in Smoking Framework

In lieu of a conclusion to this chapter, we introduce a new theoretical framework that attempts to bring together the concerns of spatial inequity, area effects on collective lifestyles and neighbourhoods and health research from a theoretical perspective. The majority of attempts to conceptualise how neighbourhoods influence health outcomes, which we saw, tended to isolate certain features of urban living, focusing on their particular roles in bringing about inequities in health. In so doing, neighbourhoods are often treated as units of analysis or exposures within which one can find correlates for the health outcomes of interest rather than areas that themselves can explain how inequities arise. 'Seldom…does location itself play a real part in the analysis; it is the canvas on which events happen but the nature of the locality and its role in structuring health status and health related behaviour is neglected' (Jones and Moon 1993, p. 515).

Our ISIS framework is concerned with this neighbourhood 'canvas', how it can differentially make available and accessible resources and how this social inequity can lead to inequities in collective lifestyles and health. Crucially, our framework examines inequity at work in two different ways: at an aggregate neighbourhood level, what others have called spatial and environmental injustice, and at an individual level (through the social class position of individuals). As mentioned earlier, marginalised populations often face a double burden: being personally socially marginalised as well as being subjected to poor-quality living environments (Masuda et al. 2010). Our framework describes the structural constraints and opportunities at both the individual and collective levels and develops the argument as to how they interact to create inequitable collective lifestyles.

Similarly to the work of Macintyre and Ellaway, our framework suggests that the geographical patterning of health inequities is linked to inequities in health-related resources available in one's immediate environment, the neighbourhood. In other words, neighbourhoods make available resources with a positive and/or negative valence for producing, in the case of the ISIS study, social inequities in smoking.

Where we begin to differ from the earlier work of our colleagues, however, is that we do not view health inequities to be a result of the inequitable distribution of resources understood as differences in the amount of resources alone. Instead, we have expanded on what is meant by 'distribution of resources'. We do not view this distribution to be an outcome understood in terms of variation in a statistical sense but as the set of processes through which resources are spread out among neighbourhoods (Bernard et al. 2007).

In order to understand the mechanisms behind this distribution, we are brought back to our initial discussion with regard to collective lifestyle, chances and choices, structure and agency. We propose that a number of contemporary social theorists can help us conceptualise how inequities come about in resource availability and access at the area level, what it is structurally that makes up spatial and environmental injustice. First, Anthony Giddens' structuration theory (Giddens 1984) provides an explanation of the relationship between structure and agency in the reproduction of health inequities at a local level. In Giddens' theory, he proposes a dialectical relationship between structure and agency. Social structures, he surmises, impose constraints and offer opportunities that shape and orient people's behaviours. Conversely, individuals are agents whose reflexive and routinised practices reproduce and transform social structures. Neither structure nor agency have predominance in his theory; they are mutually reliant. In the particular case of our ISIS study, corner stores that sell individual cigarettes provide opportunities for people to smoke cheaply, but it is the people in the area that buy the cigarettes that make their sale worthwhile. What Giddens' theory offers us is the reminder that a neighbourhood opportunity structure cannot be conceived without taking its residents into consideration. A neighbourhood is not a passive container of resources but is rather a relational structure.

While Giddens helps conceptualise this dialectical relationship between structure and agency (or what he calls recursivity), his theory is not helpful for understanding how channels through which resources are made available vary and differentially procure advantages to different people. Here, we take inspiration from Jacques T. Godbout's theory of informal reciprocity (Godbout 2000, 2003). Godbout contends that many resources are procured and exchanged outside of markets or state interventions. He suggests that there are three distinct sets of rules for the circulation of resources: market rules, states and networks within which informal reciprocity occurs. We extend on Godbout's theory and develop the idea that availability of, and access to, resources are regulated by four rules: proximity, price, rights and informal reciprocity. These rules further give rise to five interrelated domains through which residents may acquire resources influencing smoking: the physical, economic, institutional, local sociability and community organisation domains (Bernard et al. 2007; Frohlich et al. 2008). The variable configurations of these domains in neighbourhoods, we argue, lead to the local production of inequities in smoking (Fig. 3.1).

Specifically, the physical domain includes features of the natural and built environments such as air quality, the presence of buildings and open spaces, as well as their condition and cleanliness. Access and exposure to these resources is ruled by

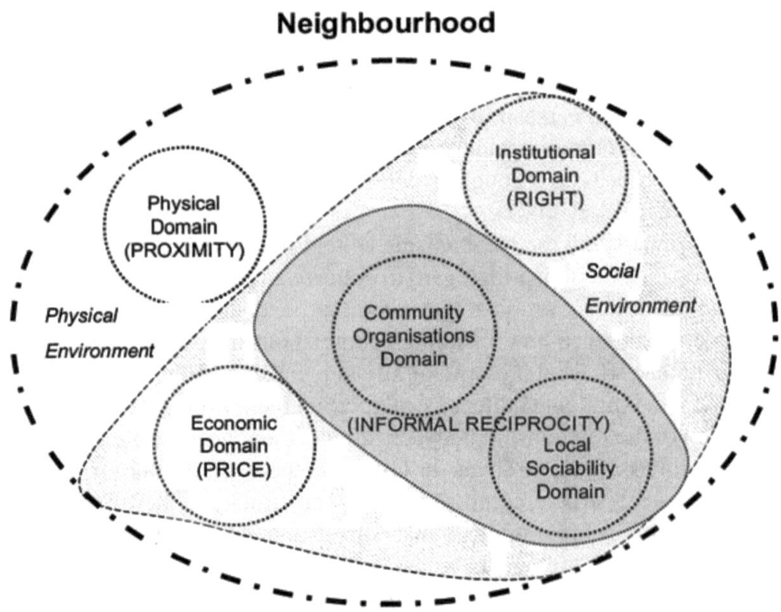

Fig. 3.1 Neighbourhood environments and rules of access (Source: Bernard P, Charrafedine R, Frohlich KL, Daniel M, Kestens Y, Potvin L (2007) Health inequalities and place: A theoretical conception of neighbourhood. Soc Sci Med 65:1839–1852, reprinted by permission of the publisher)

what we have termed proximity: people living in the same area share the same physical environment, and they are thus basically exposed to the same positive and negative resources. The economic domain is ruled by the market through price mechanisms. This domain and its rules function under the economic hypothesis that parties are presumed to seek the maximisation of their own utility. Resources within this domain can therefore only be obtained if people pay for them. In the case of the ISIS study, resources such as cigarettes sold through tobacco-selling outlets would be a prime example of a market-regulated resource. Resources made available through the institutional domain are accessed through the state via rights' mechanisms. Institutional rules regulate access to resources which citizens are entitled to according to publicly enacted rules; such entitlements are balanced against the fulfilment of citizen obligations. There is a recognised relationship between citizens who have rights and the state, which has some measure of authority. General examples of resources offered through this domain are schools, health clinics, shelters, childcare centres, etc. An example of a resource provided through the institutional domain in the case of ISIS is publicly funded smoking cessation services. The local sociability domain involves resources which can be mobilised through informal networks formed by the social links that people share. These involve noncontractual exchanges of resources outside of markets and state interventions. In this domain social relationships are explicitly engaged in gift giving which creates obligations of reciprocity that are non-specific to the contents, to the target or to the time frame of what has to be given back. Such resources include smoking-related norms. Finally, the community organisation domain follows the informal reciprocity rule but includes resources provided through formally organised collective entities such as charity groups. Many of these organisations are involved in some form of collective action. Resources offered by community organisations are normally given freely by groups or individuals to other individuals such as when community organisations organise local support groups for residents wanting to quit smoking. The critical difference between the local sociability and community organisations domains are that the former procure individuals benefits only, whereas the latter is mobilised in view of pursuing collective goals.

The discussion regarding domains and rules conceptualises how resources related to collective lifestyles can become inequitably available at a local level. A final component to our framework is an understanding of the social processes that permit the transformation of these resources into health outcomes or, in our case, into collective lifestyles. We would argue that health is produced not only with (or without) the structural constraints and opportunities offered at the local level but through individuals' capital stock which permits them to identify, access and utilise (or not) resources in neighbourhoods to their health advantage. Essentially health and behavioural outcomes at a local level are a function of both individuals' capitals and the demands and opportunities of the environment (Abel 2008). Social inequities in collective lifestyles are therefore a function of the quantity, quality and accessibility of local resources and their correspondence with the forms of capital that residents have at their disposal (Fig. 3.2).

Here, we call on the work of Pierre Bourdieu, once again. In his capital theory, Bourdieu discusses the strong link existing between different forms of capital[1], a class-specific habitus and the choices individuals have. Bourdieu understood the inequitable distribution of structurally based resources (capitals) as part of the fundamental system of inequity in a given society; it is both the result and a key mechanism of the social reproduction of power and privilege. His concept of capital was based on the distinction of three forms: social, economic and cultural capital. These three forms of capital are interrelated and inextricably linked. An important aspect to his theory was the elaborate account of the interaction between these three forms of capital in everyday life and the ways in which this interaction process contributes to the reproduction of social inequities and power distribution in society (Bourdieu 1984; Abel and Frohlich 2012).

Bourdieu's three capitals take the following forms. First, economic capital exists in the form of money and material assets (income, property, financial stocks) and is

---

[1] While capitals, according to Bourdieu, are essentially distributed by class, in order to understand how capitals can empirically influence health outcomes, we operationalise capitals at the individual level, remaining conscious that this operationalisation is but a stand-in for a collective phenomenon.

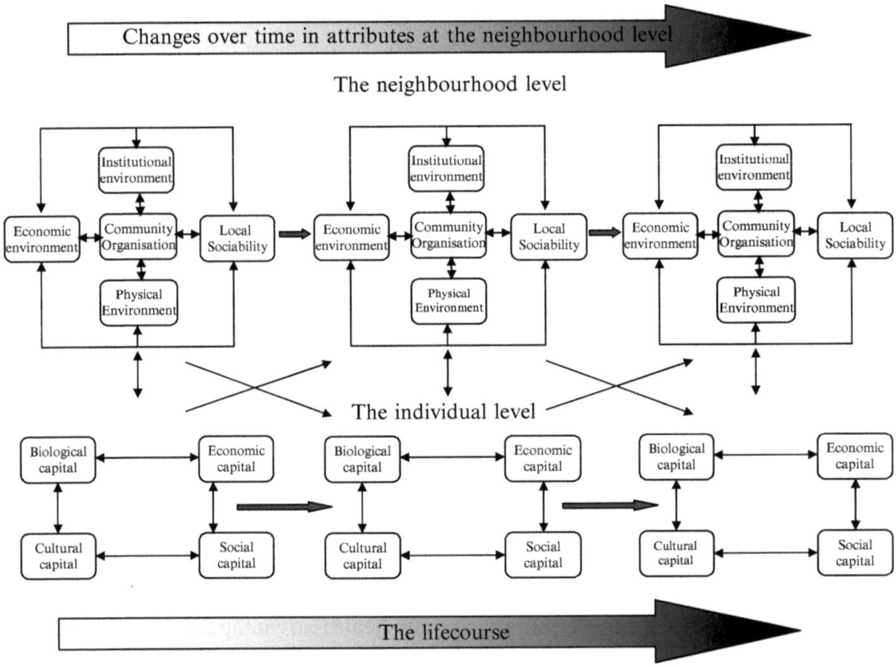

Fig. 3.2 The ISIS Framework for explaining how inequities in health are produced in neighbourhoods

a decisive factor in social advantage and disadvantage. It is also 'at the root of all the other types of capital' (p. 252). Second, social capital, from a Bourdieusian perspective, is located at the interindividual level. As such, it refers to material and nonmaterial resources which can be mobilised by virtue of many different kinds of social relationships. Lastly, cultural capital can be broadly defined as people's symbolic and informational resources for action (Bourdieu 1986; Wacquant 1992). Cultural capital exists in three different forms: incorporated (e.g. skills, knowledge), objectivised (e.g. books, tools, bicycles) and institutionalised (e.g. educational degrees, vocational certificates) (Bourdieu 1986). It is acquired mostly through social learning, with learning conditions varying across social classes, status groups or milieus (Abel 2007; Veenstra 2007; Williams 1995). A person's educational level can be understood as an indicator representing cultural capital. Yet, cultural capital refers to more than a person's formal education to include different sets of cultural competencies. Acquisition and use of these is part of a broader comprehensive social learning (socialisation) and thus depends heavily on 'total, early, imperceptible learning, performed within the family from the earliest days of life' (Bourdieu 1984, p. 66). In the form of knowledge and skills, cultural capital is a precondition for most individual action and, as such, is a key component in people's capacity for agency.

Individuals acquire and use, or do not, their capital stock in an active way. The active acquisition and development of such capital is part of individual and collective agency as is making health-relevant use of them. In other words, in order for cultural, social and economic capital to become health promoting, individuals have to actively use them. For instance, money is 'spent' on health-relevant behaviours (such as physical activity classes), support in health matters is 'sought out' (such as participating in self-help groups) and knowledge is 'applied' by individuals in order for it to function actively to engender health (for instance, decisions about what one eats).

We therefore suggest that inequity goes beyond just the unequal distribution of capital. We argue that there is considerable social inequity also in the chances and ability for people to have the different forms of capital consistently support and complement each other with the end result of their interaction being a health advantage. And this is where the two levels of inequity become of critical importance. At the individual level, capitals provide the agency potential for health. However, this potential is contingent on resources being available and accessible within a neighbourhood. So, for instance, one might have the cultural capital that would lead you to value jogging, but if your neighbourhood is too dangerous to jog in (whether this be due to traffic, stray dogs or human-caused violence), your capital may not be actualised due to structural constraints.

Conclusion

The last 20 years has seen steady and interesting developments in research focusing on area effects on behaviour and lifestyles. But there is much that needs to change if the research, and their attendant interventions, can become truly able to improve the situation of the most disadvantaged portions of our populations. First, health promotion concerned with inequities needs to dispel with the notion that health behaviour, viewed as an individual phenomenon, is the most important outcome. Individual-level interventions, and the structure-agency divide that accompanies this view of human comportment, cannot influence populations at an aggregate level and will not reduce the inequities that many of us in health promotion are so dedicated to reducing. Second, area effects research remains somewhat stymied by frameworks which, for the most part, focus on the correlates of inequalities in behavioural outcomes and/or are largely unable to explain the mechanisms that lead inequitable environments to lead to inequitable engagement in unhealthy health practices. This also needs to be pushed forward in order for us to more effectively develop interventions that will encourage and sustain change at the neighbourhood level.

How can this happen? We suggest that we move away from health behaviours as outcomes and focus more on collective lifestyles. In so doing, we bring attention to the inequitable structuring of life chances and choices and strive to understand how they interact with structural constraints and opportunities in neighbourhoods. Instead of putting emphasis on individual-level change, we turn the lens towards the societal inequities that require intervention such as the inequitable distribution of safe green spaces, good quality schools, inexpensive and healthy foods and neighbourhoods that encourage active public transit. By moving away from the individual focus that has been the trademark of health promotion for too long, the focus of health promotion can be turned, instead, towards the environmental and spatial justice issues that hark back to the wishes of the originators of the Ottawa Charter.

References

Abel, T. (2007). Cultural capital in health promotion. In D. C. McQueen & I. Kickbusch (Eds.), *Health and modernity. The role of theory in health promotion*. Berlin: Springer.

Abel, T. (2008). Cultural capital and social inequality in health. *Journal of Epidemiology and Community Health, 62*, e13.

Abel, T., & Frohlich, K. L. (2012). Capitals and capabilities: Linking structure and agency to reduce health inequalities. *Social Science & Medicine, 74*, 236–244.

Antonovsky, A. (1996). The salutogenic model as a theory to guide health promotion. *Health Promotion International, 11*, 11–18.

Berkman, L. F., & Kawachi, I. (2000). A historical framework for social epidemiology. In L. F. Berkman & I. Kawachi (Eds.), *Social Epidemiology*. New York: Oxford University Press.

Bernard, P., Charrafedine, R., Frohlich, K. L., Daniel, M., Kestens, Y., & Potvin, L. (2007). Health inequalities and place: A theoretical conception of neighbourhood. *Social Science & Medicine, 65*, 1839–1852.

Bourdieu, P. (1980). *Le sens pratique*. Paris: Les Éditions de Minuit.

Bourdieu, P. (1984). *Distinction: A social critique of the judgement of taste*. Cambridge: Harvard University Press.

Bourdieu, P. (1986). The forms of capital. In J. G. Richardson (Ed.), *Handbook of theory and research for the sociology of education*. Connecticut: Greenwood Press.

Chow, C. K., Lock, K., Teo, K., et al. (2009). Environmental and societal influences acting on cardiovascular risk factors and disease at a population level: A review. *International Journal of Epidemiology, 38*, 1580–1594.

Cockerham, W. C. (2005). Health lifestyle theory and the convergence of agency and structure. *Journal of Health and Social Behavior, 46*, 51–67.

Cockerham, W. C., Ruetten, A., & Abel, T. (1997). Conceptualizing contemporary health lifestyles: Moving beyond Weber. *The Sociological Quarterly, 38*, 321–342.

Cohen, D., Mason, K., Bedimo, A., et al. (2003). Neighborhood physical conditions and health. *American Journal of Public Health, 93*, 467–471.

Cohen, D., Spear, S., Scribner, R., et al. (2000). Broken windows and the risk of gonorrhea. *American Journal of Public Health, 90*, 230–236.

Coleman, J. S. (1990). *Foundations of social theory*. Cambridge: Harvard University Press.

COMMIT. (1995). 1. Cohort results from a four-year community intervention. *American Journal of Public Health, 85*, 183–192.

Drewnowski, A. (2009). Obesity, diets, and social inequalities. *Nutrition Reviews, 67*, S36–S39.

Duncan, C., Jones, K., & Moon, G. (1996). Health-related behaviour in context: A multi-level modelling approach. *Social Science & Medicine, 37*, 725–733.

Duncan, C., Jones, K., & Moon, G. (1999). Smoking and deprivation: Are there neighbourhood effects? *Social Science & Medicine, 48*, 497–505.

Ellaway, A., & Macintyre, S. (2009). Are perceived neighbourhood problems associated with the likelihood of smoking? *Journal of Epidemiology and Community Health, 63*, 78–80.

Fitzpatrick, K., & LaGory, M. (2011). *Unhealthy cities. Poverty, race and place in America*. New York: Routledge.

Frohlich, K. L., Bernard, P., Charafeddine, R., et al. (2008). L'émergence d'inégalités de santé dans les quartiers: Un cadre théorique. In K. Frohlich, M. DeKoninck, A. Demers, & P. Bernard (Eds.), *Les inégalités sociales de santé au Québec*. Montréal: Presses Universitaires de Montréal.

Frohlich, K. L., Corin, E., & Potvin, L. (2001). A theoretical proposal for the relationship between context and disease. *Sociology of Health & Illness, 23*, 776–797.

Frohlich, K. L., Poland, B., & Shareck, M. (2012). Contrasting entry points for intervention in health promotion practice: Situating and working with context. In M. O'Neill, A. Pederson, I. Rootman, & S. Dupéré (Eds.), *Health promotion in Canada* (3rd ed.). Toronto, Ontario: CSPI.

Frohlich, K. L., Potvin, L., Gauvin, L., et al. (2002). Youth smoking initiation: Disentangling context from composition. *Health & Place, 8*, 155–166.

Galea, S. (2007). *Macrosocial determinants of population health*. New York: Springer.

Galea, S., & Vlahov, D. (2005). Urban health: Evidence, challenges and directions. *Annual Review of Public Health, 26*, 341–365.

Giddens, A. (1984). *The constitution of society*. Berkeley: University of California Press.

Godbout, J. T. (2000). *Le don, la dette et l'identité: Homo donator Versus homo economicus*. Paris et Montréal: Éditions La Découverte et Éditions du Boréal.

Godbout, J. T. (2003). *The world of the gift*. Montréal: McGill-Queen's University Press.

Hansen, E., & Easthope, G. (2007). *Lifestyle in medicine*. London and New York: Routledge.

Higgs, G., & Langford, M. (2009). GIScience, environmental justice and estimating populations at risk: The case of landfills in Wales. *Applied Geography, 29*, 63–76.

Jones, K., & Moon, G. (1993). Medical geography: Taking space seriously. *Progress in Human Geography, 17*, 515–525.

Karvonen, S., Sipilä, P., Martikainen, P., et al. (2008). Smoking in context—a multilevel approach to smoking prevalence among females in Helsinki. *BMC Public Health, 8*, 134.

Kawachi, I. (1997). Long live community: Social capital as public health. *The American Prospect, 35*, 56–59.

Kawachi, I., & Kennedy, B. (1997). Social capital, income inequality, and mortality. *American Journal of Public Health, 87*, 1491–1498.

Kickbusch, I. (1986). Lifestyles and health. *Social Science & Medicine, 22*, 117–124.

Lalonde, M. (1974). A new perspective on the health of Canadians. http://www.hc-sc.gc.ca/hcs-sss/alt_formats/hpb-dgps/pdf/pubs/1974-lalonde/lalonde_e.pdf. Accessed 18 Dec 2011.

Lang, T., & Caraher, M. (1998). Access to healthy foods: Part II. Food poverty and shopping deserts: What are the implications for health promotion policy and practice? *Health Education Journal, 57*, 202.

Lindstrom, M. (2003). Social capital and the miniaturization of community among daily and intermittent smokers: A population-based study. *Preventive Medicine, 36*, 177–184.

Lindstrom, M. (2010). Social capital and health-related behaviours. In I. Kawachi, S. V. Subramanian, & D. Kim (Eds.), *Social capital and health*. New York: Springer.

Lindstrom, N., Moghaddassi, M., Lindgren, B., et al. (2003). Social participation, social capital and daily tobacco smoking: A population-based multilevel analysis in Malmo, Sweden. *Scandinavian Journal of Public Health, 31*, 444–450.

Macintyre, S. (2007). Deprivation amplification revisited: Or, is it always true that poorer places have poorer access to resources for healthy diets and physical activity? *International Journal of Behavioral Nutrition and Physical Activity, 4*, 32.

Macintyre, S., & Ellaway, A. (2003). Neighbourhoods and health: An overview. In I. Kawachi & L. F. Berkman (Eds.), *Neighbourhoods and health*. New York: Oxford University Press.

Macintyre, S., Ellaway, A., & Cummins, S. (2002). Place effects on health: How can we conceptualise, operationalise and measure them? *Social Science & Medicine, 55*, 25–139.

Macintyre, S., McIver, S., & Sooman, A. (1993). Area, class and health: Should we be focussing on places or people? *Journal of Social Policy, 22*, 213–234.

Masuda, J. R., Poland, B., & Baxter, J. (2010). Reaching for environmental health justice: Canadian experiences for a comprehensive research, policy and advocacy agenda in health promotion. *Health Promotion International, 25*, 453–463.

McLeroy, K. R., Bibeau, D., Steckler, A., et al. (1988). An ecological perspective on health promotion. *Health Education Quarterly, 15*, 351–377.
Mechanic, D. (1993). Social research in health and the American socio-political context: The changing fortunes of medical sociology. *Social Science & Medicine, 36*, 95–102.
Multiple Risk Factor Intervention Trial Research Group. (1981). Multiple risk factor intervention trial. *Preventive Medicine, 10*, 387–553.
Multiple Risk Factor Intervention Trial Research Group. (1982). Multiple risk factor intervention trial: Risk factor changes and mortality results. *Journal of the American Medical Association, 24*, 1465–1476.
Pabayo, R. A., Belsky, J., Gauvin, L., et al. (2011). Do area characteristics predict change in moderate-to-vigorous physical activity from ages 11 to 15 years? *Social Science & Medicine, 72*, 430–438.
Pabayo, R. A., Gauvin, L., Barnett, T. A., et al. (2012). Understanding the determinants of active transportation to school among children: Evidence of environmental injustice from the Quebec longitudinal study of child development. *Health & Place, 18*, 163–171.
Pearce, J. R., Richardson, E. A., Mitchell, R. J., et al. (2010). Environmental justice and health: The implications of the socio-spatial distribution of multiple environmental deprivation for health inequalities in the United Kingdom. *Transactions of the Institute of British Geographers, 35*, 522–539.
Pearce, J. R., Richardson, E. A., Mitchell, R. J., et al. (2011). Environmental justice and health: A study of multiple environmental deprivation and geographical inequalities in health in New Zealand. *Social Science & Medicine, 73*, 410–420.
Poland, B., Krupa, G., & McCall, D. (2009). Settings for health promotion: An analytic framework to guide intervention design and implementation. *Health Promotion Practice, 10*, 505–516.
Poortinga, W. (2006). Do health behaviours mediate the association between social capital and health? *Preventive Medicine, 43*, 488–493.
Putnam, R. D. (1993). *Making democracy work: Civic traditions in modern Italy*. Princeton: Princeton University Press.
Richard, L., Potvin, L., Kishchuk, N., et al. (1996). Assessment of the integration of the ecological approach in health promotion programs. *American Journal of Health Promotion, 10*, 318–328.
Rose, D., & Richards, R. (2007). Food stores access and household fruit and vegetable use among participants in the US Food Stamp Program. *Public Health Nutrition, 7*, 1081–1088.
Rütten, A. (1995). The implementation of health promotion: A new structural perspective. *Social Science & Medicine, 41*, 1627–1637.
Sampson, R. J. (2003). Neighbourhood-level context and health: Lessons from sociology. In I. Kawachi & L. F. Berkman (Eds.), *Neighbourhoods and health*. New York: Oxford University Press.
Sampson, R. J., & Raudenbush, S. W. (1999). Systematic social observation of public spaces: A new look at disorder in urban neighbourhoods. *The American Journal of Sociology, 105*, 603–651.
Schaefer-McDaniel, N., O'Brien Caughy, M., O'Campo, P., et al. (2010). Examining methodological details of neighbourhoods observations and the relationship to health. A literature review. *Social Science & Medicine, 70*, 277–292.
Siahpush, M., Borland, R., Taylor, J., et al. (2006). The association of smoking with perception of income inequality, relative material well-being, and social capital. *Social Science & Medicine, 63*, 2801–2812.
Soja, E. W. (2010). *Seeking social justice*. Minnesota: University of Minnesota Press.
Taylor, W. C., Poston, W. S. C., Jones, L., et al. (2006). Environmental justice: Obesity, physical activity, and healthy eating. *Journal of Physical Activity & Health, 3*, S30–S54.
Tolbert Kimbro, R., Brooks-Gunn, J., & McLanahan, S. (2011). Young children in urban areas: Links among neighbourhood characteristics, weight status, outdoor play, and television watching. *Social Science & Medicine, 72*, 668–676.

Veenstra, G. (2007). Social space, social class and Bourdieu: Health inequalities in British Columbia, Canada. *Health & Place, 13*, 14–31.

Wacquant, L. J. D. (1992). Toward a social praxeology: The structure and logic of Bourdieu's sociology. In B. Bourdieu & L. J. D. Wacquant (Eds.), *An invitation to reflexive sociology*. Chicago: University of Chicago Press.

Walker, G., Mitchell, G., Fairburn, J., et al. (2005). Industrial pollution and social deprivation: Evidence and complexity in evaluating and responding to environmental inequality. *Local Environment, 10*, 361–377.

Weber, M. (1978). *Economy and society: An outline of interpretive sociology*. Berkeley: University of California Press.

Williams, S. J. (1995). Theorising class, health and lifestyles: Can Bourdieu help us? *Sociology of Health & Illness, 17*, 577–604.

Wilson, J. Q., & Kelling, G. L. (1989). Broken windows. In R. G. Dunham & G. P. Alpert (Eds.), *Critical issues in policing: Contemporary readings*. Illinois: Waveland Press Inc.

World Health Organisation (WHO). (2008). *Closing the gap in a generation: Health equity through action on the social determinants of health. Final report of the commission on social determinants of health*. Geneva: World Health Organisation.

World Health Organization. (1986). Ottawa charter for health promotion. *Health Promotion International, 1*, 405.

Chapter 4
Sociological Perspectives on Neighbourhood Context and Health

Pernille Tanggaard Andersen

Introduction

There is a need for a better understanding of the processes through which neighbourhood environments can affect health (Andersen et al. 2011a; Raphael 2006; Macintyre et al. 2002; Diez-Roux 2001). When investigating neighbourhood context, we need to adopt a more dynamic understanding of the influence of social context on health. Here, context is mainly considered to be the collective way of life expressed by the local residents through their relations to the characteristics of the area as well as their similarities in terms of social practices. Adopting a dynamic approach, this chapter explores the ways in which sociological theory provides useful perspectives on the investigation of social context, health and human behaviour. When examining sociological theories, a variety of models of understanding neighbourhood contexts, health behaviour and lifestyles is applied for the purpose of further investigation.

The sociological subject matter and the ecological approach to health, which form the basis of this chapter, are introduced in the following. Firstly, a sociological definition of the term "local neighbourhood" is formulated based on four dimensions: actors, tasks (problems), structures and resources. This definition is followed by a presentation of various sociological perspectives that can be applied when analysing those four dimensions. The perspectives include firstly, microsociological theory concerned with behaviour and everyday life; secondly, sociological theory on local communities, social capital and empowerment processes; and thirdly, the ways in which sociological theory might be applied to exclusion mechanism research. The chapter is concluded by presenting a specific sociological analysis of Bakkedal, a deprived local neighbourhood in Denmark.

P. Tanggaard Andersen (✉)
Unit for Health Promotion Research, Institute of Public Health, University of Southern Denmark, Niels Bohrs Vej 9-10, Esbjerg 6700, Denmark
e-mail: ptandersen@health.sdu.dk

C. Stock and A. Ellaway (eds.), *Neighbourhood Structure and Health Promotion*,
DOI 10.1007/978-1-4614-6672-7_4, © Springer Science+Business Media New York 2013

Sociology and the Ecological Approach to Health

The subject matter of sociology is the theory of all social matters, including the relationship between individuals, groups and society as a human condition of life as well as a source of change (Giddens 1995). Therefore, sociology is concerned with identifying connections and patterns within those social relationships and the social interaction present within and amongst various abstraction levels (macro, meso and micro) seen from various perspectives (Aakvaag 2008).[1] The central issue within sociological theory remains the analysis of existing societies and the questions related to the relationship between individuals and societies, including the ways in which the lives of societies, groups and individuals are formed and changed (Andersen and Timm 2010). Thus, the starting point of sociology is to understand the social relations present within the complex connections, in which they arise, meaning various social contexts. With regard to understanding health and illness, sociology applies a complex viewpoint not only involving physical, psychological and existential dimensions but also, and to a similar extent, social life within small and large communities. This means that health and illness embrace the entire life and all life conditions of a person, which in turn requires a consideration of all of those interacting dimensions in order to understand action, practice and context (Andersen and Timm 2010). The approach presented by sociology of health and illness fits nicely to the perspectives within ecological health research through the shared focus on a holistic approach to the meaning of context in terms of human behaviour, health and well-being.

A Sociological Approach to Local Communities

A local community might be defined as a collection of citizens/individuals, who have organised themselves within a community through shared institutional frameworks, culture and norms. A local community is often defined by means of a geographically bound community, which all local individuals/citizens feel connected to despite any social or cultural differences (Laverack 2003; Napier 2002). Seen in this light, a local community is where people live, work and/or spend their leisure time (Nutbeam 1986). The human social relations make up the core and the development potential within each local community. The social relations/networks that exist amongst those individuals contribute to the creation of a community, of hierarchies

[1] At a macro level, factors such as those overall societal institutions that structure a society in financial, political and legal terms, but also family, health care systems, etc., are present. The meso level includes various types of everyday life experienced by people living in a society, everyday cultural life of social groups and subgroups within the local communities, organisational and institutional life, etc. The micro level is concerned with each individual life story and actual everyday life within the given cultural and societal framework.

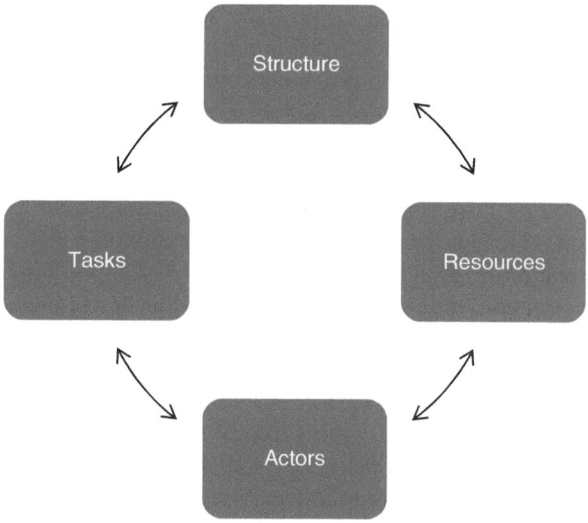

Fig. 4.1 Local community organisation

and of social structures, which directly or indirectly, amongst other things, define who we are and how we differ from others. In this way, symbolic communication often exists within such a local community boundaries.

Sociological research into local communities usually involves urban local areas, town quarters, suburbs, villages or marginalised residential areas. A general theme in loc.l community studies is the examination of community creation and the ways in which social relations work and establish behavioural structures and frameworks (Bracht 1999). Other studies focus more on the analysis of the power structure within loc.l communities, i.e. the 1963 study "Community Power Structure" by Floyd Hunter.[2]

Høgsbro speaks of four dimensions making up the local community organisation (Fig. 4.1):

As such, the local community/residential area might be considered a loosely structured organisation, in which the individuals to a small or large extent depend on each other and which involves an interaction of tasks, resources, actors and

[2]However, local community studies might also include other types of settings than local towns or rural areas. The perspective of such studies might also be the analysis of an organisation, i.e. an administrative and functional social system of individuals and groups, which was established for the purpose of achieving a certain goal. In this context, an application of the local community analysis perspective contributes to an examination of work processes, coordination, organisational culture and behaviour amongst local citizens and professionals. Thus, local community studies might also include examinations of care homes, kindergartens, school or other public or private organisations.

structures (Høgsbro 2005). The *social structure* of a local community covers, amongst other things, the grouping of citizens in terms of sex, age and occupation; geographical location; as well as the local community features with regard to environments, organisations, associations and social networks. The *resources* of a local community cover, amongst other things, the population group composition; resources pertaining to education, income, social and/or health-related issues; as well as those social resources that exist across the local community. For example, social resources might include social networks consisting of various interpersonal relationships such as family, work or leisure time connections.[3] The *actors* of a local community might be citizens, professionals, volunteers, relatives or others who are involved in/important to the specific local area. The *tasks* of a local community are related to those tasks, challenges and issues that exist within the local community (Høgsbro 2005). Therefore, a local community analysis might assist in identifying resources and needs within a local area. Such knowledge will contribute to obtaining an overview of resources, social networks, barriers and potential strategies with regard to health promotion and prevention within the area.

Because the local community makes up a central framework in people's lives, it provides a natural setting for health promotion initiatives. Previous research has shown that the local community, in which people live, influences health behaviour, health and mortality (Krueger and Chang 2008; Reijneveld 2002; Pickett and Pearl 2001; Bosma et al. 2001). The local community has the potential to provide a long range of factors and/or stress factors, which cause everyday issues and influence health (Andersen et al. 2011a; Staffort and Marmot 2003; Diez-Roux 2001). When conducting performing studies into local community and residential areas, it is therefore of vital importance to examine everyday life as it is in fact being lived, i.e. customs, routines and everyday behaviour that take place and impact the lives of the local citizens.

Sociological Theory on Health Behaviour and Everyday Life

Taking a holistic approach to everyday life and health of local citizens involves obtaining knowledge about the ways in which health behaviour and everyday life are related to each other, and the following section introduces various theories on this matter.

In general, health behaviour is defined as an overall expression of those actions that we carry out alone or with others and which influence our health in the short or long run (Kivisto 2011; Rasmussen et al. 2000). This holistic view on health behaviour stands in contrast with traditional health promotion which would narrowly

[3]Homogeneous networks, i.e. small groups of similar individuals maintaining close contact. Heterogeneous networks include a variety of people who gather because of a certain issue. Traditional networks often involve people, who have known each other for many years, e.g. family, neighbours or work colleagues.

define health behaviour mostly as smoking, diet, alcohol and physical activity. Overall, behavioural theories in social psychology consider the health behaviour of an individual to be a result of that person's subjective view of the situation as well as his or her opinions, motivations and intentions (Kivisto 2011). The theories of social psychology have been criticised for weighing the individual's perception, meaning that health behaviour comes across as always being a result of conscious and "rational" considerations. Also, they individualise the term "health behaviour" and include only to a limited extent the more society-related factors such as living conditions, upbringing and cultural environment. Such society-related factors make up the basis of sociological health behaviour theories such as social learning theory. According to this theory, social learning is a deciding factor with regard to individual behaviour. Social learning takes place through imitation of behaviour exhibited by valued persons but also by the individual reacting and adapting his or her own actions to fit the suitable behaviour defined by those valued persons.

Alfred Schultz [1899–1959] concerns himself with behaviour, lifeworld and everyday life, and amongst other things, he speaks of behaviour being taken for granted (Schutz 1967; Schutz and Luchmann 1973). One of the reasons why it is so difficult to achieve behavioural change is that it feels natural to act in a certain way. According to Schultz, we all live in our own lifeworld, which is the world that seems natural to us and is taken for granted by us. This lifeworld also involves norms, assumptions and behaviour that keep our lifeworld going. Within our lifeworld, some issues are so-called thematised or current to us; others are not (Schutz and Luchmann 1973). These themes make up the horizon or the knowledge base that we use to evaluate the world. New themes only then become relevant to us once we face a new situation that requires new knowledge or behavioural change. That makes our knowledge pragmatic. We know what we need to know. However, when facing a new situation, we will make sure to obtain the knowledge needed in order to maintain our lifeworld. Lifeworld describes the everyday life that seems so natural to us that we do not question it. Each person has a different lifeworld; whereas certain things are taken for granted by some people, others question them (Beck-Jørgensen 1994; Schutz and Luchmann 1973). You might compare this situation with a woman being admitted to hospital because of a serious allergic reaction. Before being taken to hospital, she never thought about allergies and asthma and how to avoid those problems. It was not a theme in her lifeworld; although she had heard of asthma before, it was not *relevant* to her. Now it has turned into a relevant problem for her, and this theme will become part of her lifeworld. However, being taken to hospital does not mean that a person automatically implements behavioural changes after returning home. Once we feel healthy again, we often return to the way of living that has felt natural to us so far.

Everyday life makes up our lifeworld, and it consists of a flow of social relations, norms, objects, schedules, repetitions and customs. Those generations of meaning, which structure everyday life, are, as mentioned before, so natural that we hardly notice them. When analysing everyday life, it might be relevant to examine "the symbolic order of matters of course" (Beck-Jørgensen 1994), meaning an examination of everyday life's matters of course exhibited through routines, traditions and rituals that provide continuity and clarity. Analysing the everyday life of an individual, it might be relevant to partly look at the conditions (individual, interpersonal and societal) that make up the everyday life and partly analyse the ways in which the individual handles, understands and manages those conditions (Beck-Jørgensen 1994). Conditions of everyday life could include the ways in which the individual reacts to his or her environment, participates in communities and is affected by social norms and behavioural rules and how institutional and societal conditions influence everyday life and how it is being lived within the local area.

Local Community, Integration and Well-Being

As mentioned earlier, the idea of a local community and setting is based on the assumption of a bound and social community in which social relations, exchange of experience as well as shared structures/frameworks make up the basis for integration.

Local integration is seen from one of two perspectives: either focusing on community and cultural elements or on integration through social capital. The community perspective is inspired by Emile Durkheim's [1858–1917] ideas about mechanical solidarity as the basis of local integration (Røiseland et al. 1999). According to Durkheim, the cohesion factor of premodern society was a simple division of tasks and a large degree of conformity. A certain level of consensus with regard to stable values and norms existed, which fostered a clear-cut morale that was internalised into the shared collective soul through religion and tradition. A sense of community and collective awareness made each individual experience a feeling of belonging—of having some type of identity (Durkheim 1984; Andersen 2002). In modern society, life is characterised by a higher degree of pluralism, mobility and task division, which affects the creation of close and binding local communities. People still participate in a long range of communities; however, they are no longer as closely attached to shared local residential areas as before (Røiseland et al. 1999). Local residential areas are no longer homogeneous but often characterised by many different cultural backgrounds, religions and different ways of living everyday life. Therefore, it is often impossible to define a shared cultural element (community) when analysing the issue of integration within residential areas.

Social capital is another term also concerned with integration processes. Pierre Bourdieu [1930–2002] was the first person to compile a thorough development and comprehensive application of the concept. In his early work, Bourdieu emphasises that social capital is a product of durable relationships and that it is upheld by these relationships.[4] In continuation hereof, Kawachi and Berkman (2003) suggest that social capital must be viewed as the cohesion factor, norms about mutual assistance, trust and other social structure features, which provide resources to the community and to each individual.

---

[4]Bourdieu defines social capital as "the aggregate of the actual or potential resources which are linked to possession of a durable network of more or less institutionalised relationships of mutual acquaintance or recognition" (Bourdieu 1985, p. 248).

Another important theorist, when working with social capital, is Robert Putnam. His definition is developed on the basis of a study of the development of democratic political culture in Italy. Social capital is seen as the ability of actors to secure benefits through membership in networks and other social structures (Putnam 2000; Andersen et al. 2011b). Originating from social relations based on networks, norms and trust, the term "social capital" often reflects some type of cohesion factor within a group or a local area. By creating social capital, each individual gains access to resources that surpass the mere sharing amongst individuals. Network participation often has a positive impact on the individual in the form of social capital, and by being part of a social network, the individual will find it easier to reach both individual and shared goals (Putnam 1995, 2000).

When investigating social capital, it is important to consider the different forms of social capital and the distinction between bonding, bridging and linking social capital (Putnam 2000; Szreter and Woolcock 2004). Bonding social capital refers to strong ties between members of a network who view them as being alike and as having a mutual social identity, e.g. age, class, ethnic group, whereas bridging social capital refers to weaker ties between individuals who are unalike in terms of social identity. Linking social capital constitutes a refinement of bridging social capital and refers to ties between individuals in different formal or institutionalised power or authority hierarchies (Szreter and Woolcock 2004).

In this way, the local community profile itself influences the social networks and the amount of social capital fostered within such social networks. Amongst other things, Cattell examined poor and worn down residential areas in London, and he concluded that residential areas with a low level of social capital witnessed more social exclusion, a higher crime rate, scattered networks and only very limited contact amongst the residents (Cattell 2001). Cattell has helped identifying that living in certain local areas can be so distressing that it affects people's well-being and health behaviour negatively. In that connection, Frohlich et al. (2001), amongst others, have suggested that health behaviour is affected by and must be considered part of social practice, which is developed within the environment in which the individual lives and moves. When studying local areas, analysing social capital on that basis might provide useful knowledge about community establishment (inclusion and exclusion mechanisms, etc.) as well as shared norms and values.

Putnam (1995, 2000) states that development of social capital is closely related to participation in civil organisations such as voluntary organisations and interest groups. Putnam's theory on social capital has been criticised within social epidemiology for its romanticised view on communities that have no social conflicts. Furthermore, it has been debated if there is evidence that social capital is a determinant of better health or not. This debate also relates to the definitions we use, e.g. if we analyse social network, social support and social coherence (Muntaner et al. 2010; Muntaner and Lynch 2002). This takes us to a different term, which might be of vital importance when studying integration in local residential areas: empowerment. Empowerment is defined as "enabling or providing others with the abilities to gain control of their own life situation" (Minkler 2005; Rappaport 1984). The strength of this term lies in the ability of empowerment to develop individual competencies whilst creating a more proactive approach to changing one's life conditions

(Kieffer 1984; Rodwell 1996). At a local community level, empowerment ideally "establishes the basis for participation in shared political initiatives, which can lead to increased psychological and individual empowerment and more decision-making competence within the local area" (Laverack and Wallenstein 2001; Bracht 1999). In continuation hereof, the basic idea behind this term is that empowerment can assist in minimising the impact of the professionals/"the system" on the local citizens, instead of opening up for more personal responsibility and taking more direct charge of one's own life (Tengland 2008). It is often said that empowerment processes can play a vital role with regard to redistribution of power, society goods and social fairness (Swift and Levin 1987). When analysing empowerment, however, one should not forget that the term is often applied in different ways depending on the ideological strategy behind the initiatives in questions. Seen from a liberalistic point of view, empowerment strategies often provide the individual with a higher degree of autonomy and ability to pursue personal goals. The viewpoints of social criticism and solidarity take a different approach to empowerment strategies, often focusing on the dialectics between living conditions and rights as well as an adjustment of structures that create inequality (Andersen and Timm 2010).

Sociological Theory on Exclusion Mechanisms and Stigma

Whereas the above examined integration and well-being issues, the following section deals with theories regarding lack of inclusion and a variety of exclusion mechanisms.

Various conflicting political and scientific perceptions of the term "social exclusion" exist, and there is *no* approved definition (Levitas 1998). There is, however, a general consensus that social exclusion in general refers to *a lack of participation* in society (Larsen 2009), and the multidimensional and dynamic aspects of this term are often highlighted. Social exclusion is *multidimensional* because it is not only concerned with income but also with a long range of other living standard and living condition indicators. Social exclusion is *dynamic* because when analysing social exclusion, the underlying processes must be considered, and those factors responsible for causing the individual to become marginalised must be identified. In this way, the multidimensional dimension not only describes deprivation caused by a lack of personal resources but also by insufficient community resources (local area dimension). Therefore, social exclusion analyses often focus on discontinuity between the individual and the surrounding environment (Larsen et al. 2012).

In general, social exclusion is concerned with those people, who are poor (excluded) within not only one but several vital living condition areas, e.g. having a low income, no work, immigrant background, no education and/or bad health. Social exclusion happens when bad living conditions and a lack of participation within a range of society areas start to accumulate (Levitas 1998). As an example, this is concerned with maintaining a reasonable living standard, being part of a family network or another social network, participating in professional and political initiatives or taking part in leisure time activities (Larsen 2004, 2009). The combination of bad living conditions might lead to a range of "vicious circles" that increase the risk of social exclusion and marginalisation. Thus, exclusion is not a situation that suddenly arises but rather the result of a process typically involving some type of marginalisation that turns into social exclusion.

In order to be able to understand the complexity of the mechanisms behind social exclusion, it is necessary to examine both living conditions, cultural marginalisation and participation as well as maintain focus on subjectively experienced social exclusion. When performing a more detailed examination of social exclusion and housing conditions, three areas can be analysed according to Larsen and Kristensen (2007): (1) few or no social relations, (2) low or no participation in professional and political initiatives and (3) low or no participation in leisure time activities. Actual analyses will often paint a picture of various combinations of inclusion and exclusion at various levels (Larsen et al. 2012). Social inclusion and exclusion mechanisms can, e.g. vary, because they are both determined by overall society structures and at the same time influenced by everyday life and local community culture. Specifically, this means that one can be socially marginalised because of unemployment and at the same time feel included in a subgroup or a neighbourhood because unemployment is the norm in the local community and everyday life (Larsen et al. 2012). It is often the local norms and values that are crucial for what is characterised as being normal or "deviant" (Jenkins 1997).

However, whether a person feels connected to and part of the local society or not is also about the extent to which the surrounding society either assigns symbolic capital to this person (Bourdieu 1990) or stigmatises him or her as being different/aberrant compared to the local society norms. Lacking approval within social communities can cause a social exclusion process and stigmatisation. According to Erving Goffman [1922–1982] (1963), stigma is defined as a characteristic that is deeply miscrediting and reduces the stigmatised person from being whole and ordinary to becoming distressed and excluded. Stigma occurs through social interaction when a group has certain features that are different to the established norms (Larsen et al. 2012). The decision as to which individuals or groups are included in society depends on a basic principle of categorisation inherent in human beings. This principle of categorisation establishes and maintains borders between identities, and its design depends on place and time (Jenkins 1997). The inclusion and exclusion process contains a basic power perspective. According to Foucault (1977), deciding what is normal and what is not constitutes an exercise of power in its own right. Defining normality is thus a decision as to which values are valid in a society. A dominating group's categorisation of a less powerful group defines both the existence conditions and possibilities for that group. This is not merely an act of neutral and passive categorisation but rather an *intervention* in the social world, which determines options and limits (Larsen et al. 2012; Jenkins 1997). In this sense, social exclusion should be considered a relation and interaction between the decision-making and norm-defining groups and those groups that differ from those norms, which means that it is often relevant to examine intersections between dimensions of inequality in order to gain an in-depth understanding of exclusion.

The Case of Bakkedal

The residential area of Bakkedal is located in a quite large provincial town in Denmark. A health profile from 2007 shows that resident health profiles vary significantly depending on the resident address. Amongst other things, the local health profile points out that Bakkedal residents often feel stressed, smoke more, display more unhealthy eating habits and are more frequently physically inactive compared to the residents of the municipality in question as a whole. Bakkedal houses a lot of residents that have no connection to the labour market or the educational system, and a large percentage of the residents have been convicted for offences related to the criminal law, the weapons law or the drug prohibition law. Based on the characteristics of Bakkedal, it is described as a residential area bearing the mark of concentrated social exclusion and a feeling of marginalisation from the surrounding society.

The municipality of X has been focusing on this residential area for a long time, attempting to fight social inequity in health within the municipality for several years.[5] Amongst other things, this has led to the implementation of various activities within the residential area for the periods 2008–2014.

Organisation and Promotion of Activities in Bakkedal

In the last years, several health promotion activities are stated in Bakkedal, including activities such as swimming, zumba, pilates, street dance and line dancing and the creation of a community centre, a craft club and various smoking cessation and weight control courses.

As a starting point, the initiatives in Bakkedal are coordinated by a project manager, who implements and coordinates a range of health-promoting initiatives within the area in cooperation with the residents. At the same time, one of the project aims is that the project manager must hand over more and more project management tasks to the residents themselves with a view to withdrawing the project manager completely when the project ends in 2014. The project strategy has been characterised by resident involvement and the municipality administration wanting to slowly withdraw from the organisational tasks. As early as during the project start-up phase, the residents were invited to café meetings where decisions on a range of activities were made and a number of task groups were formed for the purpose of promoting health and well-being in the local area. Since then, the task groups have cooperated with the project manager in terms of planning and implementing various activities such as a café and film club; fitness activities such as

[5] Three strategies have been defined as a means of promoting social equality in health issues: (1) high level of resident involvement, (2) differentiated offers adapted to fit the needs of various target groups and (3) multipronged initiatives in the immediate environment.

zumba, pilates and line dancing; and the establishment of a drop-in centre, a needlework club and courses on how to stop smoking and lose weight, as well as swimming courses for women. Most of the projects were initiated by the residents themselves and are run by a task group formed by the residents in cooperation with the project manager.

In 2009 the former local care home was turned into a community centre. This community centre is home to most of the activities related to the health project. In addition, a café was established, which is run by volunteers in the evenings and makes up a daily meeting point for many local residents. Another initiative, which has assisted in establishing a framework for physical activity and allowing residents to "meet up" outdoors, is the establishment of a funcourt that hosts a variety of sports activities such as basketball, volleyball, football, handball and hockey. This initiative is particularly aimed at children and youngsters living in the area.

The mentioned initiatives illustrate in various way how the establishment of the right physical surroundings in the local area provides a positive means of offering activities that promote local communities. In this way, the physical surroundings foster well-being and healthy habits. Existing research work in Bakkedal also shows, however, that the expansion and improvement of the physical surroundings comprise no miracle cure when it comes to the well-being and health of the local residents (Andersen and Timm 2010). During the implementation of the project within the local area, several barriers had to be dealt with. The following presentation discusses two such barriers: the aspect of resident involvement and the aspect of inclusion/exclusion.

Lessons Learned in Bakkedal

The municipality has been very interested in resident involvement and the idea of making the local residents own the project. Some of the local residents have played an active role during the development of the neighbourhood project and the establishment of the community centre, amongst other things. However, one of the barriers experienced has been a lack of task division between professionals and volunteers. From the very beginning, several questions remained unanswered: To what extent are the residents to be included, when and how? Who is responsible for decision-making? Which role will the professionals and the municipality play? The lack of role definition has led to a vast amount of internal discussions and caused quite some conflicts on an ongoing basis. The turbulent community centre establishment period has, amongst other things, caused the volunteers to feel short of decision-making authorisation, which in turn has made them reduce their level of involvement. The establishment of the community centre is, however, dependent on professional assistance, and whereas in a perfect world, the professionals would only take on an active role in terms of servicing and counselling, as it has also happened in Bakkedal, there is always a risk of them dominating the processes. Furthermore, the professionals represent "the system", and as many of the residents depend on social security and are subject to public power and authority administration through the municipality in their everyday lives, a too dominating position of the professionals can lead to opposition to the project as a whole (Minkler 2005). The experience gained in Bakkedal shows that a precise role definition for professionals and volunteers is vital if resident involvement and empowerment processes are to succeed (Andersen and Timm 2010).

The municipality also focused on doing something active to improve social equity in health, and the improvement of the physical surroundings has at least provided the possibility for a healthier lifestyle to develop amongst the residents. This means that the local area has experienced a boost in terms of physical surroundings and activities within the area, thereby placing itself on a more equal footing with wealthier neighbourhoods in town. The question is whether or not the project has managed to alter the internal structures of inequality? The answer to this question is complex. On the one hand, the establishment of a funcourt and the community centre, amongst other things, has meant that more residents participate in various activities and leave their personal imprint on the local area and that the residents meet across the former groups. On the other hand, the project has also caused a higher level of polarisation. Overall, a large part of the residents participate and make their influence count within the local area; however, at the same time, another group of residents do not participate, and this group feels powerless with regard to all the new initiatives that are changing their local area. Finally, a small group of residents still feels isolated and not at all targeted by the various activities on offer.

Thus, the experiences gathered in Bakkedal suggest that whereas health-promoting initiatives in loc.l areas bring about "positive development", they also carry the risk of increasing resident polarisation. One of the main reasons for this is that such projects often carry embedded conceptions about what "the good neighbour" and "the healthy residential area" mean and must be. Such conceptions produce ideals about how one is supposed to behave, how to maintain neighbour relations and how intensely to get involved in the surrounding environment (Larsen 2009, 2010). It is often difficult to fulfil such ideals—particularly if one's own life is characterised by a problematic everyday life with a low socioeconomical standard. When establishing local health projects, it is therefore essential to work with a range of strategies in order to reach different target groups and to be aware of the criteria of success. There is no doubt that the local area constitutes a central framework for health initiatives, and experience suggests that working with various strategies for various groups of residents is vital. So far, various partial evaluations are conducted both within the municipality and the consulting companies, but unfortunately there has been no economic resources and political priority to implement a systematic and thorough evaluation of the entire project.

Concluding Remarks

This chapter has illustrated the way in which sociological theory is concerned with identifying connections and patterns within social relations and social interaction seen from different perspectives. Sociological analysis is applicable because this perspective is able to bring about knowledge about actors, structures, resources and problems (tasks) of a local community/residential area by means of examining the residents' everyday life, social practices and terms for local interaction. Often, an important result of sociological research turns out to be knowledge of hidden social structures that influence actions and behaviour. Therefore, one of the vital strengths of sociology is the theoretical and methodological sensitivity, which puts into perspective our sometimes unfounded assumptions about how our world is structured.

Local community or neighbourhood's role is on the agenda in many contexts, because civil society is one of the cornerstones of a functioning society. It is in civil society that we create social networks, relationships and communities, and it provides a key platform for the development of active citizenship. Therefore, there is a need for research and knowledge about the frameworks and mechanisms that affect the neighbourhood and how the interaction between citizens and neighbourhoods takes place. This knowledge is essential in creating and implementing health promotion activities, so that they meet citizens' needs and are sustainable in the future.

References

Aakvaag, G. (2008). *Moderne sociologisk teori [Modern sociological theory]*. Oslo: Abstrakt Forlag.

Andersen, P. T. (2002). *Retten til at vælge fællesskab [The right to choose community]*. Doctoral thesis, Aalborg Universitets Forlag, Aalborg.

Andersen, P. T., Bak, C. K., Vangsgaard, S., Dokkedal, U., & Larsen, P. V. (2011a). Self-rated health, ethnicity and social position in a deprived neighbourhood in Denmark. *International Journal for Equity in Health, 10*, 5. http://www.equityheaqlthj.com/content/10/1/5.

Andersen, P. T., Jørgensen, S. K., & Larsen, E. L. (2011b). For the sake of health! Reflections on the contemporary use of social capital and empowerment in Danish health promotion policies. *Social Theory and Health, 9*, 87–107.

Andersen, P. T., & Timm, H. (2010). *Sundhedssociologi [Health sociology]*. København: Hans Reitzels Forlag.

Beck-Jørgensen, B. (1994). *Når hver dag bliver hverdag [When each day get everyday]*. København: Akademisk Forlag.

Bosma, H., Van den Mheen, H. D., Borsboom, G. J. J. M., & Mackenbach, J. P. (2001). Neighborhood socio-economic status and all-cause mortality. *American Journal of Epidemiology, 153*, 363–371.

Bourdieu, P. (1985). The forms of capital. In J. Richardson (Ed.), *Handbook of theory and research for the sociology of education* (pp. 241–258). New York: Macmillan.

Bourdieu, P. (1990[1980]). *The logic of practice*. Oxford: Polity Press.

Bracht, N. (Ed.). (1999). *Health promotion at the community level: New advances*. Thousand Oaks: Sage Publications.

Cattell, V. (2001). Poor people, poor places, and poor health: The mediating role of social networks and social capital. *Social Science & Medicine, 52*, 1501–1516.

Diez-Roux, A. V. (2001). Investigating neighborhood and area effects on health. *American Journal of Public Health, 91*(11), 1783–1789.

Durkheim, E. (1984[1883]). *The division of labour in society*. Hong Kong: Macmillan.

Foucault, M. (1977). *Discipline and punish*. New York: Random House.

Frohlich, K. L., Corin, E., & Portvin, L. (2001). A theoretical proposal for the relationship between context and disease. *Sociology of Health and Illness, 23*, 776–797.

Giddens, A. (1995). *Politics, sociology and social theory: Encounters with classical and contemporary Social thought*. Cambridge: Polity Press.
Goffmann, E. (1963). *Stigma: Notes on the management of spoiled identity*. Harmondsworth: Penguin.
Høgsbro, K. (2005). Lokalsamfundet – struktur og intervention [Local community – structure and intervention]. In F. Kamper-Jørgensen & G. Almind (Eds.), *Forebyggende sundhedsarbejde [Health promotion work]*. København: Munksgård Danmark.
Jenkins, R. (1997). *Social identity*. London: Routledge.
Kawachi, I., & Berkman, L. (2003). *Neighbourhoods and health*. Oxford: Oxford University Press.
Kieffer, C. (1984). Citizen empowerment: A development perspective. *Prevention in Human Services, 3*, 9–36.
Kivisto, P. (2011). *Social theory. Roots and branches*. New York: Oxford University Press.
Krueger, P. M., & Chang, V. W. (2008). Being poor and coping with stress: Health behaviors and the risk of death. *American Journal of Public Health, 98*, 889–896.
Larsen, J. E. (2004). *Fattigdom og social eksklusion – Tendenser i Danmark over et kvart Århundrede [Poverty and social exclusion – tendency in Denmark]*. København: Socialforskningsinstituttet.
Larsen, J. E. (2009). Marginalisering og levekår [Marginalization and living conditions]. In J. E. Larsen & N. Mortensen (Eds.), *Udenfor eller indenfor: Sociale marginaliseringsprocessers mangfoldighed [Outside or inside]* (pp. 122–154). København: Hans Reitzels Forlag.
Larsen, E. L. (2010). Community participation in health promotion: Perspectives of participation and everyday life in a multi-ethnic and socially deprived neighbourhood. Ph.D. series no. 1, forskningsenheden for Sundhedsfremme, Syddansk Universitet.
Larsen, E. L., Andersen, P. T., & Bak, C. K. (2012). Fortællinger om et liv som arbejdsløs og socialt ekskluderet [Tales of life as unemployed and socially excluded]. *Tidsskrift for forskning i sygdom og samfund 16*, 83–103.
Larsen, J. E., & Kristensen, J. (2007). Fattigdom, social eksklusion og boligforhold [Poverty, social exclusion and housing conditions]. *Dansk Sociologi, 18*, 9–28.
Laverack, G. (2003). Building capable communities: Experiences in a rural Fijian context. *Health Promotion International, 18*, 99–106.
Laverack, G., & Wallenstein, N. (2001). Measuring community empowerment: A fresh look at organizational domains. *Health Policy and Planning, 15*, 255–262.
Levitas, R. (1998). *The inclusive society? Social exclusion and new labour*. London: Macmillan.
Macintyre, S., Ellaway, A., & Cummins, S. (2002). Place effects on health: How can we conceptualize, operationalize and measure them? *Social Science & Medicine, 55*, 125–139.
Minkler, M. (Ed.). (2005). *Community organizing and community building for health*. New Brunswick: Rutgers University Press.
Muntaner, C., & Lynch, J. (2002). Social capital, class gender and race conflict, and population health: An essay review of Bowling Alone's implication for social epidemiology. *International Journal of Epidemiology, 31*, 261–267.
Muntaner, C., Lynch, J., & Smith, G. D. (2010). Social capital and the third way in public health. *Critical Public Health, 10*, 107–124.
Napier, A. J. (2002). *Lessons for community capacity building: A summary of the research evidence*. Australia: Mount Isa Centre for Rural and Remote Health.
Nutbeam, D. (1986). Health promotion glossary. *Health Promotion, 1*, 113–125.
Pickett, K. E., & Pearl, M. (2001). Multilevel analyses of neighbourhood socioeconomic context and health outcomes: A critical review. *Journal of Epidemiology and Community Health, 55*, 111–122.
Putnam, R. (1995). Bowling alone. America's declining social capital. *Journal of Democracy, 6*, 65–78.
Putnam, R. (2000). *Bowling alone*. New York: Simon & Cluster.
Raphael, D. (2006). Social determinants of health: Present status, unanswered questions, and future directions. *International Journal of Health Services, 36*, 651–677.
Rappaport, J. (1984). Studies in empowerment: Introduction to the issue. *Prevention in Human Services, 3*, 1–7.

Rasmussen, M., Due, P., & Holstein, B. K. (2000). *Skolebørnsundersøgelsen for 1998 [Investigation on schoolchildren from 1998]*. København: Komiteen for sundhedsoplysning.
Reijneveld, J. (2002). Neighbourhood socio-economic context and self reported health and smoking: A secondary analysis of data on seven cities. *Journal of Epidemiology and Community Health, 56*, 935–942.
Rodwell, C. (1996). An analysis of the concept of empowerment. *Journal of Advanced Nursing, 23*, 305–313.
Røiseland, A., Andrews, T., Eide, A. H., & Fosse, E. (Eds.). (1999). *Lokalsamfund og helse [Local community and health]*. Oslo: Fagbokforlaget.
Schutz, A. (1967[1932]). *The phenomenology of the social world*. Evaston: North Western University Press.
Schutz, A., & Luchmann, T. (1973). *The structures of the life world*. Evaston: North Western University Press.
Staffort, M., & Marmot, M. (2003). Neighbourhood deprivation and health: Does it affect us all equally? *International Journal of Epidemiology, 32*, 357–366.
Swift, C., & Levin, G. (1987). Empowerment: An emerging mental health technology. *Journal of Primary Prevention, 7*, 242–265.
Szreter, S., & Woolcock, A. (2004). Health by association? Social capital, social theory and the political economy of public health. *International Journal of Epidemiology, 33*, 650–667.
Tengland, P. A. (2008). Empowerment: A conceptual discussion. *Health Care Analysis, 16*, 77–96.

Chapter 5
People and Place: The Interrelated Connections Between Interactions, Perceptions and Space

Eva Ladekjær Larsen

Introduction

Geographical variations in health outcomes have been a research topic in public health for more than 150 years. Overall two explanations for these variations have dominated this research field. The composition explanation, which refers to the concentration of individuals with similar socio-economic status in specific residential locations, is used to explain why certain neighbourhoods are characterised by, for example, high mortality and morbidity. The context explanation, on the other hand, approaches geographical health variations as if it is *place* itself that affects health. For example, poor neighbourhoods comprised of worn-down buildings, a high crime rate, an insecure social environment, and lacking green outdoor spaces, children's playgrounds, public benches, etc. can have a negative effect on health. The context explanation is however a blurry conception that seeks to capture:

> those factors influencing human behaviours or health which remain once every imaginable individual characteristic is taken into account. It is indeed a black box, an unspecified "miasma" which somehow, but we don't know how, influences some aspects of health, health related behaviour or health risk in some population groups. (Macintyre et al. 2002, p. 129)

Exploring the contents of the "black box" has opened the way for introducing concepts originating in the social sciences. Social capital, defined by various theorists like Bourdieu (1985), Coleman (1990) and Putnam (1993), is, for example, commonly used as explaining differences in ill health (Carpiano 2006), although critics stress that the relationship between social capital and health is too difficult to determine due to the complex interaction between social status and health status (Ziersch et al. 2005; Kennelly et al. 2003; Hawe and Shiell 2000). Moreover, a high

E. Ladekjær Larsen (✉)
Unit for Health Promotion Research, University of Southern Denmark,
Niels Bohrs Vej 9-10, 6700 Esbjerg, Denmark
e-mail: elarsen@health.sdu.dk

C. Stock and A. Ellaway (eds.), *Neighbourhood Structure and Health Promotion*,
DOI 10.1007/978-1-4614-6672-7_5,

level of social capital does not necessary lead to good health. Portes (1998) draw our attention to the negative side effects of high levels of social capital, e.g. restricted individual freedom and increased social control and group closure. There is thus a need to further explore what is going on in "contexts", e.g. what are the ideals, norms and values being practised and how are these practices related to health.

The debate of whether it is either context or composition that causes ill health leads nowhere. A more fruitful approach may be to acknowledge that there is a reciprocal relationship between people and place that potentially co-determines health behaviour, risk behaviour and/or health status (Bernard et al. 2007; Cummins et al. 2007; Macintyre and Ellaway 2003; Macintyre et al. 2002).

This chapter attempts to shed light on the content and characteristics of this relationship by turning to sociological and anthropological disciplines, which have a long tradition in the study of the interaction between people and place. The body of literature concerning this relationship is huge (see, e.g. Morill et al. 2005; Lofland 1998; Williams 2007 for overviews). In this chapter, I will focus mainly on the research tradition embedded in the theoretical orientation of *symbolic interactionism*. In brief, social interactionism evolves from American pragmatism, a philosophic tradition focusing on the interactional nexus of social relationships (Kurtz 1984). It explores primarily how individuals and groups negotiate, (re)construct and engage in social interactions within a wider social and cultural context (Blumer 1969). The value of conceiving people and place from the perspective of social interactionism is threefold: (i) it allows us to explore how people use place, e.g. how residents practise everyday life activities in the neighbourhood and the meanings they attach to places; (ii) it turns our focus towards social relationships in specific places and finally (iii) it addresses how place structures social behaviour. Before addressing these three interconnected relationships, I will briefly introduce the historical background of how the relationship between people and place has evolved in the social sciences. The chapter draws on discussions and case illustrations first appearing in my Ph.D. thesis: *Community participation in health promotion: Perspectives of participation and everyday life in a multi-ethnic and socially deprived neighbourhood* (2010).

Background and Definitions

The Detachment of Social Relations from Geographical Space

The sociological classic writers such as Emile Durkheim, Max Weber, Ferdinand Tönnies and Georg Simmel were concerned with how modern society changed social relationships. In their work, modern society increasingly transforms and characterises social relationships as being detached from geographical space. Durkheim (1893/1984) introduced the distinction between *mechanical* and *organic solidarity*, the former referring to the nature of social ties in small-scale societies and the latter to modern societies. To Durkheim, premodern and "primitive" societies were based on *conscious collective* that captures the individual's consciousness and regulates social norms and behaviour so it matches the needs, norms and values of the community as an entity. Tönnies (1887–1973) introduced *Gemeinschaft* (community), representing social relationships in traditional societies, and *Gesellschaft* (association), characterising contractual relationships in modern societies of bureaucracy and commercial organisations. According to Weber, bureaucracy and capitalism is the driving force leading to loss of freedom and meaning for the individual (Weber 1970). In a disenchanted world *(die Entzauberung der Welt)* that modern society is, the individual is confronted with many different forms of values, which he/she must choose, but is not capable of. Individual agency is therefore predominantly motivated by utilisation values rather than inherent community-based and loyalty values (Ritzer 2008). Simmel (1998) presents the idea that urban modern life creates a psychological condition that insists on the development of the intellect, protecting the individual from hectic city life with its diversity of stimuli and superficial relationships. Moreover, social relations are unimportant per se and only gain importance if they are considered to have a utilisation value. These theorists shared the idea that premodern communities were geographically based, homogeneous and concerned with duties and values that served the community rather than the individual. This assumption led to concerns that modernity caused social chaos and disruption. These assumptions were challenged already in the 1920s by what later became known as the Chicago School. The Chicago School specialised in urban sociology and was particularly interested in working class neighbourhoods and how they were socially organised. These studies, most notable, Park's *The City* (1925) and *Human Communities* (1952), Wirth's *Urbanism as a way of life* (1938) and Whyte's *Street Corner Society* (1943), illustrated the social order of neighbourhoods, and social relationships also in modern society entail intimacy and place attachment rather than superficiality and geographical detachment. However, the concern that modernity causes social disruption is still valid today and to be found in current theoretical perspectives of local communities. For example, Zygmunt Bauman, Richard Sennett, Amitai Etzioni and Manuel Castells have been labelled "pessimists", due to their characterisation of late modern society as based on socio-geographical segregation, social disintegration and increasing inequity (Jørgensen 2008).

Place, Space and Neighbourhoods

Concepts of space and place have varied through history of human geography. Altman and Low (1992, p. 4) define place referring to space: "that has been giving meaning through personal, group or cultural processes". In this sense space is more abstract than place and deprived of any human thought or action (Tuan 1977). The concept of place, as Agnew (1987) notes, has been used within social science and has three main orientations: "locale" refers to settings where social relations are constituted; "locations" represent geographical areas, defined by social and economic processes and encompassing the settings for social interaction; whereas "sense of place" refers to the subjective feelings associated with particular places. The phenomenological discipline has divided place into objective dimensions (the naturalistic qualities of place) and subjective dimensions (individualistic meanings attached to place) (Saar and Palang 2009). Criticising this binary opposition for distinguishing two inseparable spheres, a third space is introduced: the betweenness of places, where the subjective and the objective spaces meet and where objective reality and cultural meanings are fused (Entrikin 1991). Following Gustafson (2001), this chapter uses a definition of place that considers its meaningfulness:

> Meaningful places emerge in a social context and through social relations, they are geographically located and at the same time related to their social, economic, cultural etc. surroundings, and they give individuals a sense of place, a subjective territorial identity. (Gustafson 2001, p. 6)

This concept of place embraces the material circumstances, the social identities and subjective experiences, enabling an approach that considers three interconnected layers of place: that of societal structures, of local social interactions and of subjective emotions of attachment, or what can be termed as the *intersubjectivity of space* (Pranikoff and Low 2007).

As already noted, our era of modern society has developed with increasingly cultural de-territorialisation and been replaced by what Appadurai calls flows of ethno-, media-, techno-, finans- and ideoscapes (Appadurai 1996). In this sense it seems fair to ask if it is even possible to draw geographical boundaries and term them, for example, "neighbourhoods". A geographical territory consists, namely, of one or several centres, peripheries and borderlands. People who settle in sub-territories do not necessarily share cultural ideas as people in centres. When a geographical localisation does not reflect a cultural and social entity, how then do we conceptualise neighbourhood as a social place and something that people may identify with? The studies of the social structure and orders of neighbourhoods have been approached in various ways (see, e.g. Chaskin 1997; Day 2006). Cohen's work *The symbolic construction of community* (1985) may enable us to understand how a neighbourhood's identity is constructed. Cohen was inspired by the Norwegian anthropologist Fredrik Barth who presented the theory of ethnic boundaries (1969), whose major concern was to explore the demarcation between social boundaries rather than the cultural substance embedded within them. The theory views the cultural substance embedded within a particular community as being under a process of being reshaped by social interactions and negotiations. Moreover, the theory enhances that culture is unevenly distributed within communities, urging us to investigate the differences *within* communities. To Cohen, communities are distinct cultural entities applying simultaneously similarities and differences. Community is thus a relational idea opposed to other communities or cultural entities and is executed by the exigencies of social interaction, making use of particular frameworks such as kinship, religion, ethnicity or place (Cohen 1985).

Finally it should be mentioned that neighbourhoods do not exist as isolated islands but are part of wider society and that neighbourhoods are constructed on the basis of political and social histories of those societies. Poor neighbourhoods and their residents have, for example, been associated with social stigma and moral degradation across time and space (Reidpath et al. 2005; Warr 2005). The process of stigmatisation happens over time, following unequal power distributions in society and where cultural, social and economic forces determine and maintain human differences, linking them to negative stereotyping (Goffman 1963). Stigma is thus a way of governance, of maintaining a specific social order and of justifying social, political and economic exclusion (Reidpath et al. 2005). The relationship of unequal power distribution and its consequences for poor neighbourhoods enable us to include in our neighbourhood approach its relation to wider society. However, if wider power structures in society are neglected in neighbourhood regeneration programmes, there is a risk that "outside agents" continually stigmatise poor neighbourhoods.

Place Attachment: Meanings of Place and the Creation of Home Territories

So far I have argued that place is space embodied with meaning. However, not all places are sites of place attachment. Rather, place attachment occurs as emotional bonding to a place when it cannot be substituted by other places from the perspective of the individual who experiences this attachment (Milligan 1998). Connections between people and "their places" may be conceptualised as *home territories*, a term first coined in a study by Cavan (1963) and represents *the relative freedom of behaviour and the sense of intimacy and control of the area* (Cavan 1963, p. 18). Home territories are created in public spaces by people who use these places regularly and together with other people with whom they have relationships, such as friends, family or neighbours. The process of place attachment is enabled by the creation of these home territories as will be demonstrated below.

Case Study: Sønderbro

Sønderbro, a public housing area in a Danish provincial town, is in an ongoing process of neighbourhood regeneration. As a consequence of the neighbourhood's high percentage of residents receiving welfare (78 %), combined with the high percentage of migrants (60 %), in addition to a poor reputation for crime and drug abuse, the area has for decades been characterised as "socially deprived" and undesirable to live in. To change this reputation, to improve neighbourhood security and to support health and well-being of all residents, a development initiative was launched in the mid-1990s. The aim of the development initiative was to organise and develop the neighbourhood in ways that considered the needs and resources of its residents. The physical appearance of Sønderbro had been improved, the buildings renovated and settings to encourage social interactions have been constructed.

Such settings include green areas, benches, children's playgrounds, the laundry house, the community house and the snack bar (Larsen 2010; Larsen and Stock 2011; Larsen and Manderson 2009). These settings can be defined as places; they are no longer abstract spaces deprived of human thought but constructed with the purpose of being grounds for human interactions.

It may not always be obvious which places can be characterised as "home" territories and which are merely grounds for social interactions nor is there necessary consensus among residents which territories belong to which group of residents. It does however become explicit as certain territories are contested:

> Bodil: "Usually we sit down here in the evenings drinking coffee and playing trivial pursuit, but now our bench has gone missing. It has been moved down to the fire place, I don't know who did it, but Jens [a community worker] does not care and will tell us to sort it out by ourselves.....You see the benches over there? I call them the gossip benches. Every night they [The Turkish women] sit there gossiping, sometimes scowling at us. Maybe they took it. Or their kids did" (17 July 2007).

The removal of "her bench" challenged her control of the area, and she clearly felt provoked by the fact that somebody had taken "her bench" as if somebody had entered her personal home. She also explained that she felt intimidated by a neighbour, who she felt observed her movements and who was not a person she desired to include in her home territory.

Likewise another resident, Ulla, a retired female, who frequently used a particular area also known in the neighbourhood as "the drunks' area", expressed her emotional bond to the place. She complained that drunken teenagers used their benches during night time, making loud noise and messing up the area with empty beer bottles, broken glass, cigarette buds and trash. The worst part in Ulla's point of view was that she herself and her own crowd were being blamed for both the noise and the rubbish scattered around. She herself described the area as her own garden and nursed the place by cleaning up after herself. Her sense of "ownership" of certain benches was strengthened by bringing in personal items such as ashtrays. That somebody else was using their bench and messing it up challenged her control of the bench, not that she didn't want somebody else using it but that she could not control "their" behaviour and that she might be blamed for misbehaviour she was not responsible for.

The relationship between people and places, exemplified by *home territories,* is an important component in place attachment. According to theory of place attachment: "people develop attachment bonds with certain places, thereby entering into meaningful relationships with these places and ultimately incorporating them as part of their self-identity" (Leith 2006, p. 318). The creation of emotional links to places is constituted by meaningful interactions, having two related components: the *interactional past* and the *interactional potential* of a place (Milligan 1998). Past events, practices and routines associated with a specific place or memories of a place form the *interactional past.* When, for example, residents recall past events in their *home territories*, they construct and express a sense of belonging like Bodil's story of "my bench" illustrates. The *interactional potential* of a site is on the other hand what is imagined or expected to happen at the site. This is connected to routine behaviour such as coming to the same bench every day or to planning future events, like arranging a picnic or community festival. The experiences of interactional past and potentials can be coined to *experiences of continuity*, meaning that residents experience coherence between the neighbourhood's past, present and future.

Social Interactions at Specific Places: Relationships in Neighbourhoods

Looking into the literature of social relationships in public places, such as street corners, parks and neighbourhoods, several typologies that capture the nature of these relationships have been constructed. Representing the interactionist perspective, Lofland distinguishes between *public*, *parochial* and *private realms* (Lofland 1989, 1998). Realm differs from place and can be described as a social territory in which a certain type of relational form dominates and thus captures the nature of social interactions in places. The *public realm* refers to the public domain such as street corners, parks, coffee shops and plazas. Relationships in these places are characterised by brief encounters and impersonal and superficial relationships, where people typically are unknown to each other or only known to each other by category by performing a specific role, such as a postman, a police officer or similar. These relationships are characterised as a *stranger relational form.* Similarly, the urban anthropologist Hannerz terms these kinds of brief encounters as *traffic relationships* (Hannerz 1980). The *private realm* belongs to the intimate domain such as private homes in which the relational form is long term or durable like family or close friends. The *parochial realm* refers to a communal relational form represented by places such as neighbourhoods or workplaces. The point is that each realm is tied to a set of norms and behaviours that only applies within that specific realm. Lofland argues that the benefits of this trichotomous distinction are an improved understanding of social territories, their boundaries, structures and inherent qualities formed by social interactions.

Kusenbach (2006) develops this distinction in her exploration of neighbouring patterns in the parochial realm. She distinguishes between four different practices that individuals engage in to treat each other as neighbours: *friendly recognition, parochial helpfulness, proactive intervention* and *embracing and contesting diversity.* Within each practice are distinct behavioural patterns. *Friendly recognition* ranges from a friendly nod when greeting to small talk of weather conditions, to cheerfulness and to flirting. *Parochial helpfulness* is represented by small services such as borrowing a cup of sugar, accepting package delivery or watering plants while one's neighbour is away on vacation. *Proactive intervention* goes beyond the parochial helpfulness since neighbours in this practice are taking action without having negotiated first. They are small favours initiated in situations to prevent one's neighbour getting into trouble. Finally in Kusenbach's terms, the last neighbouring practice is *embracing and contesting diversity.* These are acts of inclusion or exclusion of neighbours who differ from oneself and extend beyond other culturally defined boundaries. She demonstrates how residents tolerate cultural diversities and even express that they prefer diversity above homogeneity. Other examples illustrate hostility towards residents who differ distinctively from oneself, and these acts are ranging from withholding friendly recognition to anonymously complaining to the housing authorities of what they consider as inappropriate neighbouring behaviour.

Kusenbach's distinction between types of neighbouring behaviour is useful in exploring how residents treat each other as neighbours or to explore which kinds of relationships are predominant in the parochial realm. This pattern of neighbouring behaviour was highly recognisable in the neighbourhood of Sønderbro, but I also found that residents were treating each other in other ways than being merely neighbours. Here a neighbour was sometimes described as "the anonymous" person living upstairs or next door, one you can hear move around, but never speak to other than muttering a "hello" when bumping into him/her in the stairways. A neighbour can thus be geographically close but socially distant. I call this a *geographical neighbour*. Attached to this category is a set of ideals of how to perform "good neighbouring behaviour". A positive feature associated with the *geographical neighbour* was described as "one who does not get into other people's businesses". It was highly valued that neighbours did not interfere, asking personal questions, gossiping or telling people what to do (Larsen and Manderson 2009).

A neighbour was also described as one you have a relationship to. I call this a *social neighbour*. In contradiction to the *geographical neighbour*, a *social neighbour* is one that cares and shows interest, helps out and interferes if problems occur or support is needed. Treating one as a *social neighbour* included exchanging favours and objects, much like Kusenbachs' categories of *parochial helpfulness* and *proactive intervention*.

Finally, the majority of residents were categorised as "non-neighbours". Acts that fall into this category are "indifference", not necessarily in negative terms, but rather as an expression of not having any needs or desire to engage. This form is characterised by "no social contact" other than the awareness of other people's physical presence and managing this presence, for example, the unwritten rules that apply when passing each other on the pavement or when a resident chooses to sit at another bench than the bench already occupied by a fellow resident. In these situations residents treat other residents as *strangers*, that is, patterned ways of interaction that structure and maintain a specific social order, in this case residents that share social space, but no social relation (see also Lofland 1973; Goffman 1963). Residents expressing this norm most often had their networks outside of the community and considered the neighbourhood as a place to live, rather than a place to have a life.

On the other hand, a very different type of "non-neighbour" was close relationships such as relatives or close friends. Several of the residents had relatives living in the neighbourhood or residents had formed close bonds. In this sense they no longer defined each other as neighbours but rather as friends or family members. Close relationships advantage the individual in that they feel emotionally, practically and even financially supported. But the bonds may also have side effects. One is that individuals might feel restricted in their individual freedom and even monitored.

Exclusion and restricted individual freedom are what Portes (1998) refers to as negative aspects of social capital; those strong, social bonds, although having embedded resources, carry the potential of controlling social behaviour that are not expedient for the individual's social and mental well-being.

Neighbouring interactions are therefore only one part of the social interaction pattern in neighbourhoods. The point is that the social realms, Lofland and Kusenbach distinguish between, which in each way inform social interactions, are multiplex in neighbourhoods. People are not just neighbours. They are also relatives, close friends, enemies, strangers and long-term acquaintances. In determining relationships in neighbourhoods, it may then be fruitful then to distinguish between *types* of neighbours and how residents categorise neighbours and non-neighbours.

Places and Social Behaviour

The final issue brought up here is the relationship between place and social behaviour and of how the physical surroundings of public life can be manipulated to enable or enforce certain social behaviours. The built environment does certainly not rigidly determine how people should socially behave, the kind of relationships they should have or how they should socially interact with each other. Rather, the built environment structures, enable and constrain interactional options between people and between people and place. Following Morill et al. (2005), it is fruitful to distinguish between *framing of a place* and *regulation of a place.* The framing of a place includes how space is defined concerning its use, accessibility and visibility and refers to the interpretive processes that occur when people interact with each other or with places. The interpretative process allows people to categorise, identify and perceive the meaning of a place and enable them to make sense of what a place is for, who it is for and how one should behave in it. In order to make sense of place, people draw on different frames that are embedded in historical and cultural circumstances. A place may be constructed for certain intentions, such as a public playground or an urban park. In this sense a place can be more or less *institutionalised* for specific interactions and relations. On the other hand, these intentions may be challenged by different groups of people. Urban parks, for example, may be used for recreation, picnic and family get-togethers or for more nefarious activities such as prostitution, drug trafficking or illegal camps for homeless people.

The regulation of place is closely related to the framing of a place but refers to the normative rules that regulate social behaviour, including processes of social control that are found in particular places. Public sociality, or to use Lofland's term: social interactions in the public realm, is characterised by brief encounters and is governed by norms that require individuals to maintain certain social distances from each other, although being physically close. Observing social behaviour in a London underground train, one finds that people rarely start conversations or look at co-passengers. These norms of behaviour may naturally be challenged by different groups of people. The *principles* of public sociality are described as "repertoires" that individuals use when navigating in public places (Morill et al. 2005, p. 234). To see them as *principles* acknowledges that individuals have different skills and expectations as they interact in public places.

Furthermore, we may distinguish between open-placed frames and close-placed frames. The latter refers to places designed with specific intends, for example, places arranged with fixed seatings, tables or walls that restrict accessibility and purpose. Some benches situated in public parks have, for example, been designed in ways that don't allow people to lie down in order to prevent homeless people from "staying over". Close-placed frames thus define behaviour in a restricted manner. Open-placed frames are on the other hand designed to allow human creativity and freedom to decide how specific places should be used and thus refer to "permissive" behaviour. In this sense, city councils, governments or housing agencies construct and design physical surroundings to control social behaviour in a more or less restricted manner. Space then, how it is being used and by whom, is reflecting power relations in society and is the potential site for contesting societal hegemony (Altman and Low 1992). A further example from Sønderbro will be used to illustrate this argument.

When the outdoor areas of Sønderbro were renovated, residential meetings were held in order to discuss and accommodate the residents' needs and wishes. At that time, there had been some complaints that alcoholics were occupying the benches at the main entrance of the neighbourhood and some residents felt insecure. But instead of desiring to exclude the alcoholics and ban them from the outdoor areas, the residents agreed that a shelter should be built for them in a less visible area, where alcohol consumption was allowed. The residents named this shelter *The Tea House*; however, the tea house was often empty. The alcoholics preferred to sit outside at nearby benches. Only in rainy weather they would enter the hut for shelter. Their choice of not using the hut for the intended purpose was related to how the alcoholics *framed* the place. To them it was not just a matter of having a place to drink alcohol; it was a hang-out, a place to be seen and observe the comings and goings of residents in the neighbourhood. The walls of the hut restricted these activities by blocking the view. Moreover, being in the hut was associated with being "locked up". In this sense the *non-use* of the tea house was both a way of maintaining their everyday routines and an act of resisting what other residents had decided for them.

So far I have illustrated how space restricts and permits specific social interactions to occur and how places are used. While this theoretical orientation is careful not to explicitly define a causal relation between certain places and behaviour, other theoretical orientations demonstrate that place indeed *does* something to people's behaviour and well-being. The *Broken Windows Theory* is a criminological theory that argues that disorder incites to more disorder (Wilson and Kelling 1982). For example, it is argued that if a building with broken windows is left unfixed, vandals will break a few more windows and eventually break into the building and perhaps even turn it into a shelter. The *Broken Windows Theory* has been integrated in urban and preventive crime policies in various Western countries for several decades now and has recently been empirically demonstrated in a study by Keizer et al. (2008).

Architectural design and the built environment surrounding our everyday life may control, stimulate or enforce certain types of behaviour, but it may also stimulate healing processes or promote health and well-being. Recent research trends in health geography have developed the concept of *therapeutic landscape*, which provides an analytical framework for exploring how the natural, built, social and symbolic landscapes contribute to human health. A therapeutic environment is one that has *positive person-environment interaction—where improvements in the physical setting are complemented by improvements in the social environment* (Pranikoff and Low 2007). The evolution of the concept is closely related to criticisms of the idea that rehabilitation is bound to institutionalised places of healing such as hospitals or recreation homes and instead suggests that practices of healing, health promotion or illness prevention can take place in everyday life settings such as neighbourhoods, workplaces or schools, reflecting a socioecological approach towards health (Williams 2007). The concept is however not restricted to everyday settings but is also applied in hospitals and long-term care settings. For example, spaces designed for delivering health services have been investigated in relation to interior, selection of colours and design of the furniture and of how these elements contribute to a therapeutic environment (Crooks and Evans 2007).

Conclusion

This chapter has addressed people and place interactions at three different but interrelated levels: the construction of meaningful places, the social relationships in places and the influence of places on social behaviour. From a symbolic interactionist perspective, I have explained the process of place attachment through the use of the concept of *home territories*. In this process it becomes evident that by people's frequent use of places, they develop a sense of ownership towards the place, which is overt as the territory is contested by other people. Moreover, I have demonstrated the various ways in which residents relate to each other in a neighbourhood. Relationships may vary broadly in intimacy, from treating each other as strangers to being as close as family as well as there are different ways of conceptualising what a good neighbour is and how he/she should behave. Finally I have discussed how space structures social behaviour and interactions. There are different perspectives of how rigidly spaces influence behaviour. Spaces may be designed to encouraging performing specific activities, to restricting certain actions and to determining a specific outcome like the broken windows theory suggests. By investigating this relationship, we further learn that spaces are arenas for contesting power. While authorities may design spaces for specific intentions, these intentions may be challenged by people's use of them and thus transform them into something else.

So how then are these perspectives relevant for investigating the relationship between neighbourhood and health? As I began this chapter I introduced the concerns over community loss. Some reactions to this concern have put forward a nostalgic view of community as a coherent unit, sharing needs, norms and values, a view that is replicated in the health literature (Larsen and Stock 2011). It has been argued elsewhere that this romantic view is inherent in Scandinavian housing policies, particularly concerning socially deprived areas (Pløger 2002). This perception of neighbourhood implies that its residents are always interested in and connected with each other. As this chapter has shown, this is not always the case. This dominant perception may not always reflect neighbourhood relationships but is rather a normative prescription of how things *ought* to be. Acknowledging that residents in neighbourhoods have different relationships with each other, and use the places of neighbourhood in ways that may not always be intended, increases our understanding that neighbourhoods are complex and continuously changing in form, content and qualities. It underscores the point that there are no ready-made recipes of how to construct healthy neighbourhoods. Instead, working with human-made places requires that we begin with investigating who people are and what their relations are to the places they are attached to.

References

Agnew, J. A. (1987). *Place and politics: The geographical mediation of state and society*. Boston: Allen & Unwin.

Altman, I., & Low, S. M. (Eds.). (1992). *Place attachment*. New York: Plenum.

Appadurai, A. (1996). *Modernity at large: Cultural dimensions of modernity*. London: University of Minnesota Press.

Barth, F. (1969). Introduction. In F. Barth (Ed.), *Ethnic groups and boundaries: The social organisation of culture difference* (pp. 9–39). Bergen, Norway: Universitetsforlaget.

Bernard, P., Charafeddine, R., Frohlich, K. L., Daniel, M., Kestens, Y., & Potvin, L. (2007). Health inequalities and place: A theoretical conception of neighborhood. *Social Science & Medicine, 65*, 1839–1852.

Blumer, H. (1969). *Symbolic interactionism; perspective and method*. Englewood Cliffs, NJ: Prentice-Hall.

Bourdieu, P. (1985). The forms of capital. In J. Richardson (Ed.), *Handbook of theory and research for the sociology of education* (pp. 241–258). New York: Macmillan.

Carpiano, R. M. (2006). Toward a neighborhood resource-based theory of social capital for health. Can Bourdieu and social capital help? *Social Science & Medicine, 62*, 165–175.

Cavan, S. (1963). Interaction in home territories. *Berkeley Journal of Sociology, 1963*, 17–32.

Chaskin, R. J. (1997). Perspectives on neighborhood and community: A review of the literature. *The Social Service Review, 71*(4), 527–548.

Cohen, A. P. (1985). *The symbolic construction of community*. New York: Ellis Horwood Limited and Tavistock Publications Limited.

Coleman, J. S. (1990). *Foundations of social theory*. Cambridge, MA: Harvard University Press.

Crooks, V. A., & Evans, J. (2007). The writings on the wall: Decoding the interior space of the hospital waiting room. In A. Williams (Ed.), *Therapeutic landscapes* (pp. 165–181). Hampshire, England: Ashgate Publishing Limited.

Cummins, S., Curtis, S., Diez-Roux, A. V., & Macintyre, S. (2007). Understanding and representing 'place' in health research: A relational approach. *Social Science & Medicine, 65*, 1825–1838.

Day, G. (2006). *Community and everyday life*. New York: Routledge.

Durkheim, E. (1893/1984). *The division of labour in society*. London: MacMillan.

Entrikin, J. N. (1991). *The betweenness of place: Towards a geography of modernity*. Baltimore: John Hopkins University Press.
Goffman, E. (1963). *Stigma: Notes on the management of spoiled identity*. Harmondsworth: Penguin Books.
Gustafson, P. (2001). Meanings of place: Everyday experience and theoretical conceptualizations. *Journal of Environmental Psychology, 21*, 5–16.
Hannerz, U. (1980). *Exploring the city. Inquires toward and urban anthropology*. New York: Columbia University Press.
Hawe, P., & Shiell, A. (2000). Social capital and health promotion: A review. *Social Science & Medicine, 51*, 871–885.
Jørgensen, A. (2008). Lokale fællesskaber i den senmoderne by [Local communities in the late modern city]. *Dansk Sociologi, 3*(19), 9–24.
Keizer, K., Lindenberg, S., & Steg, L. (2008). The spreading of disorder. *Science, 322*(5908), 1681–1685.
Kennelly, B., O'Shea, E., & Garvey, E. (2003). Social capital, life expectancy and mortality: A cross-national examination. *Social Science & Medicine, 56*(12), 2367–2377.
Kurtz, L. R. (1984). *Evaluating Chicago sociology. A guide to the literature, with an annotated bibliography*. Chicago: University of Chicago Press.
Kusenbach, M. (2006). Patterns of neighboring: Practicing community in the parochial realm. *Symbolic Interaction, 29*(3), 279–306.
Larsen, E. L. (2010). *Community participation in health promotion. Perspectives of participation and everyday life in a multi-ethnic and socially deprived neighbourhood*. Ph.D. series No. 1, Unit for Health Promotion Research, Institute of Public Health Faculty of Health Sciences, University of Southern Denmark.
Larsen, E. L., & Manderson, L. (2009). "A good spot": Health promotion discourse, healthy cities and heterogeneity in contemporary Denmark. *Health & Place, 15*, 606–613.
Larsen, E. L., & Stock, C. (2011). Capturing contrasted realities: Integrating multiple perspectives of Danish community life in health promotion. *Health Promotion International, 26*(1), 14–22.
Leith, K. H. (2006). "Home is where the heart is...or is it?" A phenomenological exploration of the meaning of home for older women in congregate housing. *Journal of Aging Studies, 20*, 317–333.
Lofland, L. H. (1973). *A world of strangers. Order and action in urban public space*. New York: Basic Books.
Lofland, L. H. (1989). Social life in the public realm: A review. *Journal of Contemporary Ethnography, 17*(4), 453–483.
Lofland, L. H. (1998). *The public realm*. New York: Aldine de Gruyter.
Macintyre, S., & Ellaway, A. (2003). Neighborhoods and health: An overview. In I. Kawachi & L. F. Berkman (Eds.), *Neighborhoods and health* (pp. 20–45). New York: Oxford University Press.
Macintyre, S., Ellaway, A., & Cummins, S. (2002). Place effects in health: How can we conceptualise, operationalise and measure them? *Social Science & Medicine, 55*, 125–139.
Milligan, M. (1998). Interactional past and potential: The social construction of place attachment. *Studies in Symbolic Interaction, 1*, 1–33.
Morill, C., Snow, D. A., & White, C. H. (Eds.). (2005). *Together alone. Personal relationships in public places*. Berkeley: University of California Press.
Park, R. E. (1925). The city: Suggestions for the investigation of human behaviour. In R. E. Park, W. Burgess, & R. D. McKenzie (Eds.), *The city* (pp. 1–46). Chicago: University of Chicago Press.
Park, R. E. (1952). *Human communities*. Glencoe: Free Press.
Pløger, J. (2002). Det senmoderne nærmiljø—livsformer og bykultur. En sammenligning af teori of praksis i Danmark og Norge [The late-modern community—forms of life and urban culture. Comparing theory and practice in Denmark and Norway]. NIBR—rapport 2002:16. Norsk Institutt for By- og Regionsforskning, Oslo, Norway.

Portes, A. (1998). Social capital: Its origins and applications in modern sociology. *Annual Review of Sociology, 24*, 1–24.
Pranikoff, J., & Low, S. (2007). Introduction: Understanding therapeutic landscapes from the perspectives of medical anthropology and environmental psychology. In A. Williams (Ed.), *Therapeutic landscapes* (pp. 291–297). Hampshire, England: Ashgate Publishing Limited.
Putnam, R. (1993). *Making democracy work*. New Jersey: Princeton University Press.
Reidpath, D. D., Chan, K. Y., Gifford, S. M., & Allotey, P. (2005). 'He hath the French pox': Stigma, social value and social exclusion. *Sociology of Health & Illness, 27*(4), 468–489.
Ritzer, G. (2008). *Sociological theory*. Boston: McGraw-Hill.
Saar, M., & Palang, H. (2009). The dimension of place meanings. *Living Reviews in Landscape Research, 3*, 1–24.
Simmel, G. (1998). *Hvordan er samfundet muligt? Udvalgte sociologiske skrifter [How is society possible? Selected sociological essays]*. København, Denmark: Samlerens Bogklub.
Tönnies, F. (1973/1887). *Community and association*. London: Routledge and Paul Kegan.
Tuan, Y. F. (1977). *Space and place: The perspective of experience*. Minneapolis: University of Minnesota Press.
Warr, D. J. (2005). Social networks in a 'discredited' neighborhood. *Journal of Sociology, 41*(3), 285–308.
Weber, M. (1970). In H. Gerth & C. W. Mills (Eds.), *From Max Weber.* London: Routledge.
Whyte, W. F. (1966/1943). *Street corner society. The social structure of an Italian slum*. Chicago: University of Chicago Press.
Williams, A. (Ed.). (2007). *Therapeutic landscapes*. Hampshire, England: Ashgate Publishing Limited.
Wilson, J. Q., & Kelling, G. L. (1982). Broken windows. http://www.manhattan-institute.org/pdf/_atlantic_monthly-broken_windows.pdf. Accessed 29 Dec 2011.
Wirth, L. (1938). Urbanism as a way of life. *The American Journal of Sociology, 44*, 1–24.
Ziersch, A. M., Baum, F., MacDougall, C., & Putland, C. (2005). Neighborhood life and social capital: The implications for health. *Social Science & Medicine, 60*(1), 71–86.

Part II
Measuring and Monitoring Neighbourhood Structure

Chapter 6
Methods to Measure Neighbourhoods and Analyse Their Impact on Health: An Overview

Sven Voigtländer, Oliver Razum, and Ursula Berger

Introduction

Studying the influence of neighbourhood conditions on health outcomes with empirical methods has several challenges. The most important are that (a) neighbourhoods are not predefined or natural units of observation, (b) neighbourhoods have to be measured in terms of their sociodemographic composition as well as the quantity and quality of resources they offer, (c) the distribution of individuals across neighbourhoods is not random regarding factors such as social position or individual preferences, (d) the health impact of neighbourhood conditions may differ according to certain individual or household characteristics, (e) people might live in different neighbourhoods throughout their life and (f) neighbourhoods change over time. In this chapter, we will discuss methods to respond to these challenges. As empirical analysis ideally follows theory, we begin with presenting a conceptual framework which links social position, neighbourhood environment and health. We will then use this framework to illustrate various methods to (a) define and delineate neighbourhoods including administrative and ego-centred boundaries, (b) measure

S. Voigtländer (✉)
Section on Quality of Health Care, Health Economics, Health System Analysis,
Bavarian Health and Food Safety Authority, Eggenreuther Weg 43, 91058 Erlangen, Germany

Department of Epidemiology and International Public Health, School of Public Health, Bielefeld University, P.O. Box 10 01 31, 33501 Bielefeld, Germany
e-mail: sven.voigtlaender@lgl.bayern.de

O. Razum
Department of Epidemiology and International Public Health, School of Public Health, Bielefeld University, P.O. Box 10 01 31, 33501 Bielefeld, Germany
e-mail: oliver.razum@uni-bielefeld.de

U. Berger
Department of Medical Informatics, Biostatistics and Epidemiology (IBE), Ludwig-Maximilians-University Munich, Marchioninistr. 15, 81377 München, Germany
e-mail: berger@ibe.med.uni-muenchen.de

C. Stock and A. Ellaway (eds.), *Neighbourhood Structure and Health Promotion*,
DOI 10.1007/978-1-4614-6672-7_6,

neighbourhood exposures referring to derived and integral neighbourhood variables as well as specific ecometric methods, (c) model neighbourhood effects on health outcomes based on a mixed model framework and its potential extensions, e.g. interaction effects, non-linear effects as well as spatial models and (d) incorporate time as well as timing in the analysis by using methods of panel data analysis and concepts of life course epidemiology. More detailed information for some of these methods is provided by the following chapters in this book, e.g. Chaps. 8 and 10.

Theoretical Considerations Preceding Empirical Analysis

Before giving an overview of methods to study neighbourhood effects on health, we will present a conceptual framework which will help to outline the various methodological challenges. Basically, a framework explaining neighbourhood health effects has to fulfil two requirements: First, it has to integrate "neighbourhood" in the discourse about social inequalities in health, i.e. to link the issues social position, neighbourhood and health. Second, it has to conceptualise neighbourhood as a social system comprising different kinds of health-related resources.

Our conceptual framework linking neighbourhood to social inequalities in health is illustrated in Fig. 6.1. The framework is based on the idea that the position of the individual in the structure of social inequality (Macro Level) influences individual health (Micro level) through differential exposure to stressors and resources within specific social contexts (Meso level) (Steinkamp 1993). These contexts can be family, peer group or workplace. Neighbourhood—as we now argue—is one of these contexts at the Meso level in which people live their daily lives (Voigtländer et al. 2012).[1] Referring to Richter and Wächter (2009, p. 22), we define neighbourhood as "the structure of the social ties of residents in an area who live in proximity to each other and who—to some extent—use the same facilities or participate in the same organisations" (English translation by the authors). Neighbourhood context (Meso level) is dependent on the structure of social inequality (Macro level) in two ways: firstly, that the social position of an individual influences his or her choice of residential locations and as such the potential neighbourhood and its characteristics. Secondly, that neighbourhood contexts reflect social inequality meaning that social inequality "spatialises" itself resulting in spatial concentrations of specific people, facilities, organisations and other contextual characteristics (Bourdieu 1999).

Figure 6.1 also shows that neighbourhood is, on the one hand, characterised by the specific sociodemographic composition in terms of residents' factors like age,

[1]This conceptualisation differs from the one of Chap. 15 in this book. This chapter refers to the theory of Steinkamp and regards neighbourhood as part of the Meso level including family, peer group and workplace, while Chap. 15 refers to the "Social-Ecological Model" as proposed by Bronfenbrenner and conceptualises neighbourhood as part of the exosystem which lies between the mesosystem and the macrosystem.

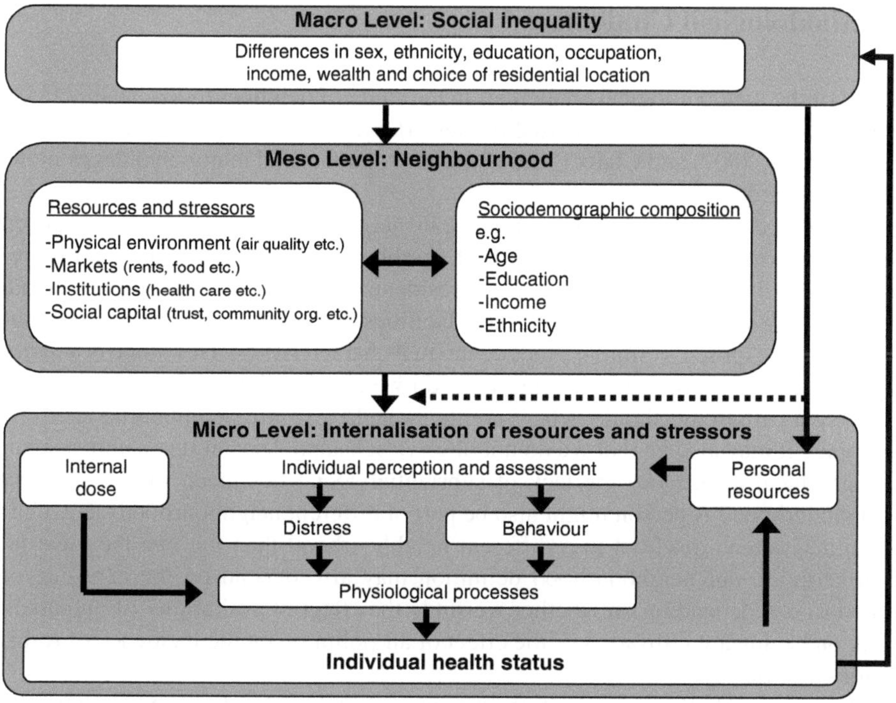

Fig. 6.1 Conceptual framework linking social inequality, neighbourhood context and health (Source: based on Voigtländer, S., Mielck, A., & Razum, O. (2012). Die Bedeutung des kleinräumigen Kontexts für Gesundheit: Entwurf eines Erklärungsmodells. *Gesundheitswesen*, *74*, 702–709 with permission by the publisher)

income and ethnicity. Some authors point out that factors related to the change in sociodemographic composition such as residential stability are important as well (e.g. Galster 2008). On the other hand, neighbourhood is characterised by its resources and stressors, which can be grouped into specific resource domains, i.e. physical environment, markets, institutions and social capital (cf. Bernard et al. 2007). Neighbourhood sociodemographic composition both shapes the resources accessible within a neighbourhood and is influenced by these, e.g. a particular composition might help to improve neighbourhood resources while low neighbourhood resources may be a reason for an individual to change residential location. Furthermore, Fig. 6.1 shows that the influence of neighbourhood (Meso level) on health (Micro level) works through three pathways: (a) a direct pathway related to direct health effects of hazardous environments; (b) an indirect pathway of neighbourhood resources through individual coping resulting in distress or behavioural change, e.g. smoking initiation or increased physical activity; and (c) a personal resources pathway describing the influence of neighbourhood on identity and following from this on individual coping.

Methodological Challenges

Most of the methodological challenges in the study of neighbourhood health effects can be derived from the conceptual framework presented in Fig. 6.1. Besides, Diez Roux (2001, 2007) and Chaix (2009) have also summarised major challenges in the existing literature.

The first challenge is to define or delineate neighbourhood. Ideally—as proposed by our previous theoretical definition of neighbourhood—a neighbourhood represents a small geographical entity whose residents are linked to each other by social ties and—to some extent—use the same facilities, participate in the same organisations or are exposed to similar other contextual characteristics. This alone is a major challenge because of the following: How do we define neighbourhood social ties? Is there a certain threshold? Where are the boundaries? Are neighbourhoods overlapping? It may also be that we do not observe substantial social ties within a small geographical area. Does the lack of substantial social ties mean that there is no neighbourhood? A person might also be part of different neighbourhoods, e.g. children may attend a school in a different neighbourhood than the one they live in. Furthermore, our neighbourhood definition may also depend on the exposure of interest, e.g. depending on whether we study the effect of availability of outpatient care on healthcare utilisation or the effect of air pollution on the incidence of respiratory disease.

The second challenge is the measurement of neighbourhood context including its sociodemographic composition as well as the nature of accessible resources and environmental exposures within that neighbourhood. Here, we have to consider that measurement of such characteristics is at the neighbourhood level, i.e. above the level of individuals or households. Relevant questions in this context include the following: What data sources exist to describe the social composition at this level as well as the distinct resource domains? How valid and precise is the available data? In cases where there is no data available, how can we collect the data? Regarding neighbourhood resources, it is also important that we measure not only their quantity, e.g. area of green space or number of healthcare providers, but also their quality, e.g. type and accessibility of green space or quality of healthcare provision. Another issue for clarification is whether it is sufficient to analyse one specific type of resource (or exposure) or it is essential to study the overall neighbourhood structure including other relevant characteristics.

The third challenge in the study of neighbourhood health effects is that we have to include information on individuals and households, i.e. residents within neighbourhoods. The conceptual framework shown in Fig. 6.1 indicates that these characteristics may act as confounders, effect modifiers or intermediary steps. For example, income and individual preferences clearly act as confounders because they influence residential location and with it neighbourhood context. At the same time they can have an effect on health outcomes independent of neighbourhood. Social position and individual preferences can modify the effect of neighbourhood exposures on health outcomes, e.g. the effect of neighbourhood social cohesion may be modified by individual social ties beyond the neighbourhood (Voigtländer et al. 2012) or the effect of neighbourhood walkability may be modified by preferences related to living in a specific neighbourhood type (Frank et al. 2007). Furthermore, individual or household characteristics can also act as intermediary steps as they may be part of the pathways between neighbourhood exposures and health outcomes. According to our model, individual coping mechanism, (health) behaviour and personal resources are among these factors. Diez Roux (2001) points out that factors related to social position such as education and income may themselves be dependent on the neighbourhood context and also that neighbourhood characteristics may modify the effect of individual characteristics. This is certainly true for children who are born into the neighbourhood which has been chosen by their parents.

This leads us to the fourth challenge which is how to best model neighbourhood effects on health statistically. This is a complex endeavour because information from different data sources (e.g. primary data, survey data, census data and administrative data) related to different levels of observation (e.g. individual, household, neighbourhood) might have to be linked. The resulting data set is hierarchical in the sense that it comprises a certain number of observed geographical neighbourhoods and nested within each neighbourhood observations on households and individuals. The modelling approach has to be capable of analysing such a data structure. Further questions that have to be answered when choosing a modelling approach are the following: Is it sufficient to treat neighbourhoods as independent entities, or should the modelling also take care of spatial correlations between neighbourhoods? Can we assume that the effects of neighbourhood exposures under study are linear or should we allow for more flexible non-linear effects? What can we do to deal with individual or household level confounders, i.e. the non-random selection of individuals or households into neighbourhoods based on their social position and preferences? Apart from statistical modelling techniques, the latter may be overcome by making use of natural experiments, i.e. quasi-random assignments of households to different neighbourhoods, when possible (Galster 2008).

The fifth and last challenge we want to describe here is related to the issue of time. As already noted, neighbourhoods and individuals change over time and the majority of people will live in different neighbourhoods during the course of their lives. Most of the existing studies so far are cross-sectional and as such they do not include data at different time points or changes over time in either individuals or neighbourhoods. A cross-sectional study design, however, makes the (implicit) assumption that the current health status of individuals depends on the present neighbourhood conditions. This assumption is unlikely to be correct and may lead to biased estimates of neighbourhood health effects because it ignores the fact that health and disease, especially chronic disease, develop over the life course (Ben-Shlomo and Kuh 2002). The question is here: How can concepts of life course epidemiology, i.e. accumulation, critical periods and trigger effects (Kuh and Ben-Shlomo 2004), be operationalised in order to estimate the full effect of neighbourhood upon health?

Delineating Neighbourhoods

The aim of delineating neighbourhoods is to define areas in which individuals reside, use facilities and interact with other residents. According to Chaix (2009), neighbourhoods are best delineated by viewing them as “exposure areas” that capture the (potentially heterogeneous) conditions of one’s local environment. This view is based on the idea of “interaction space”.

Exposure areas, however, are loose on the social element of our previously noted definition that a neighbourhood comprises the structure of social ties of residents. The definition of neighbourhood as an exposure area does not necessarily take the quantity and quality of local social ties into account. Here, the structure of local social ties is merely another exposure to the local environment which can be measured. Thus, the structure of neighbourhood social ties (including their intensity) is no precondition for delineating and defining neighbourhoods. Regarding our questions posed in the methodological challenges section, we can conclude that everybody—in terms of quantitative empirical studies—is a member of a neighbourhood.

Operationalising neighbourhood exposure areas in quantitative empirical studies is mainly conducted on the basis of administrative boundaries, e.g. census tracts/wards, postcode sectors, blocks, city-specific boundaries, school districts and so-called ego-centred boundaries, which consider neighbourhood from the viewpoint of an individual or household. Choice of type of operationalisation has to be based on theory, i.e. the considered pathway linking specific neighbourhood exposures with a specific health outcome. This is also true for the spatial scale. For instance, recreational walkability will operate on a smaller spatial scale than employment market characteristics (Chaix et al. 2009).

Administrative Boundaries

Using administrative boundaries means that we refer to official classifications of geographical units to partition space into discrete units, i.e. to delineate neighbourhoods. Thus, we can make use of information available from official statistics. In many countries it is relatively easy to link individuals to administrative areas because in the primary data we only need information about the location of study participants matched to the administrative boundaries used, e.g. wards and postcode sectors. We may use the participants’ addresses to create this information if it is not already on the data set. Due to data protection rules, obtaining access to participants’ location is usually more difficult at smaller spatial scales in most countries. At this level, however, neighbourhood effects may be stronger (Galster 2008; Woods et al. 2005). A problem with the use of administrative areas is that they may not properly reflect the interaction space of individuals, either because the interaction space of an individual cuts across administrative boundaries or the spatial scale is too large so that existing differences in neighbourhood exposures are dissolved (Chaix et al. 2009).

Ego-Centred Boundaries

Ego-centred neighbourhoods aim to better approximate neighbourhood by drawing a buffer around individuals' residences (Chaix et al. 2009; Frank et al. 2005). The latter have to be georeferenced. The term "georeferenced" essentially means that an object (with certain attributes) or information is also characterised by its geographical location (Werneck 2008). This may be given by latitude and longitude coordinates. Thus, ego-centred neighbourhoods are supposed to reflect the interaction space of individuals, i.e. the accessible area around their residence. The two basic types of buffers are circular buffers, e.g. creating a radius of a particular straight-line distance (e.g. 1 km) around an individuals' residence (regardless of street or roads), and the other type of buffers are street network-based buffers. The latter takes into account the fact that not every part of the buffer area may be equivalently accessible due to the local street network or physical barriers such as rivers, railways and highways. In contrast to fixed boundaries, e.g. in the case of administrative areas, ego-centred neighbourhoods differ according to residence and they may also overlap so that, for instance, two individuals with different residences share parts of their respective ego-centred neighbourhood. When we want to delineate ego-centred neighbourhoods, we need to both make use of geographic information systems (GIS) and have detailed georeferenced exposure data available. This is more complex than the use of existing administrative boundaries. There are several other variants of ego-centred neighbourhoods that have been proposed to more accurately capture the true exposure area, e.g. neighbourhoods with fuzzy instead of sharp boundaries, individual-specific instead of uniform neighbourhood boundaries and multi-scale instead of single-scale neighbourhoods (Chaix et al. 2009). For instance, with fuzzy boundaries, exposures that are further away from one's residential location weigh less, while multi-scale neighbourhoods take into account that there are exposures acting at larger scales, i.e. characteristics of the employment market.

We might also consider ways of delineating neighbourhoods other than using administrative or creating ego-centred boundaries. For example, the investigators themselves might define boundaries, i.e. partition space into discrete units. This may be done on the basis of local knowledge or information provided by residents (Diez Roux 2001), which can be collected by methods such as interviews, photographs, drawings and maps (Coulton et al. 2001; Nicotera 2007). However, there are drawbacks to this approach as delineating neighbourhoods in this way is very time-consuming and not always feasible, for example, for a large nationally representative study. Investigators may also choose to define boundaries based on other criteria such as the spatial distribution and accessibility of the local infrastructure, e.g. the catchment areas of schools and healthcare facilities.

Measuring Neighbourhood Exposures

According to our conceptual model presented in Fig. 6.1, neighbourhoods are characterised by their sociodemographic composition in terms of factors such as age, education, income and ethnicity as well as specific resources and stressors related to the physical environment, local markets, institutions and social capital. All of these neighbourhood exposures ought to be measured to fully understand the health impact of neighbourhoods. Furthermore, Diez Roux (2001, p. 1785) claims that "The development of valid and reliable measures of relevant area characteristics that can be obtained in a systematic fashion across many areas is an important need in this field".

Derived and Integral Variables

Diez Roux (2002) distinguishes between derived and integral neighbourhood variables. Derived neighbourhood variables refer to the summary (or average) characteristics of individuals in the same neighbourhood such as mean income, the number of unemployed persons as a proportion of the labour force, the migration balance or the standard deviation of the household income distribution in the neighbourhood. Derived variables may describe distinct neighbourhood-level constructs; for example, mean neighbourhood income describes overall wealth within a neighbourhood which has a different meaning compared to individual-level income. Several authors have also combined information on derived variables, e.g. income, unemployment and housing, to construct a so-called deprivation index which aims to measure overall neighbourhood socioeconomic context (e.g. Messer et al. 2006; Morris and Carstairs 1991).

Integral neighbourhood variables do not summarise individual-level characteristics but instead describe neighbourhood-level characteristics such as the quantity and quality of neighbourhood infrastructure and green space as well as social cohesion within a neighbourhood. Diez Roux (2002, p. 589) also points out that "Derived variables often operate by shaping certain integral properties of the group [neighbourhood, authors' note]", an issue that is also reflected in the conceptual model in Fig. 6.1. For instance, migration balance as a measure of residential stability influences the level of social cohesion as well as trust within a neighbourhood, and the mean neighbourhood income may influence the power of community organisations to influence political decisions related to the neighbourhood. The latter example also illustrates the difference in meaning between derived variables and their individual-level equivalents because individual income is both a health determinant in itself with low income being a risk factor for many kinds of diseases, and it is one among many individual incomes within a neighbourhood that, on an aggregate level, shape local resources (e.g. the power of community organisations to influence political decisions) affecting all inhabitants (e.g. siting of waste transfer stations and transportation systems) (Schulz and Northridge 2004).

Data sources for derived and integral neighbourhood variables differ. Derived variables can be constructed based on administrative sources such as census data and population registries (or they can be estimated from the data). The number and type of such data sources differ between countries. Moreover, data availability in terms of richness and degree of (possible) geographic disaggregation also differs substantially between countries and in some cases even between cities of the same country. For example, the United Kingdom conducts a census every 10 years which covers a wide range of topics including age, gender, marital status, household composition, housing tenure, nationality, ethnicity, religion, language, education, occupation and health (cf. http://www.ons.gov.uk). This census data is available for various area levels ranging from municipal areas down to small-area units, e.g. “Lower Layer Super Output Areas”, which are geographical areas containing on average 1,500 residents (cf. http://www.neighbourhood.statistics.gov.uk). In contrast to this, in Germany derived neighbourhood variables can rely on population registries and other municipal data comprising age, sex, household composition, nationality and welfare beneficiaries. However, Germany has no uniform classification of small-area geographical units for which data is reported (Maier et al. 2011). For instance, in Berlin, the smallest geographical units are so-called planning areas (“Planungsräume”) with an average population size of 7,500 inhabitants (Bömermann et al. 2006). This size is rather far from our before-mentioned definition of neighbourhood, comprising residents living in proximity to each other.

Ecometrics

Integral variables refer to characteristics of the neighbourhood itself (influencing health outcomes) such as air quality, availability of healthcare providers and certain stores as well as social cohesion and walkability. Administrative data do—apart from some public agencies (see below)—not offer information on these characteristics, which are, however, necessary for a more complete description of neighbourhoods. Therefore, researchers like Raudenbush and Sampson (1999) propose a quantitative assessment of neighbourhoods (and other ecological settings) called “ecometrics”. The three most important and complementary ecometric methods are the following: (a) systematic social observation (SSO), (b) survey of residents and (c) estimation of density and distance measures based on georeferenced data. SSO as well as a survey of residents require fixed neighbourhood boundaries, i.e. a discrete partitioning of space. If we want to use this information in a study based on ego-neighbourhoods we will have to transform the SSO or survey data, e.g. by calculating a weighted average exposure for the fixed areas covered by an ego-centred neighbourhood.

Systematic Social Observation

We may use SSO in cases when we assume that survey respondents are not able to provide a valid and objective description of certain aspects of the social and physical environment, which we are interested in (Raudenbush and Sampson 1999). SSO aims to provide information that is independent of the individuals in the neighbourhoods under study by means of direct observation and videotaping.

The data collected in this way is then coded by trained raters based on predefined criteria. Nicotera (2007) calls SSO a "windshield survey" because the position of the observer is—literally speaking—behind the windshield of a car; the observers do not interact with residents. In one of the first SSO studies, Raudenbush and Sampson (1999) analysed social disorder as well as physical disorder in the neighbourhoods of Chicago, USA, based on indicators such as "people selling drugs" and "needles/syringes on the sidewalk". The authors emphasise that SSO is limited to theoretical constructs which do not require residents' perspectives. According to Chaix (2009) SSO may be less useful regarding aspects of the social environment compared to the physical environment because some of the indicators are intermittently observable or equivocal, e.g. graffiti may not indicate social disorder.

Surveys Among Residents

Surveys of residents can provide information on theoretical constructs such as neighbourhood identity, social cohesion and social control which are not observable through SSO (Chaix 2009; Raudenbush and Sampson 1999). In such surveys, residents may evaluate distinct dimensions of their neighbourhood based on multiple items (Chaix 2009). The individual results are then, similar to the before-mentioned derived variables, aggregated to the neighbourhood level to serve as neighbourhood-level variables. There appears to be no consensus whether it is best to collect survey-based neighbourhood data from the primary study participants or a separate sample. Using data from the participants of the primary study has the advantage that the information collected can be used not only to generate neighbourhood-level variables but also to include it in the analysis as an indicator of individual neighbourhood experience. The disadvantage is that this approach might lead to same-source bias, such that using self-reported information on neighbourhood characteristics as well as self-reported health or health behaviours may result in spurious associations (Auchincloss et al. 2008).

Georeferenced Data

Georeferenced data offers a third option to construct specific neighbourhood measures. Availability of such data, including georeferenced data provided by public agencies, has increased in recent years and covers different aspects of neighbourhoods such as air quality, noise, green space, land use, healthcare institutions and food stores. Georeferences can be used to construct distance measures, e.g. the distance between the location of residence and the location of the next general practitioner (GP) based on the street network, as well as density measures, e.g. the density of green space within a certain area (Diez Roux 2001). Chaix (2009) suggests combining georeferenced data with information on destination attributes such as the quality of the available green space. Other authors try to combine several georeferenced measures to construct an index for a specific neighbourhood dimension. For instance, Buck et al. (2011) construct a "moveability" index including the number of accessible objects for physical activity (as a weighted sum) for each geographical location within the area under study. Their index is based on street connectivity, density of destinations related to physical activity and level of urbanisation, which they operationalise by multiple variables each. Apart from distance and density measures, we can use georeferenced data (point data), e.g. concentration of air pollutants measured at a limited number of ambient air monitoring sites, to produce estimated values for locations where data is unavailable (Werneck 2008), i.e. concentration of air pollutants at a point somewhere between two or more monitoring sites.

Georeferenced data is of particular relevance in studies based on ego-centred neighbourhoods. Here some of the previously noted methods to measure specific neighbourhood exposures, i.e. density measures, geographic distributions and indices, are also being used to measure the sociodemographic composition of neighbourhoods. Schräpler (2009), for example, uses geoinformation to determine the geographic density of welfare recipients as a socioeconomic measure of school neighbourhoods.

Modelling Neighbourhood Effects on Health Outcomes

In analyses of the impact of neighbourhood conditions on health outcomes, we can distinguish between different types of studies: Besides the comparison of a small number of pre-selected neighbourhoods, which are analysed in depth, we can either employ ecological studies or multilevel studies. Ecological studies are based on aggregated data of a geographic entity, e.g. data aggregated at the neighbourhood level. We might, for example, study the mortality rate of neighbourhoods dependent on the proportion of women as well as on the age and income composition of the population living in this neighbourhood. However, studies of this kind do not allow us to distinguish between effects operating on the individual level and neighbourhood effects. Effects of certain variables, which we find in aggregated data at the neighbourhood level, may or may not be the same as the corresponding effects at individual level. This problem is known as the "ecological fallacy" (Gordis 2004). In the following section, we give a short introduction to multilevel analyses as an alternative to ecological studies and sketch some useful extensions of this modelling method. While this chapter provides an overview on multilevel modelling, Chap. 10 in this book explains multilevel linear regression and multilevel logistic modelling in step by step procedures.

Multilevel Modelling

We can overcome the problem of ecological fallacy by analysing the health impact of neighbourhoods on an individual level while accounting for various individual characteristics such as age, gender and socioeconomic status. This means that in a neighbourhood study of this type, we combine information measured at different levels, e.g. personal characteristics measured at the individual level and contextual information measured at the neighbourhood level. Data with a multilevel structure is also referred to as hierarchical data (Leyland and Groenewegen 2003). When analysing the contextual effect of neighbourhoods on an individual's health, we implicitly presume that persons living in the same neighbourhood are more alike with respect to health than persons living in different neighbourhoods. This is because they are exposed to the same social and physical environment, they use the same local facilities and they face the same neighbourhood social structure. Thus, we assume a cluster structure, where individual data is clustered within neighbourhoods. For those neighbourhood characteristics, which are explicitly measured, i.e. contextual data, persons from the same neighbourhood will have the same value. In addition, a correlation structure between persons living in the same neighbourhood is assumed, capturing the latent (not measured) similarities between them. This underlying correlation has to be taken into account in the statistical analysis to ensure unbiased, reliable results.

To analyse clustered data, e.g. individuals living in different neighbourhoods, we can employ a multilevel modelling approach. This allows us to jointly model data from different levels, such as data measured on individuals (individual level), e.g. age, gender and socioeconomic status, as well as data describing neighbourhood characteristics (neighbourhood level), e.g. sociodemographic composition of neighbourhoods and accessibility of healthcare facilities. At the same time, it adjusts for the underlying correlation between individuals of the same cluster, i.e. the latent neighbourhood effects. The approach relies on the assumption that the observed neighbourhoods are a sample from a larger population.

Mixed Model Framework

Multilevel models can be embodied in the framework of mixed regression models, which are an extension of ordinary linear regression models. They consist of a mixture of fixed effects and random effects. The fixed effects are the typical coefficients of a linear regression model, which quantify the effect of a specific predictor, e.g. age, gender and type of neighbourhood, on the outcome. Random effects are linked to the units of the higher levels, such as the neighbourhood level. They allow for neighbourhood specific deviations from the overall mean, e.g. average physical health, which remained unexplained by the neighbourhood characteristics in the model. Here, it is not the actual effect that is of interest but rather their variation across neighbourhoods, i.e. the heterogeneity between neighbourhoods.

Consider a metric outcome, such as a person's physical health score based on the Short Form-12 Health Questionnaire (SF-12) (Jenkinson and Layte 1997). A simple linear mixed model linking the outcome to a number of predictor variables measured on the two levels, the individual level (level 1) and the neighbourhood level (level 2), has the following form:

$$y_{ij} = \beta_0 + \beta_1 x_{1ij} + \beta_2 x_{2j} + (u_j + \varepsilon_{ij}), \tag{6.1}$$

where i indexes the individual person (level 1 unit) and j indexes the neighbourhood (level 2 unit), in which individual i lives. x_{1ij} is a predictor variable measured at the individual level, e.g. income, and x_{2j} is a predictor variable measured on the level 2 unit, e.g. rurality/urbanity of a neighbourhood. Coefficients β_1 and β_2 are the fixed effects of the predictors x_1 and x_2 on the outcome y_{ij}, e.g. the mean change of the physical health score with every additional unit of income (e.g. one Euro) or the mean difference in health between individuals living in an urban to those from a rural neighbourhood. The intercept of the regression β_0 is the overall mean, e.g. of physical health, when all predictors are zero. Moreover, u_j is the random effect, which is an effect of the jth neighbourhood shared by all individuals within that neighbourhood. Thus, u_j captures the correlation between observations clustered within one neighbourhood and hence accounts for the similarity of individuals from one neighbourhood. The random effect can be seen as the residual at the neighbourhood level and is usually assumed to be independently normally distributed with zero mean and a common variance: $u_j \sim N(0,\sigma_u^2)$. In our model the variance σ_u^2 mirrors the neighbourhood specific heterogeneity of health. Finally, $\varepsilon_{ij} \sim N(0,\sigma_\varepsilon^2)$ is the typical, independently normally distributed residual (error term) of the linear regression, which is associated with individual i of neighbourhood j, and σ_ε^2 is the residual variance.

With the mixed model approach (Formula 6.1), we can partition the total variation of the outcome measure, in our example the variation of individual physical health, into variation on the neighbourhood level, σ_u^2, and variation on the individual level, σ_ε^2, such that the total variation decomposes into the following: $\sigma_{\text{tot}}^2 = \sigma_u^2 + \sigma_\varepsilon^2$. By doing so, we can explore what part of the unexplained variation is due to differences between neighbourhoods and what part is due to individual differences. Often the proportion of the neighbourhood variance σ_u^2 on the total variance $\sigma_u^2 + \sigma_\varepsilon^2$ is used to quantify the cluster effect. In a simple mixed model as in our example, this proportion is equal to the correlation between two observations of the same neighbourhood and therefore also referred to as the intra-class correlation coefficient.

Extensions of the Hierarchical Data Structure

In general, we have always a clustered data structure with an underlying correlation when observations of one cluster are more alike than observations randomly chosen from two different clusters. So in certain data we might find more levels of clusters. For example, the household might be considered as an additional level between individual level and neighbourhood level resulting in a 3-level hierarchy with individuals nested within households which are themselves nested within neighbourhoods. In this case we can extend the 2-level model by including, for each additional level, a further random effect, which captures the correlation between the observations of a unit of this level.

In this way, the mixed model approach allows us to jointly examine specific effects of predictor variables from any level of a hierarchical data set. It implicitly accounts for the underlying correlations structure at each level and provides efficient, unbiased estimates for the effects of predictor variables. Moreover, it assures correct standard errors for these estimates and with that correct confidence intervals and p-values. A further advantage of the approach is that it is parsimonious in the sense that it only requires the estimation of the variance of the random effect: we have one additional parameter per level, independent of the number of units of this level. In this way the approach can deal with a large number of level 2 units, e.g. neighbourhoods. At the same time it is able to deal with even a small number of observations per cluster, as it might, for example, be the case when defining households as level 2 units. Mixed models do not require balanced samples, i.e. they do not require the same number of level 1 observation for all level 2 units.

The data structure of clustered data is in certain cases not strictly hierarchical. We can conceive data where different types of hierarchies exist in parallel form and individuals are belonging to different types of clusters simultaneously. In a study on teenagers, we might, for example, consider the health impact of the residential neighbourhood together with the neighbourhood of the school. In this case, we speak of a cross-classified data structure. Another situation where we face a more complex hierarchical data structure arises when a person is member of more than one cluster, i.e. when we have multiple memberships. This might, for example, be the case when we study neighbourhood effects on health over the course of a time period during which individuals might change from one neighbourhood to another. Also data with cross-classified and multiple membership structures can be analysed within the framework of mixed models (Goldstein and Fielding 2006; Rasbash and Browne 2008).

Effect Modification and Interaction Effects

In the simple linear mixed model (Formula 6.1) defined above, the fixed effects of a predictor are assumed to be the same for all individuals. We might, however, assume that the effects of certain predictors vary according to other predictors of the same level, e.g. the impact of walkability on health might differ according to the social connectedness of a neighbourhood (Kaczynski and Glover 2012). In this case, social connectedness is regarded as an "effect modifier". This modifying effect can be included in the model by an interaction term of the form $\beta x_1 x_2$, where the effect of a predictor x_2 is multiplied by the effect modifier x_1. Also cross-level analyses investigating interaction effects between individual and neighbourhood variables are modelled in that way. For instance, Franzini and Spears (2003) use interaction terms to investigate a cross-level interaction between neighbourhood wealth and individual educational attainment on years of life lost to heart disease.

The Random Coefficient Model (Random Slope Model)

The model described above (Formula 6.1) assumes that the effect of a predictor, e.g. the physical health impact of individual income, is the same in all neighbourhoods. This is described by the fixed effect β. However, the relationship between individual characteristics and health may vary between neighbourhoods. We might, for example, assume that in some neighbourhoods the health benefit for persons with a higher income is more distinct. To account for such neighbourhood variation in the relationship between a predictor and the outcome, we can add "random coefficients" (also called "random slopes") in our model, which are allowed to differ between neighbourhoods. This leads us to "random coefficient models" ("random slope models"):

$$y_{ij} = \beta_0 + \beta_1 x_{1ij} + (u_{0j} + u_{1j} x_{1ij} + e_{ij}), \tag{6.2}$$

where $u_{0j} \sim N(0, \sigma^2_{u_0})$ is again the neighbourhood residual as described above and u_{1j} is the additional random coefficient (random slope) of predictor x_{1ij} in neighbourhood j. This random coefficient allows us to include a neighbourhood specific departure from the average (fixed) effect β_1 of the predictor x_{1ij}. Again, the main interest is not in the actual difference in the relationship for a single neighbourhood but in capturing this neighbourhood variation in order to obtain reliable estimates. Hence, these random coefficients are again typically assumed to be normally distributed with zero mean. The variance matrix of the random effect and the random coefficient describes the variation between the neighbourhoods.

Random coefficients are also added to a model when we aim to explore if the impact of the neighbourhood differs for different kinds of people. For example, we might presume that the neighbourhood effect on an individual's health is stronger for poor people than for rich people, i.e. the variation of health between neighbourhoods is larger for people with a low income.

Interpreting Neighbourhood Residuals

In mixed modelling (multilevel modelling), the major focus is not on quantifying an actual departure of a specific neighbourhood from the average level of the health outcome or from the overall effect of a certain predictor but on accounting for this neighbourhood variation in order to obtain reliable estimates. However, it is possible to obtain the neighbourhood specific residuals for each single neighbourhood of the data set as a by-product of model estimation, i.e. estimates for the actual values of u_0 or u_1. These residuals capture neighbourhood differences, which remained unexplained by the individual or contextual predictors of the model. Thus, their further analysis can provide additional insight into undiscovered neighbourhood mechanisms. In particular it might be helpful to plot neighbourhood residuals in a map where different shadings of colours represent different values. This would allow the exploration of potential geographical structures. A more sophisticated way to explore geographical structures in hierarchical data is the use of spatial methods, as provided by geo-additive models (see below).

Non-linear Effects and Varying Coefficient Models

The embedding of mixed models in the framework of regression models allows for a wide variety of extensions. One is the inclusion of non-linear effects. The models above assume that the fixed effect of a predictor is linear. In some situations this assumption can, however, be too restrictive. We might instead wish to allow that the effect of a continuous predictor varies dependent on its values in a non-linear form. For example, the impact of an additional Euro of income might have a higher effect on individual health for a person, which has a very small total income, while the effect will be smaller for someone whose total income is very high. So instead of assuming the effect of additional income will be the same for all values, we might assume that it is higher for small values and smaller for high values. For the model formula, this means that instead of describing the relation between the predictor and the outcome by the multiplicative term βx, the income effect is represented by the function $\beta(x)$.

The simplest way to include a non-linear effect function into a regression model is to split the values of the predictor x into a number of categories and estimate a separate coefficient for each of these categories, resulting in a step function for $\beta(x)$. Reichman et al. (2009), for example, used this method when studying the impact of neighbourhood ethnic composition on birth weight while adjusting for maternal age, which is known to have a non-linear, U-shaped association with birth weight. This method requires, however, that we prespecify cut-points for the values of predictor x to define categories.

When the continuous nature of a predictor should be preserved, we would rather choose a smooth function $\beta(x)$ to describe the relation between this predictor and the outcome. If prior knowledge of the functional form of the effect is available, we can directly include this in the model by transforming the predictor accordingly. For example, we might log-transform the income and include the term $\beta \times \log(\text{income})$ in our model formula, obtaining a function that rises steeply for small values of income and levels out for higher levels of income. If we do not have any knowledge on a possible form of the effect function $\beta(x)$, a suitable transformation can be searched by fitting a series of different transformations and selecting the best fitting model. Royston and Altman (1994) and Sauerbrei and Royston (1999) propose such an approach using a number of flexible polynomial transformations which they call "fractional polynomials". Even more flexible are non-parametric approaches leading to additive models (Hastie and Tibshirani 1990). Here $\beta(x)$ is just assumed to be any smooth function which remains unspecified in its form and is fully estimated from the data. In the mixed model context, this extension leads to additive mixed models (e.g. Ruppert et al. 2003). Different methods for a non-parametric estimation of $\beta(x)$ have been proposed, where the p-spline approach (Eilers and Marx 1996) is particularly favourable. First, it is shown that with p-splines one attains a good fit even if the true effect function has an awkward form. Second, p-splines can be reformulated in a mixed model representation, which enables the use of the same estimation procedures, making the estimation more efficient (Kauermann 2006).

Also when analysing interactions in the relationship of two predictors, the linearity assumption might at times be too restrictive, and a more sophisticated, non-linear approach might be preferred. This leads to varying coefficient models (Hastie and Tibshirani 1993), where the effect of a predictor, e.g. rurality/urbanity, is allowed to vary with the value of another modifying variable, e.g. individual income, described in the function $\beta(x_1) \times x_2$. These models can be further extended to allow for spatially varying or time-varying coefficients (see below).

Spatial Models

Mixed models in the form described above allow us to jointly analyse the impact of contextual and individual characteristics on health while accounting for the correlation structure of observations *within* a neighbourhood. A weakness of this approach is that it treats neighbourhoods as independent units and does not take the correlation *between* neighbourhoods into account. It is, however, reasonable to assume that adjacent neighbourhoods are more similar than neighbourhoods further apart. Recent developments in spatial statistics make use of the geographic information on the location of an observation to incorporate the spatial correlation structure in the analysis. This is based on the assumption that people might be affected not only by their own neighbourhood but also by surrounding neighbourhoods.

Geo-additive models (Kammann and Wand 2003) extend classical mixed models by adding a spatially correlated effect:

$$y_{ij} = \beta_0 + \beta_1 x_{1ij} + \beta_2 x_{2j} + (u_{0j} + u_{\text{geo}}(s_i) + \varepsilon_{ij}). \tag{6.3}$$

Thus, in this model, we add to the neighbourhood specific residual u_{0j} a smooth spatial effect function $u_{\text{geo}}(s_i)$ based on the geographical information s_i of observation i. This smooth, spatial function is estimated from the data. It mirrors the latent geographic structure of the data which remained unexplained by the predictors considered in the model. We can plot the estimated spatial effects in maps to visualise its geographic structures.

The geographical information on the location of an observation s_i can have two forms: (a) either we have discrete lattice data considering information about adjacent neighbourhoods or (b) it is continuous, e.g. given by geographical coordinates of the place of a person's residence. In the case of discrete lattice data, the space is discretely partitioned into a fixed number of mutually exclusive (nonoverlapping) units.

For example, a territory might be partitioned into a certain number of neighbourhoods and in model (Formula 6.3) $s_i=j$ denotes the neighbourhood of observation i. Here the adjacency must be defined for all location units. Two location units are considered to be adjacent when they share a common border. The spatial neighbourhood effect $u_{geo}(s_i)$ can then be estimated, for example, following the seminal work of Besag (1974) based on a Markov random field approach (see also Rue and Held 2005). The resulting spatial function $u_{geo}(s_i)$ can be seen as a "spatially structured" residual accompanying the "unstructured" neighbourhood residual u_{0j}. This approach can be extended considering more elaborated functions to define the adjacency of two neighbourhoods. For example, Chaix et al. (2006) take the distances between central points (centroids) of the neighbourhoods into account.

If the geographical information of an observation is continuous, i.e. given by coordinates, the adjacency between two observations can be measured by the (Euclidean) distance of their location points. Here two-dimensional smoothing techniques can be employed to obtain a smooth spatial function $u_{geo}(s_i)$ (see, e.g. Ruppert et al. 2003), such as bivariate p-splines (Brezger and Lang 2006). Alternatively the spatial effect $u_{geo}(s_i)$ can be constructed as an additional, spatially varying residual on the observation level, which is subject to a spatial correlation structure. Here it is usually assumed that the correlation between two observations decreases with increasing distance. Chaix et al. (2005) employed this approach to examine healthcare utilisation in France, where the spatial correlation structure was specified by an exponentially decreasing function of the distance.

Spatial models can be employed in different ways. First they are useful when exploring unexplained regional heterogeneity in health of geographical referenced data while controlling for individual and neighbourhood predictors, which have been shown to be associated with health. Secondly, they can also be used to map spatial distributions, e.g. of poor health, incidences of specific diseases or of any health-related neighbourhood component such as air pollution or medical facilities. In addition, they are particularly advantageous when we investigate effects of small areas such as neighbourhoods. Here they may help to compensate for small numbers of observation in each area, as the spatial smoothing has the effect of pooling data from adjacent areas. Furthermore, geo-additive models can be extended by spatially varying coefficients which describe the effect of a predictor varying smoothly over space.

Heteroscedasticity

Besides extensions to more flexible predictors, the mixed model framework also allows us to explore more complex variance structures. For certain examples, it might be too stringent to assume that the variation between neighbourhoods is the same throughout all types of neighbourhoods. For example, in an international study it might be of interest to explore if the variation of health on neighbourhood level differs between different countries. In other words, we might want to allow for heteroscedasticity of the neighbourhood residuals. This can be done by estimating separate standard deviations of the neighbourhood residuals for each country. Heteroscedasticity can be included at any level of a multilevel analysis (e.g. Pinheiro and Bates 2009 or Faraway 2005).

Generalised Mixed Models

So far, we regarded only models for continuous outcome, e.g. a continuous physical health score, assuming (approximately) normally distributed residuals on the individual level. The mixed model framework with all its extensions described above can be generalised to deal with binary or categorical response or count data. This is done by extending generalised linear models (McCullagh and Nelder 1989) to generalised mixed models including random effects to capture the correlation structure of clustered data. As in generalised linear models, generalised mixed models link the outcome variable to predictor variables via a link function. For more details we refer to McCulloch et al. (2008) or Berridge and Crouchley (2011).

Incorporating Time

In addition to the modelling issues we have just described, an analysis of neighbourhood effects on health should consider the role of time as well as timing. This has rarely been done to date because of lack of adequate data. Thus, most of the existing studies use a cross-sectional design. The implicit claim made in such studies is that the observed health status of individuals depends on current neighbourhood conditions, and this claim may be way too simple.

Concepts of Life Course

Kuh and Ben-Shlomo (2004) list three different concepts how chronic disease risk may be influenced by exposures acting across the life course of an individual: (a) accumulation of risk, (b) critical or sensitive periods and (c) trigger effects. The first concept argues that disease risks may accumulate over time. For example, exposure to neighbourhood deprivation over long periods of life stages may increase the risk of coronary heart disease (CHD). If this were the case for neighbourhood exposures, a cross-sectional study would underestimate neighbourhood effects because it does not consider the cumulative exposure (in years) including early or earlier life neighbourhood circumstances. In contrast to this, the concept of critical or sensitive periods suggests that certain exposures may have long-term health effects only if they occur in specific periods of development. For example, neighbourhood deprivation may increase the risk of CHD if someone is being exposed during a certain age bracket in childhood. If this would be a relevant pathway, a study among adults would have to also collect data on the participants' exposure to neighbourhood deprivation during their childhood. Otherwise, the study will most likely estimate a biased effect for current neighbourhood deprivation on CHD risk because only a certain proportion of participants will currently be exposed to neighbourhood deprivation that is similar to the one to which they were exposed during childhood. Trigger effects describe a chain of risk where only the final link has a health effect. For example, neighbourhood deprivation may via low educational status lead to smoking, which in turn increases the risk of lung cancer. Here the effect of neighbourhood deprivation on lung cancer would only affect those individuals for whom it triggered a chain of risk.

Næss and Leyland (2010) published one of the few empirical studies which tries to model a health outcome, i.e. mortality in Oslo, based on individuals' residential history at several life stages. Residential history is operationalised by using census information on individuals from the years 1960, 1970, 1980 and 1990. The authors develop and discuss different kinds of multilevel models, including a single time point model, a multiple membership model, a cross-classified model and finally a correlated cross-classified multilevel model, to measure the random effect of neighbourhood for different age cohorts in the years 1960, 1970, 1980 and 1990. In addition, the authors have to deal with the fact that the neighbourhood delineations changed over time. They overcome this challenge by applying the 1960 definition of neighbourhoods to the three subsequent time points using GIS. The results of the study support the hypothesis that early life neighbourhood may affect mortality independent of neighbourhood in later life. However, due to lack of appropriate data, Næss and Leyland could not analyse the reasons for the random effect of neighbourhood, whether it was due to individual- or neighbourhood-level variables.

Longitudinal Data Analysis

Incorporating information of different time points into an analysis usually requires longitudinal data, where the same individuals are observed over a certain period of time. Longitudinal data can either be collected in a panel study or it might be constructed combining data on the same individuals from different sources and time points (as done by Næss and Leyland 2010). With repeated observations on the same individual at a sequence of time points, we must assume a correlation between those observations clustered within one individual. To model data of this structure, we might make use of the mixed model approaches described above (Formula 6.1–6.3) adjusting them adequately. For instance, we can include a further level in the mixed model so that the lowest level is the level of repeated observations at the different time points; level 2 is the level of the individual, which is observed over time; and level 3 might be the neighbourhood level. The random effect of level 2 captures the correlation structure of repeated observations made on the same individual. In such a model we could also allow for updating certain predictors over time, i.e. including time-dependent variables into the model. For instance, we might include individual income or neighbourhood wealth of different time points. For other predictors, we might assume that their impact on the health changes with time or with age of the individual, and we might employ varying coefficient models as described above, which model the effect of a predictor as a function of time or age, respectively. Again, if the health outcome of interest is not continuous but, e.g. binary, we can extend generalised mixed models accordingly. Longitudinal data might also be used for analyses focussing on the time point at which certain events happen to an individual, e.g. the time at which an individual first reports poor self-rated health dependent on neighbourhood social as well as physical conditions (Voigtländer et al. 2011). Here methods of survival analysis can be used to model the time to event in a multilevel survival model (Goldstein 2011).

In conclusion, to perform longitudinal neighbourhood studies like the one by Næss and Leyland (2010) and to find out what specific individual as well as neighbourhood variables explain the identified neighbourhood random effects across the life course will be a major issue for future studies.

Acknowledgements The work for this chapter was partly supported by the German Research Foundation (DFG), grant number: RA 889/2-1.

References

Auchincloss, A. H., Diez Roux, A. V., Brown, D. G., Erdmann, C. A., & Bertoni, A. G. (2008). Neighborhood resources for physical activity and healthy foods and their association with insulin resistance. *Epidemiology, 19*, 146–157.

Ben-Shlomo, Y., & Kuh, D. (2002). A life course approach to chronic disease epidemiology: Conceptual models, empirical challenges and interdisciplinary perspectives. *International Journal of Epidemiology, 31*, 285–293.

Bernard, P., Charafeddine, R., Frohlich, K. L., Daniel, M., Kestens, Y., & Potvin, L. (2007). Health inequalities and place: A theoretical conception of neighbourhood. *Social Science & Medicine, 65*, 1839–1852.

Berridge, D. M., & Crouchley, R. (2011). *Multivariate generalized linear mixed models using R.* Boca Raton, FL: CRC Press.

Besag, J. (1974). Spatial interaction and statistical-analysis of lattice systems. *Journal of the Royal Statistical Society, Series B: Statistical Methodology, 36*, 192–236.

Bömermann, H., Jahn, S., & Nelius, K. (2006). Lebensweltlich orientierte Räume im Regionalen Bezugssystem (Teil 1). *Monatsschrift Berliner Statistik, 8*, 366–371.

Bourdieu, P. (1999). Site effects. In P. Bourdieu (Ed.), *The weight of the world: Social suffering in contemporary society* (p. 129). Stanford, CA: Stanford University Press.

Brezger, A., & Lang, S. (2006). Generalized structured additive regression based on Bayesian P-splines. *Computational Statistics & Data Analysis, 50*, 967–991.

Buck, C., Pohlabeln, H., Huybrechts, I., De Bourdeaudhuij, I., Pitsiladis, Y., Reisch, L., et al. (2011). Development and application of a moveability index to quantify possibilities for physical activity in the built environment of children. *Health & Place, 17*, 1191–1201.

Chaix, B. (2009). Geographic life environments and coronary heart disease: A literature review, theoretical contributions, methodological updates, and a research agenda. *Annual Review of Public Health, 30*, 81–105.

Chaix, B., Leyland, A. H., Sabel, C. E., Chauvin, P., Rastam, L., Kristersson, H., et al. (2006). Spatial clustering of mental disorders and associated characteristics of the neighbourhood context in Malmo, Sweden, in 2001. *Journal of Epidemiology and Community Health, 60*, 427–435.

Chaix, B., Merlo, J., & Chauvin, P. (2005). Comparison of a spatial approach with the multilevel approach for investigating place effects on health: The example of healthcare utilisation in France. *Journal of Epidemiology and Community Health, 59*, 517–526.
Chaix, B., Merlo, J., Evans, D., Leal, C., & Havard, S. (2009). Neighbourhoods in eco-epidemiologic research: Delimiting personal exposure areas. A response to Riva, Gauvin, Apparicio and Brodeur. *Social Science & Medicine, 69*, 1306–1310.
Coulton, C. J., Korbin, J., Chan, T., & Su, M. (2001). Mapping residents' perceptions of neighborhood boundaries: A methodological note. *American Journal of Community Psychology, 29*, 371–383.
Diez Roux, A. V. (2001). Investigating neighborhood and area effects on health. *American Journal of Public Health, 91*, 1783–1789.
Diez Roux, A. V. (2002). A glossary for multilevel analysis. *Journal of Epidemiology and Community Health, 56*, 588–594.
Diez Roux, A. V. (2007). Neighborhoods and health: Where are we and where do we go from here? *Revue d'Épidémiologie et de Santé Publique, 55*, 13–21.
Eilers, P. H. C., & Marx, B. D. (1996). Flexible smoothing with B-splines and penalties. *Statistical Science, 11*, 89–102.
Faraway, J. J. (2005). *Extending the linear model with R: Generalized linear, mixed effects and nonparametric regression models*. Boca Raton: Chapman & Hall.
Frank, L. D., Saelens, B. E., Powell, K. E., & Chapman, J. E. (2007). Stepping towards causation: Do built environments or neighborhood and travel preferences explain physical activity, driving, and obesity? *Social Science & Medicine, 65*, 1898–1914.
Frank, L. D., Schmid, T. L., Sallis, J. F., Chapman, J., & Saelens, B. E. (2005). Linking objectively measured physical activity with objectively measured urban form: Findings from SMARTRAQ. *American Journal of Preventive Medicine, 28*, 117–125.
Franzini, L., & Spears, W. (2003). Contributions of social context to inequalities in years of life lost to heart disease in Texas, USA. *Social Science & Medicine, 57*, 1847–1861.
Galster, G. (2008). Quantifying the effect of neighbourhood on individuals: Challenges, alternative approaches, and promising directions. *Schmollers Jahrbuch, 128*, 7–48.
Goldstein, H. (2011). *Multilevel statistical models* (4th ed.). Chichester, West Sussex: Wiley.
Goldstein, H., & Fielding, A. (2006). *Cross-classified and multiple membership structures in multilevel models: An introduction and review* (Research Report 791). Birmingham: University of Birmingham.
Gordis, L. (2004). *Epidemiology* (3rd ed.). Philadelphia, PA: Elsevier Saunders.
Hastie, T. J., & Tibshirani, R. J. (1990). *Generalized additive models*. London: Chapman and Hall.
Hastie, T., & Tibshirani, R. (1993). Varying-coefficient models. *Journal of the Royal Statistical Society, Series B: Statistical Methodology, 55*, 757–796.
Jenkinson, C., & Layte, R. (1997). Development and testing of the UK SF-12 (short form health survey). *Journal of Health Services Research & Policy, 2*, 14–18.
Kaczynski, A. T., & Glover, T. D. (2012). Talking the talk, walking the walk: Examining the effect of neighbourhood walkability and social connectedness on physical activity. *Journal of Public Health, 34*, 382–389.
Kammann, E. E., & Wand, M. P. (2003). Geoadditive models. *Journal of the Royal Statistical Society, Series C: Applied Statistics, 52*, 1–18.
Kauermann, G. (2006). Nonparametric models and their estimation. *Allgemeines Statistisches Archiv, 90*, 135–150.
Kuh, D., & Ben-Shlomo, Y. (2004). Introduction. In D. Kuh & Y. Ben-Shlomo (Eds.), *A life course approach to chronic disease epidemiology* (pp. 3–14). Oxford: Oxford University Press.
Leyland, A. H., & Groenewegen, P. P. (2003). Multilevel modelling and public health policy. *Scandinavian Journal of Public Health, 31*, 267–274.
Maier, W., Fairburn, J., & Mielck, A. (2012). Regionale Deprivation und Mortalität in Bayern: Entwicklung eines 'Index Multipler Deprivation' auf Gemeindeebene [Regional deprivation and mortality in Bavaria. Development of a community-based Index of Multiple Deprivation]. *Gesundheitswesen, 74*, 416–425.

McCullagh, P., & Nelder, J. A. (1989). *Generalized linear models* (2nd ed.). London: Chapman and Hall.

McCulloch, C. E., Searle, S. R., & Neuhaus, J. M. (2008). *Generalized, linear, and mixed models* (2nd ed.). Hoboken, NJ: Wiley.

Messer, L. C., Laraia, B. A., Kaufman, J. S., Eyster, J., Holzman, C., Culhane, J., et al. (2006). The development of a standardized neighborhood deprivation index. *Journal of Urban Health, 83*, 1041–1062.

Morris, R., & Carstairs, V. (1991). Which deprivation? A comparison of selected deprivation indexes. *Journal of Public Health Medicine, 13*, 318–326.

Næss, O., & Leyland, A. H. (2010). Analysing the effect of area of residence over the life course in multilevel epidemiology. *Scandinavian Journal of Public Health, 38*, 119–126.

Nicotera, N. (2007). Measuring neighborhood: A conundrum for human services researchers and practitioners. *American Journal of Community Psychology, 40*, 26–51.

Pinheiro, J. C., & Bates, D. M. (2009). *Mixed-effects models in S and S-PLUS*. New York: Springer.

Rasbash, J., & Browne, W. J. (2008). Non-hierarchical multilevel models. In J. de Leeuw & E. Meijer (Eds.), *Handbook of quantitative multilevel analysis* (pp. 301–334). New York: Springer.

Raudenbush, S. W., & Sampson, R. J. (1999). Ecometrics: Toward a science of assessing ecological settings, with application to the systematic social observation of neighborhoods. *Sociological Methodology, 29*, 1–41.

Reichman, N. E., Teitler, J. O., & Hamilton, E. R. (2009). Effects of neighborhood racial composition on birthweight. *Health & Place, 15*, 784–791.

Richter, A., & Wächter, M. (2009). *Zum Zusammenhang von Nachbarschaft und Gesundheit*. Köln: BZgA.

Royston, P., & Altman, D. G. (1994). Regression using fractional polynomials of continuous covariates – parsimonious parametric modeling. *Journal of the Royal Statistical Society, Series C: Applied Statistics, 43*, 429–467.

Rue, H., & Held, L. (2005). *Gaussian Markov random fields: Theory and applications*. Boca Raton: Chapman & Hall/CRC.

Ruppert, D., Wand, M. P., & Carroll, R. J. (2003). *Semiparametric regression*. Cambridge: Cambridge University Press.

Sauerbrei, W., & Royston, P. (1999). Building multivariable prognostic and diagnostic models: Transformation of the predictors by using fractional polynomials. *Journal of the Royal Statistical Society, Series A: Statistics in Society, 162*, 71–94.

Schräpler, J.-P. (2009). Verwendung von SGB II-Dichten als Raumindikator für die Sozialberichterstattung am Beispiel der "sozialen Belastung" von Schulstandorten in NRW: ein Kernel-Density-Ansatz. Band 57.

Schulz, A., & Northridge, M. E. (2004). Social Determinants Of Health: Implications for environmental health promotion. *Health Education & Behavior, 31*, 455–471.

Steinkamp, G. (1993). Soziale Ungleichheit, Erkrankungsrisiko und Lebenserwartung: Kritik der sozialepidemiologischen Ungleichheitsforschung [Social inequality, illness risk and life expectancy: Criticism of social epidemiological injustice research]. *Sozial- und Präventivmedizin, 38*, 111–122.

Voigtländer, S., Berger, U., & Razum, O. (2011). The relationship between neighbourhood resources and the risk of poor self-rated health: A hierarchical event history analysis. *European Journal of Public Health, 21*, 278.

Voigtländer, S., Mielck, A., & Razum, O. (2012). Die Bedeutung des kleinräumigen Kontexts für Gesundheit: Entwurf eines Erklärungsmodells [Impact of small-area context on health: Proposing a conceptual model]. *Gesundheitswesen, 74*, 702–709.

Werneck, G. L. (2008). Georeferenced data in epidemiologic research. *Ciência & Saúde Coletiva, 13*, 1753–1766.

Woods, L. M., Rachet, B., & Coleman, M. P. (2005). Choice of geographic unit influences socioeconomic inequalities in breast cancer survival. *British Journal of Cancer, 92*, 1279–1282.

Chapter 7
Access to Health-Promoting Facilities and Amenities

Anne Ellaway, Neil Ferguson, Karen Lamb, and David Ogilvie

Introduction

There is now good evidence that area of residence predicts health and the ability to lead a healthy life, over and above individual characteristics such as social class and income (Riva et al. 2007), and attention is now increasingly focussed on understanding the mechanisms involved. It has been suggested that aspects of the local social and physical environment such as the availability of facilities to support day-to-day life may be important (Macintyre et al. 2002). In this chapter, we will explore how such facilities can be assessed and quantified for neighbourhood research by using the example of facilities and amenities relevant for physical activity. We will firstly give a brief overview of the existing literature on the importance of the neighbourhood built environment to obesity and then focus on the distribution of physical activity opportunities, drawing on a Scotland wide study. We will then explore the issue of access to physical activity opportunities using different forms of transport.

A. Ellaway (✉) • K. Lamb
MRC Social and Public Health Sciences Unit, University of Glasgow,
4 Lilybank Gardens, Glasgow G12 8RZ, Scotland, UK
e-mail: anne@sphsu.mrc.ac.uk; klamb@sphsu.mrc.ac.uk

N. Ferguson
Department of Civil Engineering, University of Strathclyde, John Anderson Building,
107 Rottenrow, Glasgow G4 0NG, UK
e-mail: n.s.ferguson@strath.ac.uk

D. Ogilvie
UKCRC Centre for Diet and Activity Research (CEDAR), Institute of Public Health,
Forvie Site, Robinson Way, Box 296, Cambridge CB2 0SR, UK
e-mail: david.ogilvie@mrc-epid.cam.ac.uk

C. Stock and A. Ellaway (eds.), *Neighbourhood Structure and Health Promotion*,
DOI 10.1007/978-1-4614-6672-7_7,

Neighbourhood Built Environment and Obesity

A key current concern worldwide is the rising prevalence of obesity, the principal cause of which is an imbalance between energy intake and energy expenditure. Given the limited success of behavioural, educational and pharmacological interventions (House of Commons Health Committee 2004), it has been suggested that more attention should be directed towards an ecological approach to the obesity epidemic and that 'Understanding, measuring, and altering the "obesogenic" environment is critical to success' (Egger and Swinburn 1997). Obesogenic environments are those which promote excessive food intake and discourage physical activity. Obesity is more prevalent among people living in deprived areas in industrialised countries such as the UK (Department of Health Public Health Research Consortium et al. 2006). Interest in the neighbourhood of residence as a potential contributory factor in influencing body size and shape is growing; a number of studies have shown that area of residence is associated with body size and shape, independently of known correlates of obesity such as social class and income (Ellaway et al. 1997; Kahn et al. 1998; Oliver and Hayes 2005; van Lenthe and Mackenbach 2002; Wang et al. 2007). Features of the local environment such as access to shops selling healthy foods have been studied, using a range of methods. For example, in the USA, a number of studies have found fewer supermarkets in poorer, predominantly black areas (Chung and Myers 1999; Morland et al. 2002; Zenk et al. 2005). These findings contrast with those outside the USA. For example, in Brisbane, Australia, there was little difference between affluent and deprived areas in the food shopping infrastructure (Winkler et al. 2006); in New Zealand, travel (van Lenthe et al. 2005) distances to supermarkets were shorter in more deprived areas (Pearce et al. 2007); and poorer areas in the South East of the Netherlands were closer to food shops (van Lenthe et al. 2005). Some studies have found that proximity to food outlets is associated with obesity, while others have found an association only among women (Wang et al. 2007), emphasising the need to consider gender differences in the use and experience of the residential neighbourhood for health (see Chap. 18 in this book).

A number of studies have shown that the likelihood of undertaking physical activity is lower among residents of deprived areas (Ecob 1996; Ellaway and Macintyre 1996; Kavanagh et al. 2005; Sundquist et al. 1999; Yen and Kaplan 1998). One potential contributory factor is the extent to which the availability of facilities for physical activity is distributed equitably across different neighbourhoods.

In early work comparing two socially contrasting neighbourhoods in the city of Glasgow, Scotland, we found a higher number of recreational and sports facilities in the more affluent area (Macintyre et al. 1993). However, in a study looking at all neighbourhoods across Glasgow City, we found that some recreation facilities such as bowling greens and golf courses were more common in affluent areas, whereas others such as public swimming pools and public sports centres were more common in deprived areas (Macintyre et al. 2008a). Other studies elsewhere have reported a similar mixed picture across cities; for example, in Perth, Australia, lower socio-economic status (SES) areas had better access to sports/recreation centres, gyms and swimming pools, while higher SES areas had better access to golf courses and the beach (Giles-Corti and Donovan 2002), and a study in the Netherlands found there was no significant differences by neighbourhood SES in proximity to sports facilities (van Lenthe et al. 2005). However, a national study in the USA found that more physical fitness facilities, membership sports and recreation clubs, dance facilities and public golf courses were located in higher SES areas and there were fewer in areas with higher proportions of people from ethnic minority backgrounds (Powell et al. 2006). In a UK study, more facilities such as gyms, swimming pools and sports halls were present in more affluent areas across England (Hillsdon et al. 2007).

How Supportive Are Different Neighbourhoods Across Scotland for Physical Activity?

Overweight and obesity are more prevalent in Scotland than in many other European countries; approximately 70 % of men and 60 % of women are overweight, with over 25 % estimated to be obese for both genders (Scottish Executive 2009). As interventions aimed at individuals have had limited success, we wanted to examine how supportive different neighbourhoods across Scotland were for physical activity. We also wanted to examine how the distribution of facilities varied between and within the four largest Scottish cities. One of the reasons for doing this was that some studies have found differences in health and health behaviours between Scottish cities and regions (Watt and Ecob 1992; Gray and Leyland 2009).

Using a national database (sportscotland 2010), we mapped 63 different classifications of facilities, including both permanent facilities (e.g. football pitches, tennis courts, bowling greens, golf courses) and other facilities used intermittently for physical activity (e.g. school and church halls designated as 'occasional sports halls') to datazones, the key small-area statistical geography in Scotland (Scottish Executive 2004). Datazones (DZs) in Scotland are formed from groups of output areas for the 2001 Census and are nested within loc.l government boundaries. Where possible they have been defined in such a way as to respect physical boundaries and natural communities and contain households with similar social characteristics. There are 6,505 DZs in Scotland, with a mean population of 778 (range 476–2,813). For each DZ, the publicly available 2006 Scottish Index of Multiple Deprivation (SIMD) Current Income subdomain scores (Scottish Executive 2006), determined by the proportion of individuals within an area who are income deprived, and the Scottish Executive sixfold Urban Rural Classification (Scottish Executive 2008) were obtained.

One of the other issues we wanted to explore in our study was the ownership of facilities. Some are publicly owned (e.g. by the local council), and any member of the public can use them (on payment of charges if applicable), whereas other facilities are privately owned and may be restricted to those who pay a membership fee or meet other criteria. Another category of ownership is neither public nor private, e.g. facilities within schools which can only be accessed at certain times by certain groups. We therefore grouped all the facilities into public, private and 'other ownership' categories. The public physical activity facilities consisted of local authority, community enterprise, voluntary body and trust sites; the private facilities consisted of private, club, commercial and hotel facilities; and those categorised as in 'other ownership' consisted of those found within schools and churches which can only be used for physical activity at particular times, university and college facilities which can predominantly only be accessed by those with an affiliation to these establishments and facilities found within workplaces. Our analysis included 10,283 physical activity facilities across Scotland; almost a third (31.9 %) of these were publicly owned, 21.7 % were privately owned and 46.4 % were categorised as in 'other ownership'.

We also wanted to explore the distribution of facilities which were capable of being used by individuals to exercise alone (such as swimming pools, weights rooms and athletics tracks) and those for 'group' activities (football pitches, tennis courts and hockey pitches). The 'individual' and 'group' categories were created as we wished to distinguish opportunities for physical activity in which people could participate by themselves from those undertaken with others as these may appeal to different target groups. Among the public and private facilities, 1,245 (22.6 %) were classed as 'individual' facilities and 3,769 (68.4 %) as 'group' facilities. A number of amenities did not fit easily into these groupings and were therefore omitted from our analysis. We used Poisson and negative binomial regression models to investigate associations between the number of physical activity facilities relative to population size and quintile of area-level deprivation.

Although a statistically significant association between area-level income deprivation and the number of physical activity facilities was identified, there was no clear pattern (Lamb et al. 2010). This is generally consistent with the mixed picture obtained from other studies (Jones et al. 2007). Across Scotland, the most affluent and most deprived areas have fewest facilities overall. However, there is a difference when examining this by facility ownership: there are more privately owned facilities in more affluent areas and more publicly owned facilities in the more deprived neighbourhoods.

Distance to Physical Activity Opportunities and Availability of Transport Options

Although access to amenities was defined solely in terms of presence of amenities within the same datazone, this may have been sensitive to the area level chosen for analysis (the modifiable areal unit problem: (Openshaw 1984)). Moreover, the opportunity to access facilities transcends datazone boundaries. Access to suitable means of transport is likely to bring a larger range of facilities into reach. A few studies have shown that distance to physical activity opportunities and availability of transport options appears to influence use. A key aim of current UK public health and transport policy is to reduce car use and promote active travel (walking and cycling) on environmental and public health grounds, but there is little evidence on the extent to which different modes of travel facilitate access to, and use of, PA opportunities.

So building on our previous work, we then examined the distribution of facilities within walking and cycling distance in Scotland (Ogilvie et al. 2011). Unlike all other modes of transport, walking is free to all, requires no special equipment or training and is available to the majority of the population and to all ages (Ogilvie et al. 2007). However, its range is limited. Cycling, on the other hand, is also a relatively inexpensive mode of transport which brings a much larger area within a reasonable travel time without the user being dependent on the availability of public transport or the means to run a car.

To create walking and cycling networks, we used TransCAD software version 5.0 (Caliper Corporation 2011) which combines a geographic information system (GIS) with transport planning functionality. A matrix of travel times between population-weighted datazone centroids and recreational physical activity facilities was then determined, based on the assumptions that travellers would select the shortest path by distance and would travel at speeds of 5 km/h for walking (Ogilvie et al. 2007) and 14 km/h for cycling (World Health Organization 2008). We then compared access to facilities within 10-, 20- and 30-min travel time thresholds by the two modes of transport. We found that access to recreational physical activity facilities for the most affluent neighbourhoods was significantly lower for most walking and cycling thresholds tested in urban areas and for some walking and cycling thresholds tested in small towns. In general, our findings are therefore consistent with a hypothesis that the most affluent areas in Scotland have the least good access to recreational physical activity facilities within walking or cycling distance. However, the deprivation gradients in accessibility for walking were much steeper than those for cycling, demonstrating that a much larger number and variety of datazones can be reached in a given time by bicycle than on foot, giving cycling residents of poorly provided areas a greater chance of compensating for the limitations of their immediate surroundings. Indeed, a 10-min cycle ride brings more than 10 times the number of facilities within reach than does a 10-min walk, highlighting the usefulness of the bicycle as a mode of transport, particularly in large urban areas. However, a large proportion of the population in Scotland and other developed countries do not use bicycles, for a variety of reasons, and stimulating the growth of cycling for transport in such countries is a long-term project with little evidence of success to date (e.g. Department of Health and Department for Transport 2010).

Although more deprived areas across Scotland appear to have greater access to facilities, it is unclear whether and how the opportunity presented by greater access to facilities might translate into greater use, greater overall physical activity or better health. We have previously found that people may choose not to use their local facilities because they are perceived by local residents as not desirable or 'not for us' (Seaman et al. 2010; Ogilvie et al. 2010). It may be that other spaces hold more potential for physical activity, for example, urban children may be more physically active in the streets around their home (Jones et al. 2009).

It may also be that in examining the presence or otherwise of facilities per se, important differences in the type and nature of local facilities may be masked. We therefore assigned PA facilities to a physical activity intensity category (light, moderate or vigorous) based on the metabolic equivalent of task (MET) value (Ainsworth et al. 2000) attributable to the physical activity offered at the facility and then examined whether the accessibility of these facilities differed by area deprivation (Lamb et al. 2012). For example, PA facilities such as athletics tracks and swimming pools were classed as vigorous activity facilities; examples of moderate activity facilities included golf courses, cricket pitches and bowling greens. We extended our previous work on access by walking and cycling to include bus and car travel. As there were few facilities categorised as providing opportunity for light physical activity, we excluded these from our analysis. In general, those living in the most affluent neighbourhoods had reduced access to both moderate and vigorous intensity activity facilities on foot, by bike and by bus than those in less affluent areas. However, the pattern appears to differ for those with access to a car, as the most affluent areas appeared to have a higher number of moderate or vigorous intensity facilities accessible by car than more deprived areas. Therefore, it appears that having access to a car in more affluent areas could perhaps counteract the disadvantageous access in terms of other transport modes. However, this is a concern for those residing in these affluent areas who have no car access and will experience reduced local access to facilities.

Other Key Access Issues

Facilities may not be accessible for a number of reasons; Giles-Corti et al. report that although residents living in low socio-economic status areas in Perth, Australia, had equal or better access to recreational physical activity facilities, they were less likely to use facilities which charged an entrance fee, even after taking household income into account, suggesting that access alone does not determine use (Giles-Corti and Donovan 2002). Access to fixed PA facilities may not necessarily be a key factor in helping people to meet PA recommendations. Our Scottish study did not include information about green space or other spaces where PA can be undertaken free of charge. In Australia, close proximity to the coast was associated with a higher likelihood to participate in adequate activity (Bauman et al. 1999), whilst other studies have shown the importance of recreational walking and gardening (Bertrais et al. 2004) emphasising the need to explore other activity spaces, rather than simply fixed recreational PA facilities, in any analysis of the accessibility of PA sites.

Quality Issues

Some studies have found that how attractive or safe the neighbourhood is to be associated with physical activity levels. In a study in the Netherlands, for example, Van Lenthe et al. found that compared to those living in the most advantaged neighbourhoods, residents living in the socio-economically disadvantaged neighbourhoods were more likely to walk or cycle to shops or work but less likely to walk, cycle or garden in leisure time and less likely to participate in sports activities (adjusted for age, sex and individual educational level) (van Lenthe et al. 2005). The increased likelihood of almost never undertaking activities such as walking, cycling and gardening in leisure time in the most disadvantaged neighbourhoods was partly attributed to a poorer general physical design in these neighbourhoods (van Lenthe et al. 2005).

There is also the important issue of whether it is the objectively measured presence or absence of facilities that is most likely to influence behaviour or the perceived or symbolic presence or absence of facilities. For example, we found in Glasgow that answers to a question about whether a respondent lived within half a mile of a public green space did not show strong agreement with whether their home fell within an objectively measured half-mile buffer of a park; it seemed that some respondents did not feel the local park was culturally available or suitable for them (Macintyre et al. 2008b). People may not use facilities in their immediate residential environment. It might be more important for some people to have a sports centre near their place of work or their child's school. The relevance of local facilities may vary by stage in the life cycle, socio-economic status, gender, car ownership and other factors.

Geographical Scale

In our Scottish study, we used relatively small areas which are designed to respect physical boundaries and natural communities and which are widely used in administrative geography. However, as noted above, the modifiable areal unit problem (Openshaw 1984) may mean that we would have observed different results had we used larger, differently defined, types of area.

Conclusion

We have found that the distribution of amenities for physical activity is patterned by socio-spatial factors across Scotland, often in a complex manner. People who live in poor neighbourhoods are not always disadvantaged in terms of provision, for example, they have better provision of publicly owned facilities, whereas more affluent areas have more private facilities in their neighbourhood . It has been suggested that neighbourhood self-selection may be an important factor in the study of the relationship between the neighbourhood built environment and physical activity levels (McCormack and Sheill 2011). People who are disposed towards walking for transportation may seek out areas to live in which are conducive to their preferences (e.g. access to local stores and amenities). However, this issue may only be important for those who can choose where to live and the relative importance of proximity to PA opportunities (or other health-promoting amenities) in locational preferences. Our study has shown the importance of transport access, and that this and other aspects such as the quality of services need to be taken into account when planning neighbourhood amenities services which might be important for health.

References

Ainsworth, B. E., Haskell, W. L., Whitt, M. C., Irwin, M. L., Swartz, A. M., Strath, S. J., et al. (2000). Compendium of physical activities: An update of activity codes and MET intensities. *Medicine and Science in Sports and Exercise, 32*(9 Suppl), S498–S504.

Bauman, A., Smith, B., Stoker, L., Bellew, B., & Booth, M. L. (1999). Geographical influences upon physical activity participation: Evidence of a 'coastal effect'. *Australian and New Zealand Journal of Public Health, 23*(3), 322–324.

Bertrais, S., Preziosi, P., Mennen, L., Galan, P., Hercberg, S., & Oppert, J. M. (2004). Sociodemographic and geographic correlates of meeting current recommendations for physical activity in middle-aged French adults: The Supplementation en Vitamines et Mineraux Antioxydants (SUVIMAX) Study. *American Journal of Public Health, 94*(9), 1560–1566.

Caliper Corporation. (2011). TransCAD version 5.0.

Chung, C., & Myers, S. (1999). Do the Poor Pay More for Food? An Analysis of Grocery Store Availability and Food Price Disparities. *Journal of Consumer Affairs, 33*, 276–296.

Department of Health and Department for Transport, 2010. Active Travel Strategy.

Department of Health Public Health Research Consortium, Law, C., Power, C., Graham, H., & Merrick, D. (2006). Obesity and health inequalities. *Obesity Reviews, 8*(Suppl. 1), 19–22.

Ecob, R. (1996). A multilevel modelling approach to examining the effects of area of residence on health and functioning. *Journal of the Royal Statistical Society Series A Statistics In Society, 159*(Pt1), 61–75.

Egger, G., & Swinburn, B. (1997). An 'ecological approach' to the obesity pandemic. *BMJ, 315*, 477–480.

Ellaway, A., Anderson, A., & Macintyre, S. (1997). Does area of residence affect body size and shape? *International Journal of Obesity, 21*(4), 304–308.

Ellaway, A., & Macintyre, S. (1996). Does where you live predict health related behaviours? A case study in Glasgow. *Health Bulletin, 54*(6), 443–446.

Giles-Corti, B., & Donovan, R. J. (2002). Socioeconomic status differences in recreational physical activity levels and real and perceived access to a supportive physical environment. *Preventive Medicine, 35*(6), 601–611.

Gray, L., & Leyland, A. H. (2009). A multilevel analysis of diet and socio-economic status in Scotland: Investigating the 'Glasgow effect'. *Public Health Nutrition, 12*(9), 1351–1358.

Hillsdon, M., Panter, J., Foster, C., & Jones, A. (2007). Equitable access to exercise facilities. *American Journal of Preventive Medicine, 32*(6), 506–508.

House of Commons Health Committee. (2004). *Obesity*. Third Report of Session 2003–04. London: UK Parliament.

Jones, A., Bentham, G., Foster, C., Hillsdon, M., & Panter, J. (2007). *Obesogenic Environments: Evidence Review*. London: Office of Science and Technology Foresight Programme.

Jones, A., Coombes, E., Griffin, S., & van Sluijs, E. (2009). Environmental supportiveness for physical activity in English schoolchildren: A study using Global Positioning Systems. *International Journal of Behavioral Nutrition and Physical Activity, 6*, 42.

Kahn, H., Tatham, L., Pamuk, E., & Heath, C. (1998). Are geographic regions with high income inequality associated with risk of abdominal weight gain? *Social Science & Medicine, 47*(1), 1–6.

Kavanagh, A. M., Goller, J. L., King, T., Jolley, D., Crawford, D., & Turrell, G. (2005). Urban area disadvantage and physical activity: A multilevel study in Melbourne, Australia. *Journal of Epidemiology and Community Health, 59*(11), 934–940.

Lamb, K. E., Ferguson, N. S., Wang, Y., Ogilvie, D., & Ellaway, A. (2010). Distribution of physical activity facilities in Scotland by small area measures of deprivation and urbanicity. *International Journal of Behavioral Nutrition and Physical Activity, 7*, 76.

Lamb, K. E., Ogilvie, D., Ferguson, N. S., Murray, J., Wang, Y., & Ellaway, A. (2012). Sociospatial distribution of access to facilities for moderate and vigorous intensity physical activity in Scotland by different modes of transport. *International Journal of Behavioral Nutrition and Physical Activity, 9*(1), 55.

Macintyre, S., Ellaway, A., & Cummins, S. (2002). Place effects on health: How can we conceptualise, operationalise and measure them? *Social Science & Medicine, 55*(1), 125–139.

Macintyre, S., Macdonald, L., & Ellaway, A. (2008a). Do poorer people have poorer access to local resources and facilities? The distribution of local resources by area deprivation in Glasgow, Scotland. *Social Science & Medicine, 67*(6), 900–914.

Macintyre, S., Macdonald, L., & Ellaway, A. (2008b). Lack of agreement between measured and self-reported distance from public green parks in Glasgow, Scotland. *International Journal of Behavioral Nutrition and Physical Activity, 5*, 26.

Macintyre, S., McIver, S., & Sooman, A. (1993). Area, class and health: Should we be focusing on people or places? *Journal of Social Policy, 22*, 213–234.

McCormack, GR., & Shiell, A. (2011). In search of causality: a systematic review of the relationship between the built environment and physical activity among adults. *Int J Behav Nutr Phys Act, 8*, 125.

Morland, K., Wing, S., Diez Roux, A., & Poole, C. (2002). Neighborhood characteristics associated with the location of food stores and food service places. *American Journal of Preventive Medicine, 22*(1), 23–29.

Ogilvie, D., Foster, C., Rothnie, H., Cavill, N., Hamilton, V., Fitzsimmons, C., et al. (2007). Interventions to promote walking: Systematic review. *BMJ, 334*(7605), 1204.

Ogilvie, D., Lamb, K. E., Ferguson, N. S., & Ellaway, A. (2011). Recreational physical activity facilities within walking and cycling distance: Sociospatial patterning of access in Scotland. *Health & Place, 17*(5), 1015–1022.

Ogilvie, D., Mitchell, R., Mutrie, N., Petticrew, M., & Platt, S. (2010). Shoe leather epidemiology: Active travel and transport infrastructure in the urban landscape. *International Journal of Behavioral Nutrition and Physical Activity, 7*, 43.

Oliver, L. N., & Hayes, M. V. (2005). Neighbourhood socio-economic status and the prevalence of overweight Canadian children and youth. *Canadian Journal of Public Health, 96*(6), 415–420.

Openshaw, S. (1984). Ecological fallacies and the analysis of areal census data. *Environment and Planning A, 16*(1), 17–31.

Pearce, J., Blakely, T., Witten, K., & Bartie, P. (2007). Neighborhood deprivation and access to fast-food retailing - A national study. *American Journal of Preventive Medicine, 32*(5), 375–382.

Powell, L. M., Slater, S., Chaloupka, F. J., & Harper, D. (2006). Availability of physical activity-related facilities and neighborhood demographic and socioeconomic characteristics: A national study. *American Journal of Public Health, 96*(9), 1676–1680.

Riva, M., Gauvin, L., & Barnett, T. (2007). Toward the next generation of research into small area effects on health: A synthesis of multilevel investigations published since July 1998. *Journal of Epidemiology and Community Health, 61*, 853–861.

Scottish Executive. (2004). *Scottish executive Scottish neighbourhood statistics data zones*. Edinburgh: Scottish Executive.

Scottish Executive. (2006). *Scottish index of multiple deprivation 2006 technical report*. Edinburgh: Scottish Executive.

Scottish Executive. (2008). *Scottish executive urban rural classification 2007–2008*. Edinburgh: Scottish Executive.

Scottish Executive. (2009). *The Scottish health survey*. Edinburgh: Scottish Executive.

Seaman, P. J., Jones, R., & Ellaway, A. (2010). It's not just about the park, it's about integration too: Why people choose to use or not use urban greenspaces. *International Journal of Behavioral Nutrition and Physical Activity, 7*, 78.

Sportscotland. (2010). Sportscotland: The National Agency for Sport. http://www.sportscotland.org.uk.

Sundquist, J., Malmstrom, M., & Johansson, S. (1999). Cardiovascular risk factors and the neighbourhood environment: A multilevel analysis. *International Journal of Epidemiology, 28*, 841–845.

van Lenthe, F., Brug, J., & Mackenbach, J. (2005). Neighbourhood inequalities in physical inactivity: The role of neighbourhood attractiveness, proximity to local facilities and safety in the Netherlands. *Social Science & Medicine, 60*(4), 763–775.

van Lenthe, F., & Mackenbach, J. (2002). Neighbourhood deprivation and overweight: The GLOBE study. *International Journal of Obesity, 26*(2), 234–240.

Wang, M. C., Kim, S., Gonzalez, A. A., MacLeod, K. E., & Winkleby, M. A. (2007). Socioeconomic and food-related physical characteristics of the neighbourhood environment are associated with body mass index. *Journal of Epidemiology and Community Health, 61*(6), 491–498.

Watt, G. C. M., & Ecob, R. (1992). Mortality in Glasgow and Edinburgh: A paradigm of inequality in health. *Journal of Epidemiology and Community Health, 46*(5), 498–505.

Winkler, E., Turrell, G., & Patterson, C. (2006). Does living in a disadvantaged area mean fewer opportunities to purchase fresh fruit and vegetables in the area? Findings from the Brisbane food study. *Health & Place, 12*(3), 306–319.

World Health Organization. (2008). *Health Economic Assessment Tool for Cycling (HEAT for Cycling). User guide, Version 2*. Copenhagen: WHO Regional Office for Europe.

Yen, I. H., & Kaplan, G. A. (1998). Poverty area residence and changes in physical activity level: Evidence from the Alameda County Study. *American Journal of Public Health, 88*(11), 1709–1712.

Zenk, S. N., Schulz, A. J., Israel, B. A., James, S. A., Bao, S. M., & Wilson, M. L. (2005). Neighborhood racial composition, neighborhood poverty, and the spatial accessibility of supermarkets in metropolitan Detroit. *American Journal of Public Health, 95*(4), 660–667.

Chapter 8
GIS: A Spatial Turn in the Health Science?

Jasper Schipperijn, Bo Ejstrud, and Jens Troelsen

Introduction

The idea of a "spatial turn" in science has been formulated among scholars to describe a renewed interest in spatially oriented research, which has developed around the turn of the twenty-first century. The phrase is in fact a paraphrase on earlier "turns", especially in the humanities, with the "quantitative turn" being typical for the 1960s and the "cultural" or "linguistic turn" developing during the 1980s. This latest turn does not reflect that spatial problems themselves are new, and indeed geography as a discipline is taught not only at university but at all school levels in most countries. The interest in geographically related problems also traditionally extends into many other disciplines, and as most undergraduate students studying basic epidemiology will be aware that "place" is one of the three main variables in descriptive epidemiology (the other two being "person" and "time"). The spatial turn is therefore more of a broad reorientation towards otherwise classical research areas. Interestingly, it happens across a very wide range of academic disciplines, including health studies.

There are a number of reasons behind this rediscovery of "the power of maps". There is no doubt, however, that one of the predominant drivers has been the development of Geographical Information Systems (GIS). These are software systems which can handle geographically referenced data. Maps have always

J. Schipperijn (✉) • J. Troelsen
Institute of Sports Science and Clinical Biomechanics, University of Southern Denmark, Campusvej 55, 5230 Odense M, Denmark
e-mail: jschipperijn@health.sdu.dk; jtroelsen@health.sdu.dk

B. Ejstrud
Institute of History and Civilization, University of Southern Denmark, Niels Bohrs Vej 9-10, 6700 Esbjerg, Denmark
e-mail: ejstrud@hist.sdu.dk

C. Stock and A. Ellaway (eds.), *Neighbourhood Structure and Health Promotion*,
DOI 10.1007/978-1-4614-6672-7_8,

been a powerful tool, but making them digital has boosted the use of geospatial information in many academic disciplines. GIS is widely used in both research and management and therefore an important tool to master, also in the study of neighbourhoods and health.

The objective of this chapter is to discuss the potential and limitations of GIS in order to characterise different geographical areas in relation to different health aspects and outcomes (Kawachi and Berkman 2003). We will give a short overview of existing knowledge based on examples and studies of neighbourhoods and conclude with a wider discussion of possible future perspectives for the use of GIS in the study of neighbourhoods and health.

What Is Geographical Information Systems?

GIS is not one particular kind or brand of software. We are not giving an extended exposition of the subject; however, a brief and general presentation of the technology may be useful here. For a broader introduction we refer to the many textbooks and online texts on the subject (e.g. Longley et al. 2011).

There are two main types of GIS, the difference between them being how data are stored, vector-based GIS and raster-based GIS. Figure 8.1 illustrates the difference between the two types of GIS. A vector-based GIS stores data as points with a geographical coordinate, for instance, latitude and longitude. A single point can refer to a dot on the map, but points can also be combined to form open lines or closed polygons. Typically, the objects drawn on the map will connect to a database, storing information about each object in table format. Standard database operations can therefore be performed on the objects, together with the geographical operations on the map. Based on localised points, vector-based systems are therefore well suited to outline discrete geographical entities and in many respects handle like any other database management system or statistics package, with the important addition of a geographical component. Vector-based GIS are less suited where data are not discrete but form gradients. The most widely used example of such data is land elevation. Other examples with relevance to health science could be distances or emissions and fallout. For such types of data, the raster-based GIS is more appropriate. Here, the landscape is divided in a grid of cells of uniform size, and each cell assigned a value, which reflects the data value at that particular point. This approach to data gives many analytical advantages but obviously also some shortcomings, not least when it comes to data storage and analysis, which can be overwhelming. Other problems are the limited ability to represent linear features and therefore topologically coherent networks. In addition, the raster cells may have a size which is both aesthetically unpleasing and difficult to use in a specific research context.

It is possible to convert data between vector and raster formats. In fact many standard GIS maps stem from scanned paper maps, which have been vectorised by

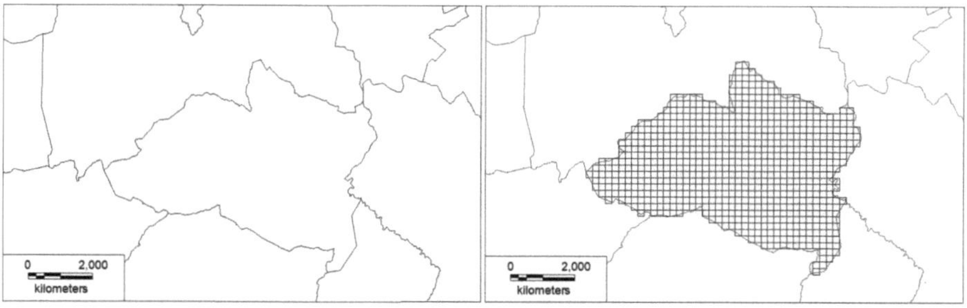

Fig. 8.1 Difference between vector-based GIS and raster-based GIS. *Left*: A parish map with one of the parishes highlighted. *Right*: The same parish in 250×250 m raster cells. The large cell size is used here for illustration. Smaller cells would obviously give a better outline of the area

either automatic or manual means (often a combination of the two), and then finally converted into raster format. Other data sources are remotely sensed data (from satellites and aircrafts) or databases with spatial information.

A normal topographical map combines many different types of information. Land use categories, road networks and elevation are all shown on the same map. This is a practical format for a paper map, because we want to compare the spatial information. But when digitising these maps into GIS format, each type of information must be separated out in its own data file, normally called a "layer" or a "theme", although different software packages use different words for these basic files. The separation of the map into its individual components enables the user to analyse each component separately; the length of a road system or the area of a certain type of land use. The layer system also makes it easy for each individual user to produce customised maps, where only the relevant layers are shown.

Although GIS has made mapmaking easier, basic cartographic deeds must still be observed, in particular with regard to scale. When working with neighbourhoods we often work with spatial relations on a very local scale. But the GIS layers that we have available may be based on maps that were originally drawn at a much less detailed scale and should therefore not be used at the chosen level of analysis. This can be difficult to recognise, especially when working with vector maps. Most GIS systems can handle digital data in many different projections and datums (a standard position or level that measurements are taken from), for the vector systems even in the same analysis. However, the pitfalls of overlaying such maps should not be overlooked. For raster maps re-projection of the data will usually be required. The endless graphical possibilities of digital mapping also require some discipline on behalf of the user: for all its virtues GIS has not made it more difficult to lie with maps (Monmonier 1996): e.g. ill-conceived graphic generalisation of data, or data classification, can either reveal meaningful spatial trends or promote misleading interpretations.

The Development of Geographical Information Systems

The early development of GIS took place around 1960 in Canada where the development of CGIS (Canada Geographic Information System) began. Other initiatives followed and these early systems ran on large mainframe systems with input and output functions, which even simple computer toys would perform today. This development took place mainly within environmental studies, in spatial planning and for military purposes. A lot of important development took place during the 1960s and 1970s. During the 1980s, the development accelerated, and several of the GIS software systems which are still used today were launched or developed (Arc/Info, GRASS, MapInfo, Idrisi). The Global Positioning System (GPS) also became operational during the 1980s. While GIS was still considered a specialist tool, many disciplines took the technology up, and it became widespread. From the late 1990s and into the twenty-first century, GIS became increasingly integrated in many aspects of public management, as well as being used for academic studies and in corporate business. GIS is now routinely integrated in landscape management at all levels and many aspects of government planning and management. With web-based mapping, GIS has also spread to the non-professional markets, although few would probably identify Google maps as a GIS. It, and most of the web-based services with it, does not have the analytical functions of an actual GIS, but the many route planning services would be a GIS technology known by many people.

In health studies, the legacy of John Snow has inspired a natural interest in spatial studies, and GIS was also taken up. While there have been applications of the technology in epidemiological disease mapping and forecasting, the majority of studies have been within what could be called environmental epidemiology, correlating the spatial distribution of health with other environmental and social factors (Gatrell and Löytönen 1998). Another important use of GIS has been the planning of emergency services and the mapping of medical care. The first studies began to appear in the late 1980s (Openshaw et al. 1987), and the development of the use of GIS within health studies has advanced in the same way as in many other disciplines. To some degree GIS can be considered relatively well integrated in management and research. Several textbooks and anthologies have emerged to offer the interested reader a deeper look into the possibilities and perspectives of GIS (e.g. Cromley and McLafferty 2012; Kurland and Wilpen 2007; Lai and Mak 2007). Journals such as the International Journal of Health Geographics and Health and Place have many and varied examples of GIS-based health research.

Defining Neighbourhoods in Geographical Information Systems

GIS is a very helpful tool to characterise geographical areas for a wide range of health-related studies. However, when data is to be extracted from GIS databases or health data is to be displayed on a map, the question arises which area unit or "neighbourhood" to use. Commonly used area units include various statistical entities, such as census tracts and census blocks in United States, and their equivalents in other countries. But also ZIP codes and school, hospital and election districts are used, as are administrative units such as parishes, municipalities and counties. In recent years, researchers frequently refer to "neighbourhoods" as their area unit. However, looking into these studies, it becomes clear that "neighbourhood" can be defined in many different ways, which makes comparing results across studies difficult (e.g. Riva et al. 2007). Furthermore, using different neighbourhood definitions can lead to different results (e.g. Haynes et al. 2008; Jones et al. 2010; Mitra and Buliung 2012; Parenteau and Swada 2011; Riva et al. 2008; Schuurman et al. 2007; Tian et al. 2010), so selecting an appropriate neighbourhood unit, both from a conceptual and mathematical perspective, is important before embarking on GIS analyses. In the following sections we shall describe commonly used neighbourhood definitions and discuss their advantages and disadvantages. Figure 8.2 shows the spatial differences between seven types of neighbourhood definitions.

Statistical or Administrative Neighbourhoods

Since the late 1980s, researchers have been using various types of statistical or administrative units to define their neighbourhoods. This is no surprise given that data are often readily available in these units. This type of studies are often the groundwork and can provide justification for more detailed investigations of neighbourhood health effects, as also stated by Diez Roux and Mair (2010). Furthermore, in studies where the exact respondent addresses are unknown, using data aggregated to statistical or administrative neighbourhoods typically is the only viable option. Using GIS data in combination with non-spatial statistical data, it becomes possible to generate various measures for a wide range of neighbourhood characteristics, for example, socio-economic status, crime-rates, number of parks or number of fast-food outlets.

However, it is not always clear how the boundaries of administrative units have been defined and whether or not these boundaries are relevant for the particular health behaviour or health outcome that is studied. Furthermore, administrative units are typically of different sizes and that makes calculating and comparing all density related measures less straight forward. In their review of this type of studies, Riva and colleagues concluded that "area effects on health, although significant in most studies, often depend on the health outcome studied, the measure of the areas exposure used and the spatial scale at which associations are examined" (Riva et al. 2007, p. 853). The review emphasises the importance of considering the spatial scale of the neighbourhood as part of the equation in health studies.

Buffers Around Home Addresses

To overcome some of the problems associated with using administrative or statistical units, researchers started assigning buffers around a respondent's home address,

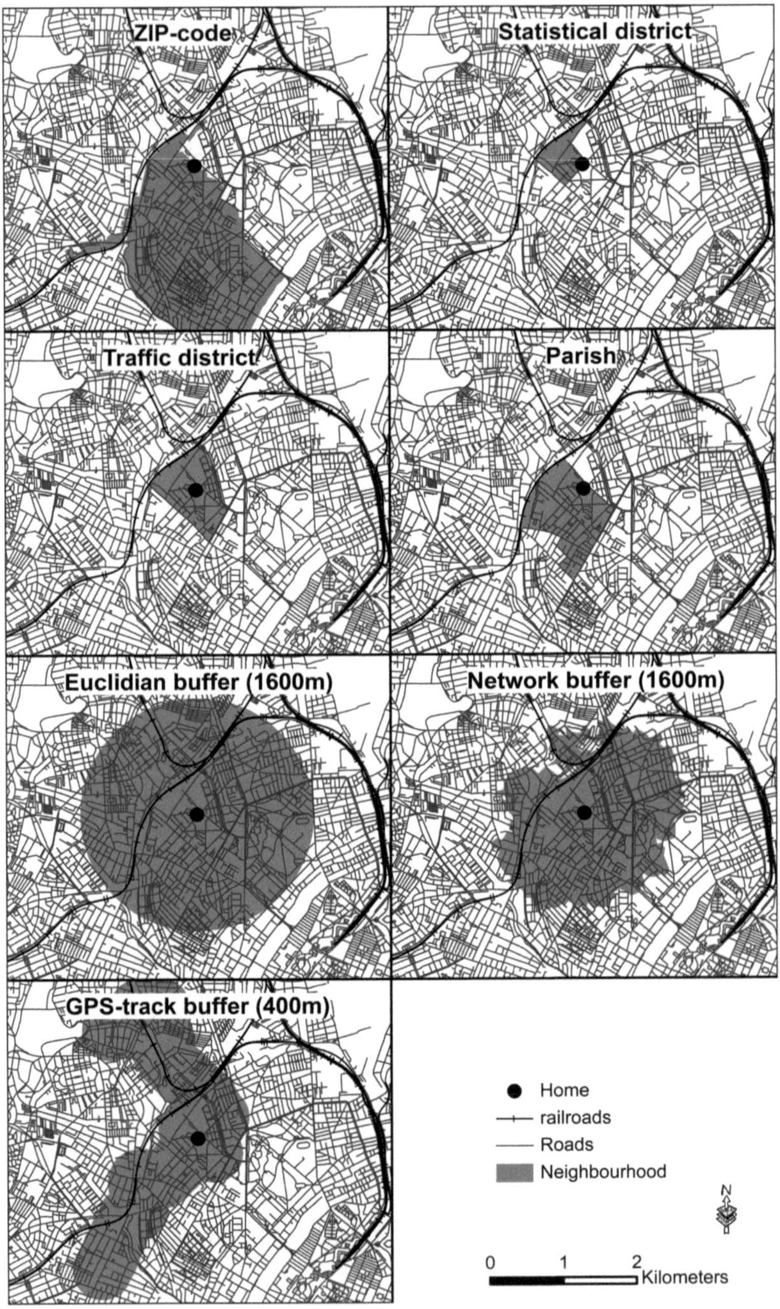

Fig. 8.2 Spatial differences between seven types of neighbourhood definitions, for the same respondent living in Copenhagen, Denmark. The GPS-track is based on 60 h of GPS data recorded during 1 week, for a 14-year-old respondent

either using a Euclidian distance (as the crow flies) or a network distance, measured using the street network. The two methods can give quite different results, and many researchers consider the network method to be more meaningful (see, e.g. Lee and Moudon 2008; Oh and Jeong 2007), especially if data on walking and biking trails are included. For both methods the threshold values are often set based on estimated travel times, e.g. a 5–10-min walk, bike or drive, which results in distance thresholds ranging from 400 m to 5 km, with 800 m (½ mile) and 1,600 m (1 mile) as commonly used values. Within these individual buffers, a range of neighbourhood characteristics can be generated in GIS (for an overview, see Brownson et al. 2009). Typical examples of neighbourhoods characteristics studied are density and accessibility of neighbourhood features that are considered relevant for the health behaviour or health outcome studied. Probably some of the most studied characteristics are related to walkability, with walking as the health behaviour in focus. A walkability index that includes street connectivity, land use mix, residential density and retail floor area ratio was developed by Frank et al. (2010) and has shown positive relations between walking and a higher walkability index score. Using individual buffers requires that respondent addresses are known and can be geocoded correctly. Geocoding is the process of matching raw address information with associated geographic coordinates (latitude and longitude) from other digital geographic data.

While using individual buffers reduces some of the conceptual problems associated with administrative or statistical units, it also has some methodological drawbacks. In a pilot study by Smith et al. (2010), 58 face-to-face interviews were carried out and participants were asked to draw their neighbourhood on a map. The results from this study show that a participant drawn neighbourhood on average represents 16 % of the commonly used 1,600 m Euclidian buffer, and 36 % of a 1,600 m network buffer. Smith and colleagues conclude that "adults" interpretation of their neighbourhood area does not appear to relate accurately to the definitions typically used in research into environmental perceptions and walking (Smith et al. 2010, p. 1).

Self-Reported Neighbourhood Characteristics

Another method frequently used, especially within the physical activity field, is to ask respondents to rate various neighbourhood characteristics in surveys. In this type of studies respondents are typically asked to individually define their neighbourhood, for example, by thinking of the area "within a 10–15 min walk" from their home. Pikora and colleagues identified four key environmental domains likely to influence physical activity behaviour: functional (walking surface, streets, traffic, permeability), safety (personal, traffic), aesthetic (streetscape, views) and destination (facilities) (Pikora et al. 2003). Data on this type of perceived environmental measures have been collected by phone interviews or self-administered questionnaires; see, e.g. the Neighbourhood Environment Walkability Survey (NEWS) tool (Saelens et al. 2003).

In its basic form, using self-reported measures does not require knowing the respondents home address, nor does it require the use of GIS. However, if self-reported data is to be combined or compared to objective measures, compiling all data in GIS seems to be useful. Combining self-reported data with objectively measured data within one study is thought to create additional strengths (e.g. Millington et al. 2009).

The main conceptual advantage of using self-reported measures is that respondents are likely to report on the area they consider their neighbourhood, and possibly for that reason, self-reported measures can be a better predictor for behaviour than objective measures. For example, the self-estimated distance to a green space is a better predictor for the frequency of use of that green space than the objectively measured distance to the same green space (Schipperijn et al. 2010). The same result can be seen for other recreational facilities (Scott et al. 2007), most likely because it reflects the respondents' opinion and knowledge of the facilities. If a facility is well known and well liked, respondents are likely to underestimate the distance; if it is less known and disliked, distance is likely to be overestimated (Scott et al. 2007). Not knowing exactly which neighbourhood respondents had in mind when answering, nor being able to directly compare answers from respondents who live close to each other, can be seen as a disadvantage of using self-reported measures.

Activity Space

Within health sciences, a relatively new way of looking at neighbourhoods is the use of Activity Spaces. Activity Space is a term describing how individuals' habitual movements interact with their environment (Sherman et al. 2005). Activity Spaces can, among other, be defined by a minimum convex polygon that contains all daily activity locations (Fan and Khattak 2008). In GIS, a minimum convex polygon can be created by drawing lines between the outer most points if at least three (self-reported) daily locations are known. Villanueva et al. (2012) used this method to look at children's Activity Space in Perth, Western Australia. They compared Activity Spaces with 800-m and 1,600-m network buffers and concluded that "children may only walk or cycle a small proportion of their traditionally defined 'neighbourhood' suggesting that studies using circular or network buffers may inaccurately capture neighbourhood environments" (Villanueva et al. 2012, ahead of print).

A different way of generating the locations needed to construct Activity Spaces is using GPS equipment to track participants' movement. A pilot study in Michigan, USA, used GPS to help determine respondents' Activity Space (Zenk et al. 2011). They derived two Activity Space measures from their GPS data, the standard deviational ellipse (SDE) and daily path area. After mapping daily trips and determining the locations of regular activities, SDEs are calculated based on distance and direction of these locations from home (Sherman et al. 2005). Zenk and colleagues constructed a daily path area by buffering all GPS points with 0.5 mile (800 m) and dissolving all buffers to one polygon. The daily path-based Activity Spaces were substantially larger than the SDE-based Activity Spaces. They concluded that "most individuals spent time in a broader space than their residential neighbourhood, and that those activity spaces differ from residential neighbourhoods in environmental features" (Zenk et al. 2011, p. 1159). The study shows that Activity Spaces are likely to be more associated with the areas people actually use on a daily basis compared to buffer zones around their home address. This finding underlines that GIS analyses focusing on factors associated with human behaviour must consider which neighbourhood definition is most relevant for that specific behaviour. More information on this approach can be found in Chap. 9 in this book.

Modifiable Area Unit Problem

The different ways of defining a neighbourhood can lead to statistical bias in analysing data. The larger the area the data is aggregated to, the less specific the results are to the population in that area, but equally there are fewer problems with small number bias and imprecision due to a reduction in sampling error. Results of aggregating data will often be modified when the area unit changes. This phenomenon is known as the modifiable area unit problem (MAUP) and is described in detail by Stan Openshaw (1984). Also within the health sciences, various researchers, looking at a wide range of health outcomes, have discussed the problem and concluded that changing the area unit did change the results of their analyses (e.g. Haynes et al. 2008; Jones et al. 2010; Mitra and Buliung 2012; Parenteau and Swada 2011; Riva et al. 2008; Schuurman et al. 2007; Tian et al. 2010). Openshaw (1977) proposed a general purpose automated zoning procedure (AZP) based on the iterative recombination of building blocks into output areas to maximise the value of an objective function. Based on this principle, Cockings and Martin (2005) presented a series of criteria for zone design for different health-related topics, depending on the research aim. For example, if the research aim is testing a hypothesis, the criteria are to maximise internal homogeneity of risk and/or confounding factors. A more explorative zone design could be achieved by similar, but conceptually different, techniques aiming at maximising the internal homogeneity of correlation between the hypothesised independent and dependent variables (Openshaw and Alvandies 1999). Using a geographically weighted regression (GWR) could also be useful to detect spatial differences (Fotheringham et al. 2002) as this technique allows parameter estimates to be location dependent, contrary to "normal" regression that assumes the parameters to be constant over space.

A quite different approach to increase the validity of neighbourhood boundaries was taken by Cutchin et al. (2011). They developed a so-called socio-spatial neighbourhood estimation method (SNEM) in which an expert, based on satellite or aerial photographs as well as field visits, decides where neighbourhood boundaries are to be drawn. Five subjective criteria are used in SNEM: street patterns, residential patterns, non-residential land use, landforms and that the neighbourhood should be relatively compact.

Cutchin and colleagues tested their method against a standard grid as well as census block groups, showing that the intra-class correlation coefficients (ICCs) generally were better for the SNEM neighbourhoods than for the census block groups or standard grid (Cutchin et al. 2011). MAUP problems should not be ignored within health sciences and can be reduced mathematically (automated) by maximising homogeneity with each area, as well as conceptually by basing the choice of neighbourhood unit on the specific health outcome or health behaviour in focus.

The Use of Geographical Information Systems in Health Research: Examples

Working with GIS, or in fact with any reasonably complex type of software, is in many respects much like playing with LEGO, the well-known toy. The software comprises of an array of relatively simple analytical functions and processes and sometimes less simple, but the actual product of a GIS analysis will be the result of a complex combination of these basic analytical building blocks. This brings the challenge to a short introductory chapter such as this, and more broadly to teaching GIS, that one has to balance between presenting the individual building blocks, while on the other hand also presenting some of the final products which can be achieved through their combination. Most importantly, the wider methodical implications of using any particular tool should not be lost in the technicalities of working the software and data. In this section we will illustrate the use of GIS in the study of neighbourhoods and health through presenting and discussing examples from specific studies where this technology was applied. Through these examples we will illustrate some of the building blocks available in a typical GIS and also discuss some of the wider methodical challenges.

Social Deprivation and Neighbourhoods

As mentioned above, the neighbourhood of a study would often be defined by the availability and organisation of data. In Denmark, the smallest administrative unit in the registers is the parish. While not an active administrative unit anymore, population data can still be aggregated to the parishes. With 2,121 parishes in Denmark, they cover relatively small areas, with an average size of 20 km^2 and a population of 2,506 persons. As such they are a convenient unit for spatial research in health.

One important spatial aspect to investigate is between-area differences in health. Many studies have demonstrated an inverse relation between health outcomes and area-level socio-economic status (SES) (for more detailed information see Chap. 2 in this book). While such associations are generally found to be smaller than associations with individual factors, the SES of the area itself still seems to describe variations in health outcomes (Pickett and Pearl 2001). Most such studies originate in Great Britain where a tradition exists of examining the health effects of relative deprivation since the 1980s and where several indices have been developed to measure deprivation (e.g. Carstairs and Morris 1999; Jarman 1983; Townsend et al. 1988). These indices, and their later developments, have become important tools for planning of health care services and interventions, as well as attempts of reducing inequalities in health. Generally, these studies have reported very high correlations between mortality and area-level SES, typically in the range of $R = 0.70–0.85$ (e.g. Carstairs 2000; Eames et al. 1993; Huff et al. 1999; Janghorbani et al. 2006; Langford and Bentham 1996; Smith et al. 2001; Soo et al. 2001).

But how do such indices transfer to other countries? In a pilot study, the Townsend index was tested against Danish mortality data using parishes as the basic geographical unit. This was done in preparation for a larger project which ran from 2006 to 2010 (Meijer et al. 2012a, 2012b; Stock et al. 2011; Stock et al. 2012).

The Townsend index (Townsend et al. 1988) measures material deprivation. The index is based on four variables: unemployment, car ownership, home ownership and overcrowding. While unemployment is measured as a percentage of the economically active population, the three other variables are measured as percentages of households. These numbers are log-transformed and standardised (into z-scores), and the final index is a summation of the four variables. There are several later developments of this index, but being among the first, the Townsend's index has been very influential in this type of research and has seen widespread use.

Demographic and socio-economic data can be obtained from Statistics Denmark. A well-recognised advantage for Scandinavian health studies is the availability of highly detailed registry data, but in this case the registers on mortality were undergoing organisational changes, so that the latest available data on annual deaths were from 2002. Because some parishes were very small with few annual deaths, mortality was calculated as an average for the years 2000–2002, while other data were as of July 1, 2001.

Mortality was calculated as a standardised mortality ratio (SMR), both for the entire population and for the 0–64-year segment. Many of the smallest parishes, however, have very few annual deaths, and this problem is only partly mitigated by using a 3-year average. This meant that the calculated SMRs for these parishes were either 0 (which is not possible) or could vary considerably with a few deaths. To ensure statistically stable data, parishes with less than five annual deaths were combined with neighbouring parishes with a similar settlement structure. This aggregation was done in GIS against a background map containing a classification of all settled areas in Denmark, which is available at high resolution (100×100 m) for the entire country (Nielsen et al. 2000). Using this classification as a guide, parishes with similar settlement types were geographically combined, focussing on local separation of urban, suburban and rural settlement types. This process left 1,591 aggregated parishes averaging 3,341 persons and 26.6 km^2. While such a reclassification could be done in a non-GIS environment, it would be very difficult to do without creating bias in data or simply nonsensical geographical units. Working from the map was all-important in this work.

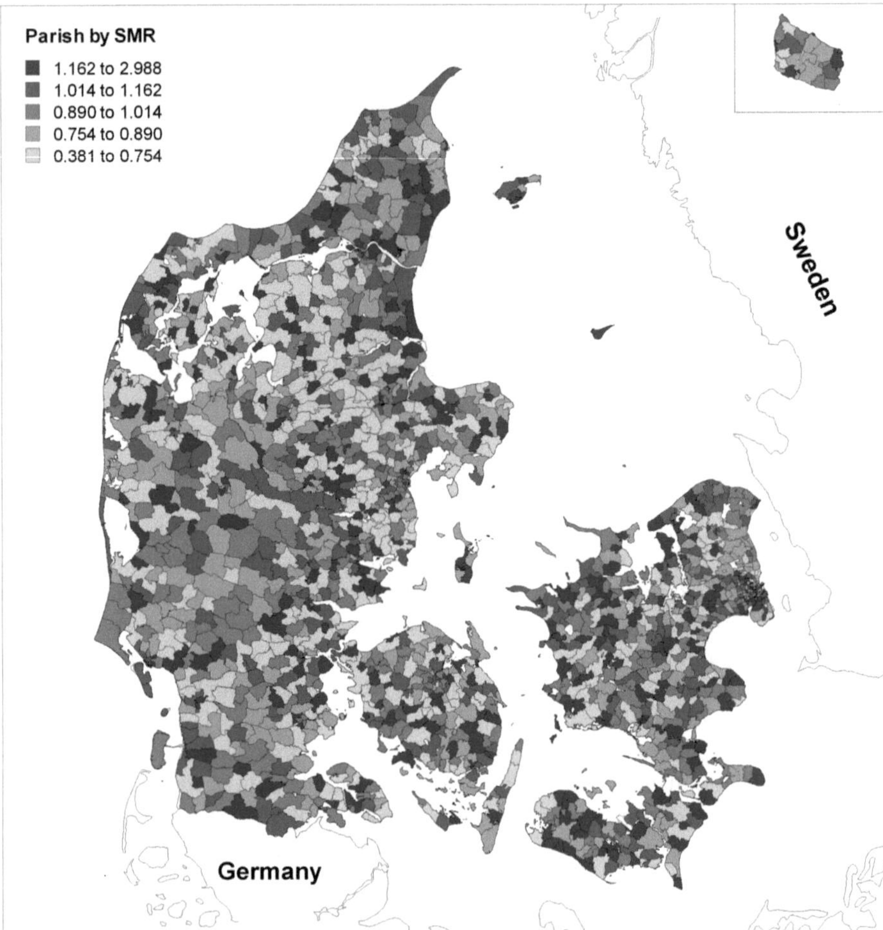

Fig. 8.3 Standardized mortality ratios (SMR) by parish, 2000–2002. The *shades* represent quintiles. Data from Statistics Denmark

Based on this revised dataset, the correlation between SMR and the Townsend index could be calculated (Fig. 8.3, Table 8.1). Statistically significant relations were found, but the correlations are considerably lower than the values reported from British studies. The Townsend index is a good descriptor of area-based health differences in Great Britain but apparently much less so in Denmark.

There are several reasons for this difference. First of all the social systems of the two countries are very dissimilar. Denmark has adopted the Nordic Welfare Model, where high taxes and a large public sector ensure a vast redistribution of wealth within the population, as well as (in principal) free and equal access to for instance

Table 8.1 Correlation of the Townsend index and its single variables with the standardized mortality ratio (SMR) for the entire population and for the 0–64 year age group. The average net income is also correlated to SMR

	SMR	$SMR_{0\text{-}64}$
Townsend	0.33	0.44
Unemployment	0.15	0.29
No car	0.34	0.44
Overcrowding	0.30	0.41
Rented accommodation	0.27	0.29
Average income	0.29	0.41

health care and education. Such basic differences between countries obviously make it difficult to transfer research results too directly across borders.

But another important reason is found on microscale, and will only be realised on very detailed maps, or in the landscape itself. Historically, the Danish settlement pattern has been socially heterogeneous. It is typical to find local areas with large houses and wealthy families patched in with government housing projects. For this reason the parishes may be too large to capture the spatial variation of social inequality, and the risk of ecological fallacy is possibly higher in Denmark than in Britain. On the other hand, some of the parishes were too small for a statistically stable calculation of SMR, so that the number of geographical units had to be reduced by 25 %. There are practical limits to the spatial scale of a given investigation, and this has an obvious effect on the results (*cf.* Schuurman et al. 2007). Data on population SES and health are now becoming available on a 100 × 100 m geographical scale, but a meaningful utilisation of data on such a level of detail will require a dedicated research effort into the spatial and societal aspects of SES on that particular level, because spatial clustering and classification is still necessary.

On a wider geographical scale, it is also important to consider the spatial properties of the ecological data with which health outcomes are compared. The socio-economic variables used to construct the Townsend index all tend to display a regional trend of high and low values. This is especially marked with the unemployment rates where the spatial autocorrelation of the data is very visible on the map (Fig. 8.4). Spatial autocorrelation has a significant impact on the calculated correlation between health outcomes and ecological variables, as it reduces the effective sample size, inflating the coefficient of determination and increasing the risk of type 1 errors (Haining 1998; Lorant et al. 2001). Virtually all statistics used in modern science assume independence between the observations, while this is visibly not the case for unemployment rates in Denmark. Autocorrelation is rarely accounted for in ecological studies, although there are techniques to mitigate the effects of spatial autocorrelation. One explanation for the limited application of such techniques is possibly that in using the well-established statistical software packages, researchers rarely see their data on a map.

Is a parish a "neighbourhood"? Historically, they probably were: dating back to the High Middle Ages, they formed the hinterland around a church in which the

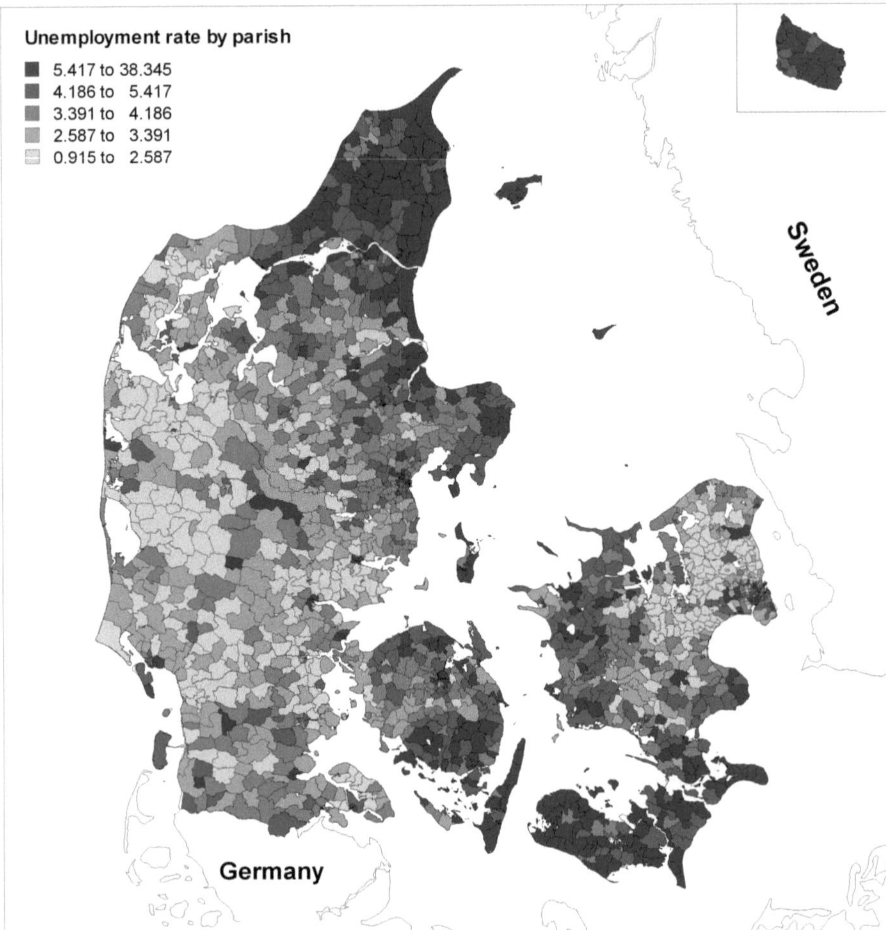

Fig. 8.4 Unemployment rates by parish from 2001. The *shades* represent quintiles. Data from Statistics Denmark

local population was bound to gather regularly. Other examples in this chapter will demonstrate how the neighbourhood today could be a much smaller unit, but most likely its daily perception and definition is fluid and context dependent. The parish is used here as a practically available unit, delineating a local area with a long administrative history, at least. Whether, and to which degree, a "local area" and a "neighbourhood" is the same is not entirely clear, as was discussed in the section above. It is clear, however, that in a book defining the neighbourhood as an important unit in health studies, geography itself inherently becomes a variable in the study. Important aspects of any analysis into the health of neighbourhoods are therefore only addressed through the study of the spatiality of the data and their context. GIS must be regarded a central tool in this process.

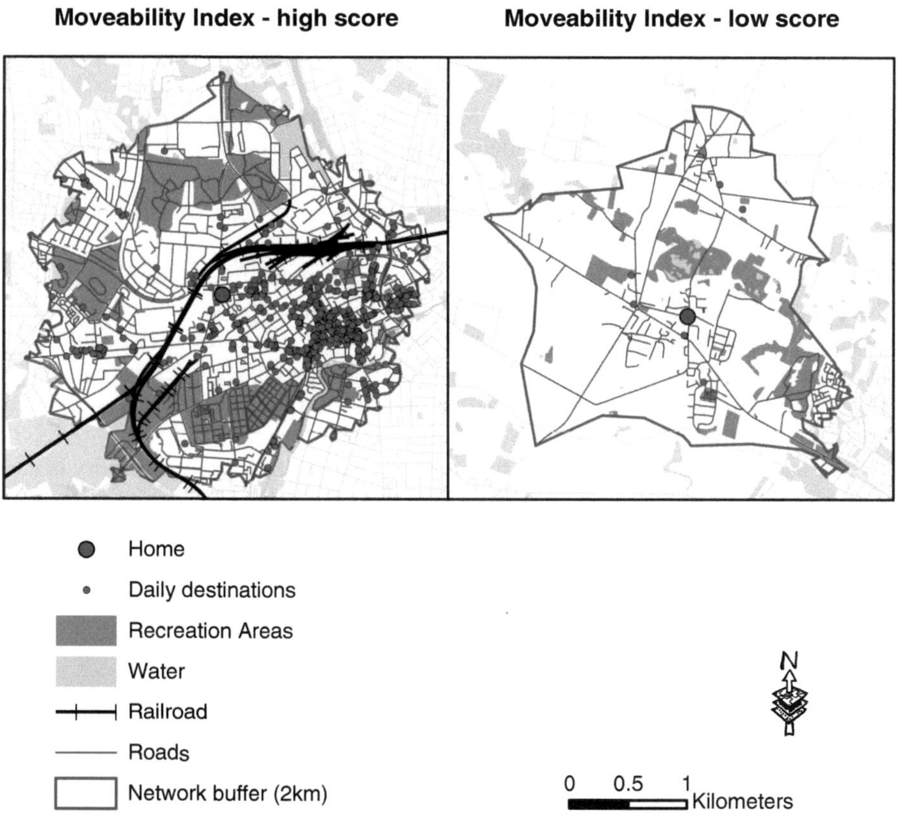

Fig. 8.5 Difference between high and low scores on the moveability index. Both areas are located within the municipality of Odense, Denmark. The respondent with a high score lives in the city centre, whereas the other respondent lives in a small residential area on the city outskirts, only 6 km from the other respondent

A Danish Moveability Index

Inspired by the walkability index developed by Frank et al. (2010) and moveability index developed by Buck et al. (2011), a moveability index is being developed for use in a Danish context. This version of the moveability index is calculated for individual network buffer zones (2 km) and includes four neighbourhood characteristics that are thought to influence overall activity levels: street connectivity, residential density, density of daily destinations and share of recreational facility area within the buffer zone. Figure 8.5 exemplifies the difference between areas with high and low scores on the moveability index.

Street connectivity was calculated based on the number of intersections with three or more connections within each buffer area. To avoid double intersections due to, e.g. two 3-way intersections near each other or double-tracked roads, 10-m buffers around each intersection were created and overlapping buffers were merged, and a new buffer centroid was used as new intersection point (for a detailed method description, see Forsyth et al. 2007). Motorways and expressways with no access for bikes or pedestrians were excluded.

Residential density was calculated based on the number of residential addresses within each buffer zone. For buildings with multiple residences, each residence was counted individually.

The Danish National Building Register contains codes for the different use of buildings. Using these codes, all building used for retail, sports clubs, schools and educational institutions and cultural facilities (libraries, theatres) were counted as daily destinations. Based on Norman et al. (2006), following facilities were included as recreational facility within the buffer area: swimming pools, fitness centres, sports clubs and stadiums, parks, woodlands and nature areas.

The usefulness of this moveability index as predictor for physical activity is currently tested using objectively measured longitudinal physical activity data from the European Youth Heart Study (EYHS). Preliminary cross-sectional analyses show an association between overall physical activity and the moveability index, adjusted for background variables.

Aggregating Health Survey Data to Meaningful Neighbourhoods

In 2007–2008, the large Danish Health Examination Survey 2007–2008 (DANHES 2007–2008) took place in 13 Danish municipalities; for an overview of the study and its design, see Eriksen et al. (2011). The aim of the study was to establish a research database for future cross-sectional and follow-up studies. To explore the possibilities for utilisation of these data in a physical planning context, the municipality of Brøndby (25,839 adult inhabitants) participated in a pilot study in 2011. The aim of the pilot study was to geocode all respondent addresses ($n=2,518$) and aggregate these data to "meaningful" neighbourhoods for use in various forms of municipal planning and policy making. Municipal employees from five departments (planning, education, sports, health and green space management) have been involved in the pilot study and have actively provided feedback during the process of identifying and delineating "meaningful" neighbourhoods.

Inspired by Cutchin et al. (2011), "meaningful" neighbourhoods were delineated by one person, based on aerial photographs as well as field visits. The five subjective criteria listed by Cutchin et al. (2011) were also used in this study: street patterns (no highways or railroads intersecting a neighbourhood), residential patterns (similarities in housing type and lot sizes), non-residential land use (e.g. schools or commercial land use), landforms (woodlands, lakes) and that the neighbourhood should be relatively compact (i.e. not elongated).

Furthermore, each neighbourhood should preferably have more than 50 respondents to assure a reasonable anonymity and reduce small sample bias. In a three-step process in which the municipality employees provided feedback and suggestions for improvement, the municipality of Brøndby was divided into 21 neighbourhoods.

To further reduce the small sample bias, for each neighbourhood, all survey data was weighted based on the respondents' representativeness within five gender-specific age groups. For example, if women between 25 and 44 years of age made up 20 % of all women within a neighbourhood but only accounted for 10 % of the women among the respondents in that neighbourhood, their answers were weighted with a factor 2.

At present, only descriptive statistics have been generated showing weighted mean values per neighbourhood, for each survey question. The 21 neighbourhoods have been used to visualise survey results on maps and give planners easy, visual access to neighbourhood specific health survey data and, as such, serve as an information base for planning and policy making. The next step is to test for neighbourhood homogeneity of independent variables, as well as for statistical significance of neighbourhood differences in health outcomes (see Figs. 8.6 and 8.7 for examples of neighbourhood-based visualisation of health survey data). These results will be used to inform municipal planning and policy making and are expected to provide guidance for strategies for future interventions or health promotion campaigns.

Schoolyard Physical Activity

A number of studies have found associations between the characteristics of schoolyards and the level of physical activity of pupils using the schoolyards (Farley et al. 2008; Ridgers et al. 2007a, b; Sallis et al. 2001). Based on these findings, it seems likely that making schoolyards more attractive will help to increase the total amount of physical activity among schoolchildren. In order to test this hypothesis, an intervention study at selected schools in Denmark will commence in 2012. The "Activating Schoolyards Study" will use combined qualitative and quantitative methods to study the effect of a series of schoolyard interventions. Before starting this intervention study, a pilot study was carried out with the objective to describe activity patterns and identify hotspots for physical activity on six schoolyards varying in size and content, located in different types of neighbourhoods.

For this pilot study, data from two separate studies was used, in which in total 745 children, 6–16 years old, enrolled at six schools were asked to wear an accelerometer and a GPS for five schooldays to determine their level of activity and movement patterns. GPS positions were recorded every 15 s and activity levels were recorded every 2 s. GPS and accelerometer data were compiled using the physical activity location measurement system (PALMS), developed by the Center for Wireless and Population Health Systems at the University of California, San Diego. GIS software was used to combine PALMS output with high-precision maps of the six schoolyards. All "land uses" of each of the six schoolyards were mapped in detail using a high-precision GPS combined with a handheld computer with mobile GIS software. To account for the reported manufacturer accuracy error of the GPS

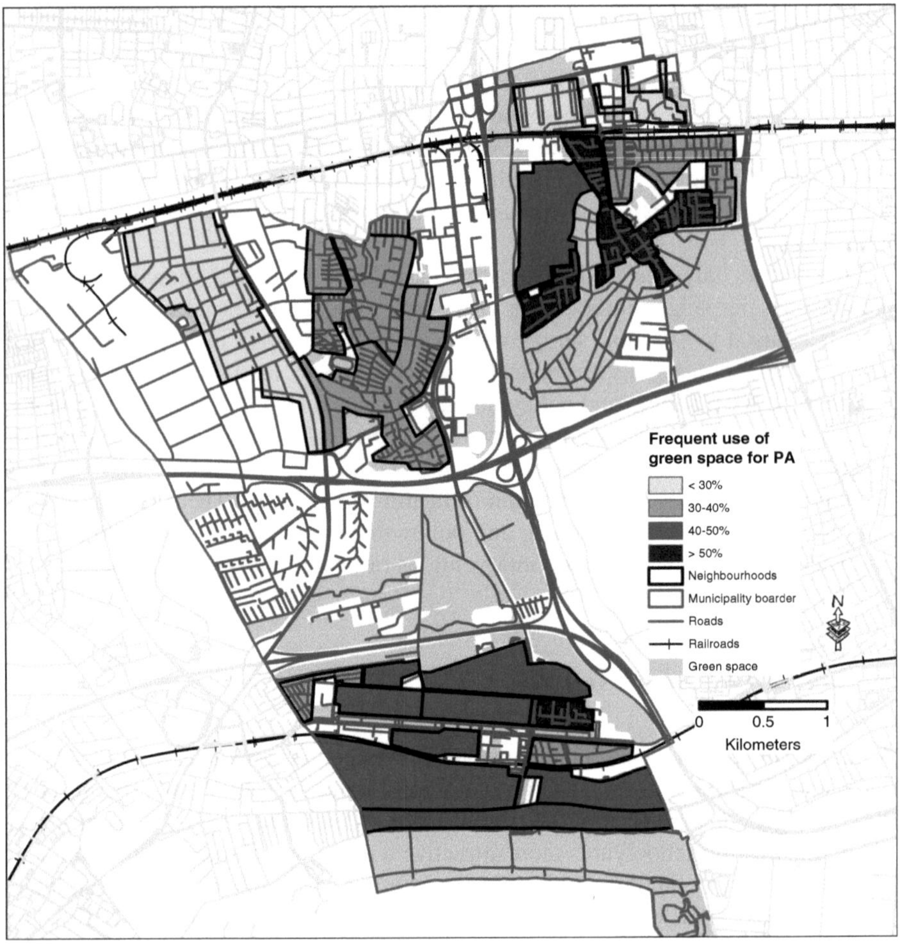

Fig. 8.6 Example of a neighbourhood based visualisation of the weighted percentage of respondents that frequently use nearby *green* space for physical activity (PA)

units worn by the participants, the detailed schoolyard maps were transformed to a raster-based map with 5×5 m cells, each cell containing a value associated with the dominant schoolyard "land use" present that cell. For each participant, average activity counts per grid cell were calculated, enabling us to determine average activity counts per schoolyard element. The initial analyses show that for these participants, artificial grass or rubber multi courts, lawn areas, grass slopes and other more natural elements were associated with schoolyard physical activity. Playground equipment, climbing frames, slides, etc. were less popular for physical activity. The initial results also show age, gender and time variances with different areas being popular for diverse age groups and at different times of the day. Figure 8.8 shows an

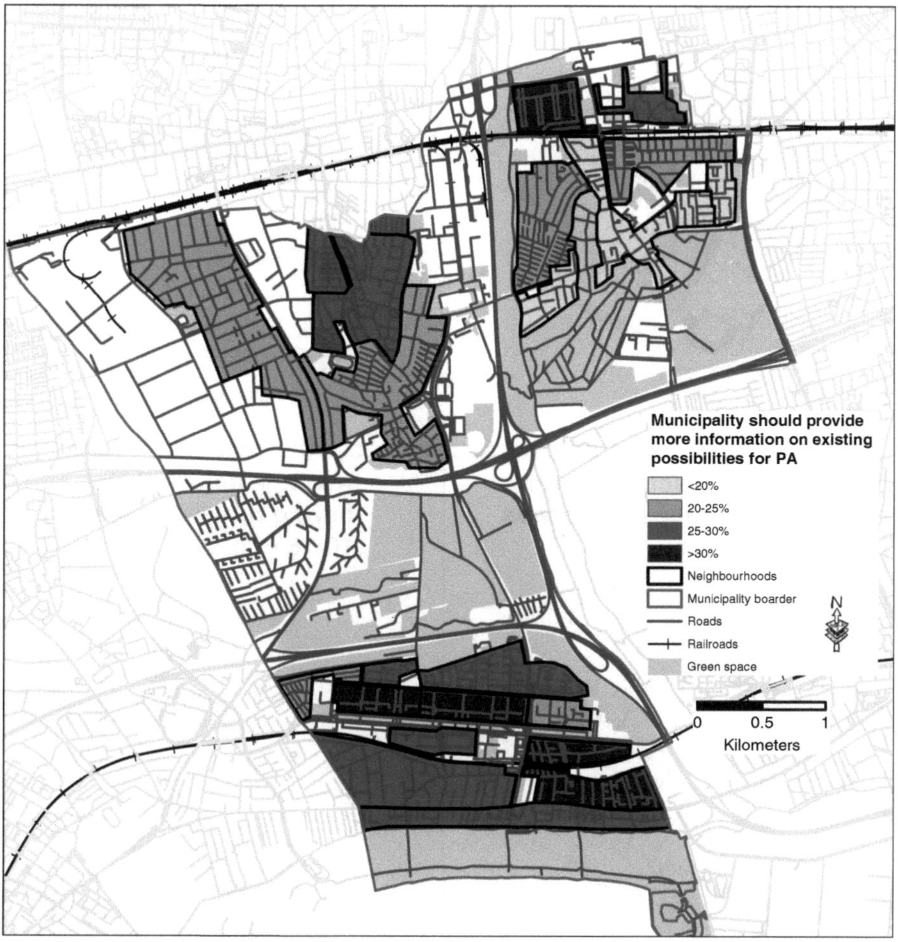

Fig. 8.7 Example of a neighbourhood based visualisation of the weighted percentage of respondents that would like to receive more information on existing possibilities for physical activity (PA)

example of a schoolyard "land use" map, a map with individual GPS points, linked to activity level data, as well as average activity levels calculated per raster cell.

Perspectives and Future Developments

When Dr John Snow in 1854 depicted a cholera outbreak in London using points to represent the locations of individual cases, he was probably among the first to demonstrate the power of a map using a geographic method to illustrate the distribution

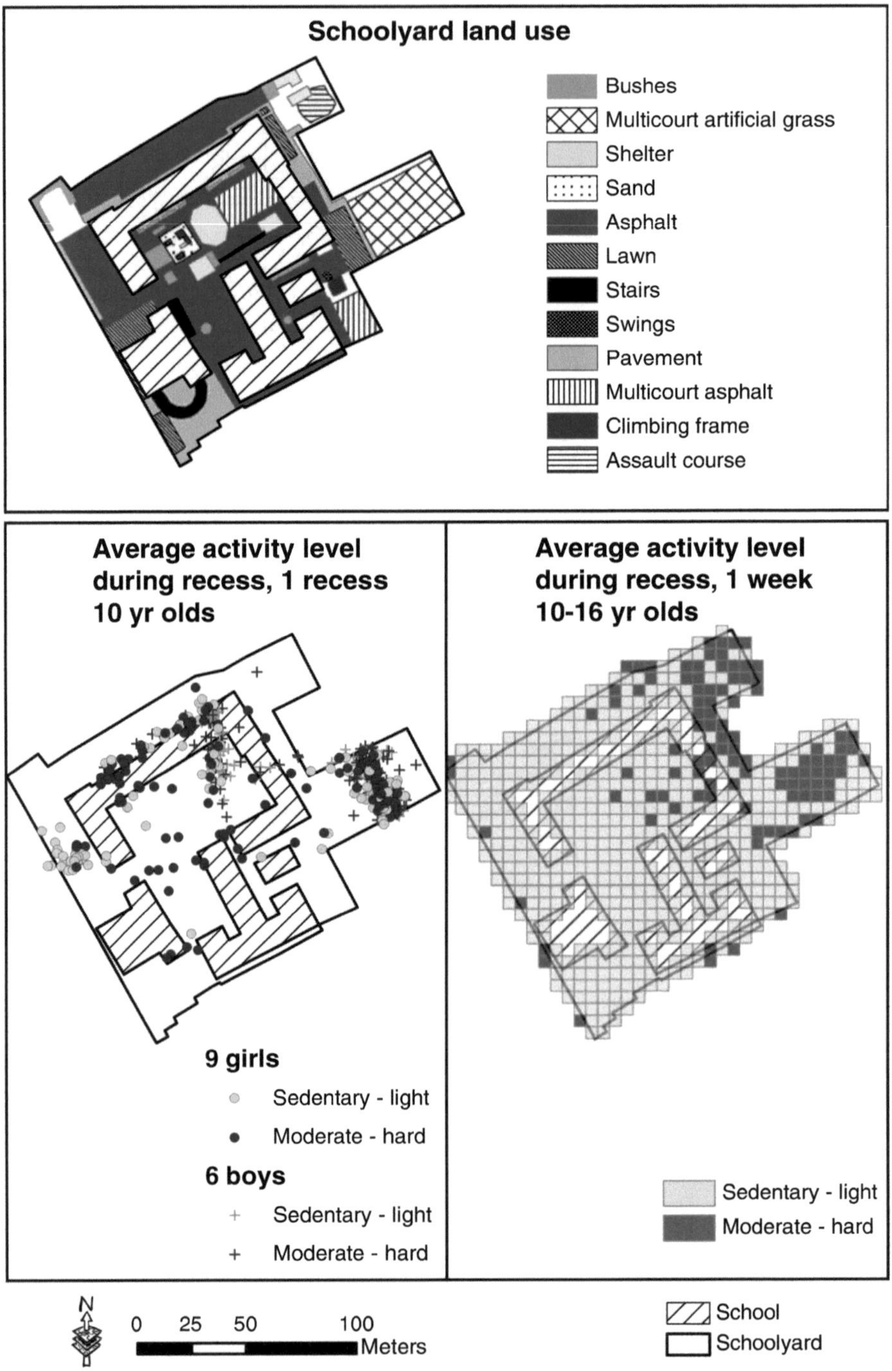

Fig. 8.8 Visualising physical activity during school recess. The schoolyard "land use" was mapped in detail. GPS and accelerometer data was combined to generate individual activity levels (one *dot* per person, per 15 s), as well as average activity levels for 5 × 5 m raster cells

of an infectious disease. His pioneer work clarified the importance of healthy neighbourhoods in preventing infectious diseases to spread, and thereby, his research paved the way for the sanitary revolution of the mid-nineteenth century. On a methodological level, John Snow's unique map is often referred to as the foundation of today's geographical public health research. The use of his cartographic methods founded analyses of geographically dependent variables in health science. As described in this chapter, there are numerous possibilities and advantages of using GIS in health research, but as discussed, there are also a number of methodological pitfalls we have to beware of when using GIS.

GIS provides great opportunities to include all sorts of environmental data in analyses. However, a first fundamental step using GIS in health science is to get a conceptual understanding of the physical environment being studied. Epidemiologist Basile Chaix proposes in this respect that "neighbourhood delimitations should capture the environmental conditions to which individuals are exposed in their local environment, i.e. that neighbourhoods should be viewed as exposure areas" (Chaix 2009, p. 93). Keeping this in mind, care should be taken when deciding on the area unit to be used in a study. Neighbourhoods can be defined in many different ways, and modifying the area unit used to delineate a neighbourhood affects the results of analyses. It is important for researchers to be aware of the effect the choice of neighbourhood can have on the analyses. Choosing the "right" neighbourhood area unit can be approached in various ways, both mathematically and conceptually.

Neither administrative units nor individual buffers are "perfect" matches for experienced neighbourhoods, and self-defined neighbourhoods are unlikely to capture all behavioural environments as frequently used destinations can be located outside people's neighbourhood.

Jones et al. (2010) have compared three neighbourhood definitions in a study on physical activity in children: enumeration districts (statistical unit), expert delineated areas with similar community characteristics and an automated zone design method based on maximum homogeneity. They found that the effect of neighbourhood characteristics on physical activity was limited and not strongly depended on the way the neighbourhoods were defined. They also conclude that "the delineation of neighbourhoods based on shared social or physical characteristics may not best capture the local influences" (Jones et al. 2010, p. 236). GPS devices with the ability to objectively track individual's locations, and thus determine their true exposure to the environment, will help improve neighbourhood definitions (Kerr et al. 2011). However, even with GPS-track buffer neighbourhoods or other conceptually valid neighbourhood units, the quality of the analyses still depends on the quality and scale of the available GIS data. If the GIS data were made for use on a municipal scale, precision will not be sufficient for use at a neighbourhood level.

The use of GPS data combined with GIS will undoubtedly strengthen future spatial analyses (see also Chap. 9). In addition to the role of GPS, we can also expect to see a continuing development in GIS per se. We envisage three future developments with the potential to enhance and refine the spatial turn in health science.

Firstly, with satellites collecting data about the condition of the Earth surface on a daily basis, or even twice a day, close to real-time environmental data could be integrated in GIS. Integrating this type of remotely sensed data creates the opportunity of adding a much more detailed time dimension to spatial analysis, e.g. investigation of active transportation in relation to road construction, traffic jams or different kinds of weather conditions. In studies on the use of urban green space, a weekly vegetation index could, for example, be added as variable to examine how the growing season influences human behaviour. Besides a better quality and a more frequently flow of high-resolution multispectral digital images, satellites are also equipped with sensors measuring climate and different kinds of thermic activity. In theory, further development of this technology opens up for tracking of human activity without using person-worn devices (e.g. accelerometer or GPS). Most likely more advanced satellite sensors will be developed in future, generating new types of data. This provides options for even more detailed analyses where GIS will be used to compile the data and form the basis for advanced modelling.

Secondly, the integration of time in GIS makes it not only possible to track and model the progress of humans throughout their daily routines but also opens up for epidemiological studies emphasising "place" in tight relation to "time" and "person". With accumulated, downloaded GIS data, it is possible to test the influence of environmental factors at a certain time in the observation period in cohort studies and other longitudinal data sets. To make comprehensive epidemiological studies, it is prospectively a matter of storing GIS data frequently for geocoding the next generation to come. Retrospectively, it is a matter of scanning historical maps, compiling geographical data and linking up these data with personal register data. New scanning techniques with automatic identification of geographical items have reduced this very time-consuming work. With the opportunity to geocode epidemiological data we have a much better scientific foundation to understand how human health behaviour relates to environmental determinants. In that perspective GIS has a huge potential to play an even more important role in epidemiology.

Thirdly, a future development that could help consolidate the spatial turn in health sciences is GIS data gathered by the general population. Such a practice of enlisting a variety of freelancers, paid or unpaid, to work on a specific task or problem is called crowdsourcing. In the endeavour to get the most detailed GIS data, it must be accepted that there are limitations with respect to which data can be derived from satellites, sensors, maps, etc. Local "experts" are, however, able to identify, interpret and verify physical objects that might be invisible to satellites due to diminished visibility or dense vegetation. Seeing GIS as an "open source", everyone can contribute to facilitate registration of physical objects at a neighbourhood level with an experienced significance for the locals. In future, this bottom-up perspective could be accomplished by following the current trend for GIS that accurate mapping and data analysis are completed while in the field. Trained local experts equipped with field-map technology make it possible to create a GIS that aligns better with the subjective perceptions of the neighbourhood.

GIS will continue to develop as tool for management and scientific research. In health science, GIS still has untapped potentials in relation to refined spatial analysis, epidemiological studies and other kinds of studies in which the physical environment is an important component. With the limitations in mind regarding neighbourhood definition and an ongoing methodical and technical advancements, the full potentials of GIS can be unleashed in the years to come.

References

Brownson, R. C., Hoehner, C. M., Day, K., Forsyth, A., & Sallis, J. F. (2009). Measuring the built environment for physical activity state of the science. *American Journal of Preventive Medicine, 36*(4), S99–S123.

Buck, C., Pohlabeln, H., Huybrechts, I., De Bourdeaudhuij, I., Pitsiladis, Y., Reisch, L., et al. (2011). Development and application of a moveability index to quantify possibilities for physical activity in the built environment of children. *Health & Place, 17*, 1191–1201.

Carstairs, V. (2000). Socio-economic factors at area level and their relationship with health. In P. Ellio, J. C. Wakefield, N. G. Best, & D. J. Biggs (Eds.), *Spatial epidemiology. Methods and applications* (pp. 51–67). Oxford: Oxford University Press.

Carstairs, V., & Morris, R. (1999). *Deprivation and health in Scotland.* Aberdeen: Aberdeen University Press.

Chaix, B. (2009). Geographic life environments and coronary heart disease: A literature review, theoretical contributions, methodological updates, and a research agenda. *Annual Review of Public Health, 30*, 81–105.

Cockings, S., & Martin, D. (2005). Zone design for environment and health studies using pre-aggregated data. *Social Science & Medicine, 60*(12), 2729–2742.

Cromley, E. K., & McLafferty, S. L. (2012). *GIS and Public Health.* New York: The Guilford.

Cutchin, M. P., Eschbach, K., Mair, C. A., Ju, H., & Goodwin, J. S. (2011). The socio-spatial neighborhood estimation method: An approach to operationalizing the neighborhood concept. *Health & Place, 17*(5), 1113–1121.

Diez Roux, A. V., & Mair, C. (2010). Neighborhoods and health. *Annals of the New York Academy of Sciences, 1186*, 125–145.

Eames, M., Ben-Shlomo, Y., & Marmot, M. G. (1993). Social deprivation and premature mortality: Regional comparison across England. *BMJ, 307*, 1097–1102.

Eriksen, L., Grønbæk, M., Helge, J. W., Tolstrup, J. S., & Curtis, T. (2011). The Danish health examination survey 2007–2008 (DANHES 2007–2008). *Scandinavian Journal of Public Health, 39*(2), 203–211.

Fan, Y., & Khattak, A. (2008). Urban form, individual spatial footprints, and travel. *Transportation Research Record: Journal of Transportation Research Board, 2082*, 98–106.

Farley, T. A., Meriwether, R. A., Baker, E. T., Rice, J. C., & Webber, L. S. (2008). Where do the children play? The influence of playground equipment on physical activity of children in free play. *Journal of Physical Activity and Health, 5*, 319–331.

Forsyth, A., D'Sousa, E., Koepp, J., Oakes, J. M., Schmitz, K. H., Van Riper, D., et al. (2007, June). Twin Cities walking study—environment and physical activity: GIS protocols version 4.1. http://www.designforhealth.net/pdfs/GIS_Protocols/MinnGIS_Ver4_1_FINAL.pdf.

Fotheringham, A. S., Brunsdon, C., & Charlton, M. E. (2002). *Geographically weighted regression: The analysis of spatially varying relationships.* Chichester: Wiley.

Frank, L. D., Sallis, J. F., Saelens, B. E., Leary, L., Cain, K., Conway, T. L., et al. (2010). The development of a walkability index: Application to the neighborhood quality of life study. *British Journal of Sports Medicine, 44*, 924–933.

Gatrell, A. C., & Löytönen, M. (1998). GIS and health research: An introduction. In A. C. Gatrell & M. Löytönen (Eds.), *Health and GIS. GISMAPS 6. European Science Foundation* (pp. 3–16). London: Taylor and Francis.

Haining, R. (1998). Spatial statistics and the analysis of health data. In A. C. Gatrell & M. Löytönen (Eds.), *Health and GIS. GISMAPS 6. European Science Foundation* (pp. 29–38). London: Taylor and Francis.

Haynes, R., Jones, A. P., Reading, R., Daras, K., & Emond, A. (2008). Neighbourhood variations in child accidents and related child and maternal characteristics: Does area definition make a difference? *Health & Place, 14*(4), 693–701.

Huff, N., Macleod, C., Ebdon, D., Phillips, D., Davies, L., & Nicholson, A. (1999). Inequalities in mortality and illness in Trent NHS Region. *Journal of Public Health Medicine, 21*(1), 81–87.

Janghorbani, M., Jones, R. B., & Nelder, R. (2006). Neighbourhood deprivation and excess coronary heart disease mortality and hospital admissions in Plymouth, UK: An ecological study. *Acta Cardiologica, 61*(3), 313–320.

Jarman, B. (1983). Identification of underprivileged areas. *BMJ, 286*, 1705–1709.

Jones, A. P., van Sluijs, E. M. F., Ness, A. R., Haynes, R., & Riddoch, C. J. (2010). Physical activity in children: Does how we define neighbourhood matter? *Health & Place, 16*(2), 236–241.

Kawachi, I., & Berkman, L. F. (2003). *Neighborhoods and health*. New York: Oxford University Press.

Kerr, J., Duncan, S., & Schipperijn, J. (2011). Using global positioning systems in health research—a practical approach to data collection and processing. *American Journal of Preventive Medicine, 41*(5), 532–540.

Kurland, K. S., & Wilpen, L. G. (2007). *GIS tutorial for Health*. Redlands: ESRI.

Lai, P. C., & Mak, A. S. H. (Eds.). (2007). *GIS for health and the environment. Development in the Asia-Pacific Region*. Berlin: Springer.

Langford, I. H., & Bentham, G. (1996). Regional variations in mortality rates in England and Wales: An analysis using multi-level modelling. *Social Science & Medicine, 42*(6), 897–908.

Lee, C., & Moudon, A. V. (2008). Neighbourhood design and physical activity. *Building Research and Information, 36*, 395–411.

Longley, P. A., Goodchild, M., Maguire, D. J., & Rhind, D. W. (2011). *Geographic information systems and science* (3rd ed.). New York: Wiley.

Lorant, V., Thomas, I., Deliège, D., & Tonglet, R. (2001). Deprivation and mortality: The implications of spatial autocorrelation for health resources allocation. *Social Science & Medicine, 53*(12), 1711–1719.

Meijer, M., Kejs, A. M., Stock, C., Bloomfield, K., Ejstrud, B., & Schlattmann, P. (2012a). Population density, socioeconomic environment and all-cause mortality: A multilevel survival analysis of 2.7 million individuals in Denmark. *Health & Place, 18*(2), 391–399.

Meijer, M., Röhl, J., Bloomfield, K., & Grittner, U. (2012b). Do neighborhoods affect individual mortality? A systematic review and meta-analysis of multilevel studies. *Social Science & Medicine, 74*(8), 1204–1212.

Millington, C., Ward Thompson, C., Rowe, D., Aspinall, P., Fitzsimons, C., Nelson, N., et al. (2009). Development of the Scottish walkability assessment tool (SWAT). *Health & Place, 15*, 474–481.

Mitra, R., & Buliung, R. N. (2012). Built environment correlates of active school transportation: neighborhood and the modifiable areal unit problem. *Journal of Transport Geography, 20*, 51–61.

Monmonier, M. S. (1996). *How to lie with maps*. Chicago: University of Chicago Press.

Nielsen, K., Stjernholm, M., Olsen, B. Ø., Müller-Wohlfeil, D. I., Madsen, I. L., Kjeldgaard, A., et al. (2000). Areal Informations Systemet – AIS Miljø- og Energiministeriet, Danmarks Miljøundersøgelser. http://www2.dmu.dk/1_Viden/2_Miljoe-tilstand/3_samfund/AIS/2_Rapport/ais_rapport.pdf.

Norman, G. J., Nutter, S. K., Ryan, S., Sallis, J. F., Calfas, K. J., & Patrick, K. (2006). Community design and access to recreational facilities as correlates of adolescent physical activity and body-mass index. *Journal of Physical Activity and Health, 3*(1S), 118–128.

Oh, K., & Jeong, S. (2007). Assessing the spatial distribution of urban parks using GIS. *Landscape and Urban Planning, 82*, 25–32.

Openshaw, S. (1977). Optimal zoning systems for spatial interaction models. *Environment and Planning A, 9*(2), 169–184.

Openshaw, S. (1984). *The modifiable areal unit problem*. Norwich: Geo Books.

Openshaw, S., & Alvandies, S. (1999). Applying geocomputation to the analysis of spatial distributions. In P. Longley, M. Goodchild, D. Maguire, & D. Rhind (Eds.), *Geographic information systems: Principles and technical issues* (pp. 267–282). New York: Wiley.

Openshaw, S., Charlton, M., Wymer, C., & Graft, A. (1987). A mark 1 geographical analysis machine for the automated analysis of point datasets. *International Journal of Geographical Information Science, 1*, 335–358.

Parenteau, M.-P., & Sawada, M. C. (2011). The modifiable areal unit problem (MAUP) in the relationship between exposure to NO2 and respiratory health. *International Journal of Health Geographics, 10,* 58.

Pickett, K., & Pearl, M. (2001). Multilevel analyses of neighbourhood socioeconomic context and health outcomes: A critical review. *Journal of Epidemiology & Community Health, 55,* 111–122.

Pikora, T., Giles-Corti, B., Bull, F., Jamrozik, K., & Donovan, R. (2003). Developing a framework for assessment of the environmental determinants of walking and cycling. *Social Science & Medicine, 56*(8), 1693–1703.

Ridgers, N. D., Stratton, G., Fairclough, S. J., & Twisk, J. W. (2007a). Long-term effects of a playground markings and physical structures on children's recess physical activity levels. *Preventive Medicine, 44*(5), 393–397.

Ridgers, N. D., Stratton, G., Fairclough, S. J., & Twisk, J. W. (2007b). Children's physical activity levels during school recess: A quasi-experimental intervention study. *International Journal of Behavioral Nutrition and Physical Activity, 4,* 19.

Riva, M., Apparicio, P., Gauvin, L., & Brodeur, J. M. (2008). Establishing the soundness of administrative spatial units for operationalising the active living potential of residential environments: An exemplar for designing optimal zones. *International Journal of Health Geographics, 7*(1), 43.

Riva, M., Gauvin, L., & Barnett, T. A. (2007). Toward the next generation of research into small area effects on health: A synthesis of multilevel investigations published since July 1998. *Journal of Epidemiology and Community Health, 61*(10), 853–861.

Saelens, B. E., Sallis, J. F., Black, J. B., & Chen, D. (2003). Neighborhood-based differences in physical activity: An environment scale evaluation. *American Journal of Public Health, 93,* 1552–1558.

Sallis, J. F., Conway, T. L., Prochaska, J. J., McKenzie, T. L., Marshall, S. J., & Brown, M. (2001). The association of school environments with youth physical activity. *American Journal of Public Health, 91*(4), 618–620.

Schipperijn, J., Stigsdotter, U. K., Randrup, T. B., & Troelsen, J. (2010). Influences on the use of urban green space: A case study in Odense, Denmark. *Urban Forestry and Urban Greening, 9,* 25–32.

Schuurman, N., Bell, N., Dunn, J. R., & Oliver, L. (2007). Deprivation indices, population health and geography: An evaluation of the spatial effectiveness of indices at multiple scales. *Journal of Urban Health, 84*(4), 591–603.

Scott, M. M., Evenson, K. R., Cohen, D. A., & Cox, C. E. (2007). Comparing perceived and objectively measured access to recreational facilities as predictors of physical activity in adolescent girls. *Journal of Urban Health, 84,* 346–359.

Sherman, J. E., Spencer, J., Preisser, J. S., Gesler, W. M., & Arcury, T. A. (2005). A suite of methods for representing activity space in a healthcare accessibility study. *International Journal of Health Geographics, 4,* 24.

Smith, G., Gidlow, C., Davey, R., & Foster, C. (2010). What is my walking neighbourhood? A pilot study of English adults' definitions of their local walking neighbourhoods. *International Journal of Behavioral Nutrition and Physical Activity, 7,* 34.

Smith, G. D., Whitley, E., Dorling, D., & Gunnell, D. (2001). Area based measures of social and economic circumstances: Cause specific mortality patterns depend on the choice of index. *Journal of Epidemiology and Community Health, 55,* 149–150.

Soo, L., Huff, N., Gray, D., & Hampton, J. R. (2001). Geographical distribution of cardiac arrest in Nottinghamshire. *Resuscitation, 48*(2), 137–147.

Stock, C., Bloomfield, K., Ejstrud, B., Vinther-Larsen, M., Meijer, M., Grønbæk, M., et al. (2012). Are characteristics of the school district associated with active transportation to school in Danish adolescents? *European Journal of Public Health, 22*(3), 398–404.

Stock, C., Ejstrud, B., Vinter-Larsen, M., Schlattmann, P., Curtis, T., & Grønbæk, M. (2011). Effects of school district factors on alcohol consumption: Results of a multi-level analysis among Danish adolescents. *European Journal of Public Health, 21*(4), 449–455.

Tian, N., Goovaerts, P., Zhan, F. B., & Wilson, J. G. (2010). Identification of racial disparities in breast cancer mortality: Does scale matter? *International Journal of Health Geographics, 9*, 35.

Townsend, P., Phillimore, P., & Beattie, A. (1988). *Health and deprivation: Inequality and the north*. London: Croom Helm.

Villanueva, K., Giles-Corti, B., Bulsara, M. K., McCormack, G. R., Timperio, A., Middleton, N., et al. (2012). How far do children travel from their homes? Exploring children's activity spaces in their neighborhood. *Health & Place, 18*(2), 263–273.

Zenk, S. N., Schulz, A. J., Matthews, S. A., Odoms-Young, A., Wilbur, J., Wegrzyn, L., et al. (2011). Activity space environment and dietary and physical activity behaviors: A pilot study. *Health & Place, 17*(5), 1150–1161.

Chapter 9
Using GPS to Measure the Interaction Between Individuals and Their Neighbourhood

Jolanda Maas, Reinier P. Sterkenburg, Sanne I. de Vries, and Frank Pierik

Introduction

There has been an increasing focus on examining the relationship between neighbourhood built environment and health and health behaviours. This is mainly due to the potential of environmental interventions for having a sustained impact on entire population groups rather than a short-term impact on individuals (Giles-Corti et al. 2005). Moreover, environmental interventions may influence population groups that are hard to reach with health education programmes, such as those with lower education levels, lower incomes and language barriers (Swinburn et al. 1999).

The relationship between where you live and health has long been recognised (Kawachi and Berkman 2003; Burton et al. 2011). In the past decade, the focus has been on the relationship between neighbourhood environment and physical activity to shed light on the potential drivers of the current overweight epidemic. Interest in the relation between built environment and physical activity has increased, mainly because many

J. Maas (✉)
Department of Public and Occupational Health, EMGO + Institute, VU Medical Center, Postbus 7057, 1007 MB, Amsterdam, The Netherlands
e-mail: j.maas@vumc.nl

R.P. Sterkenburg
Department of Urban Environment and Safety, Netherlands Organisation for Applied Scientific Research (TNO), Postbus 49, 2600 AA, Delft, The Netherlands
e-mail: reinier.sterkenburg@tno.nl

S.I. de Vries
Department of Life Style, Netherlands Organisation for Applied Scientific Research (TNO), Postbus 2215, 2301 CE Leiden, The Netherlands
e-mail: sanne.devries@tno.nl

F. Pierik
Department of Urban Environment and Safety, Netherlands Organisation for Applied Scientific Research (TNO), Postbus 80015, 3508 TA, Utrecht, The Netherlands
e-mail: frank.pierik@tno.nl

C. Stock and A. Ellaway (eds.), *Neighbourhood Structure and Health Promotion*,
DOI 10.1007/978-1-4614-6672-7_9, © Springer Science+Business Media New York 2013

prevention and intervention strategies have had limited effect at population level (American Journal of Preventive Medicine 1998; Dishman and Buckworth 1996; Marcus et al. 2000; Dollman et al. 2005; McDonald 2007; Ooijendijk et al. 2008).

Moreover, interest in this relationship has been stimulated by social–ecological models of health, which posit that changes in the natural and built environment that encourage physically active lifestyles may be as important as interventions at the individual or social level (Sallis et al. 2006; Brownson et al. 2009; Saelens et al. 2003; Giles-Corti and King 2009).

Studies have identified that neighbourhood characteristics like aesthetics, neighbourhood density, convenience of facilities for walking (sidewalks, trails), accessibility, opportunities for activity and perceptions about traffic and busy roads are associated with physical activity (Saelens and Handy 2008; Saelens et al. 2003; Clark et al. 2010). However, most studies on the relationship between neighbourhood and physical activity have used self-reported measures of physical activity and used relatively general descriptions of neighbourhood characteristics. Activity diaries, sometimes combined with map and pencil recording of routes, are probably the most frequently used method to record time-activity patterns. A main drawback of this method is that they are limited in their temporal resolution, because registration per minute would be too demanding for participants. In addition, diaries cannot provide exact information on the subject's location. Furthermore, these self-reported measures and observation are very time-consuming.

In gaining more knowledge about the exact influence of neighbourhood structure on health, we would ideally like to assess (1) the exact location of neighbourhood residents (e.g. inside, outside, near a park, in shops), (2) the level of exposure to neighbourhood characteristics and (3) how neighbourhood residents move through their neighbourhood (e.g. walking, cycling or by car). With global position systems (GPS), this kind of information can be assessed. They offer a low-cost, objective and unobtrusive monitoring device to assess the actual movement patterns of people through the environment. These devices have been shown to be more accurate than self-reported travel surveys or activity diaries (Duncan and Mummery 2007; Badland et al. 2010; Stopher et al. 2007).

A number of studies have used GPS devices to assess the association between physical activity and several aspects of the environment, some with a focus broader than the neighbourhood environment. A review by Krenn et al. (2011) found 24 studies, most of them published in 2009 and 2010, which used GPS devices to assess the relationship between physical activity and the environment. These studies focused on children, adults or older adults and assessed the association between physical activity and the built environment around home or work, the feasibility of different combinations of GPS, accelerometer and geographical information systems (GIS), trip purpose, analyses of locations where transport-related physical activity took place and validation of travel diaries using GPS (Krenn et al. 2011). GPS devices have also been used in studies assessing the exact exposure to pollutants (Morabia et al. 2010), such as air pollution (Adams et al. 2009), or for indicating the exposure to sunlight which is needed to produce vitamin D (Lauretani et al. 2010).

The aim of this chapter is to provide the reader with a theoretical background and practical advice for applying GPS in research. The second section of this chapter describes what a GPS device is and what kind of information can be gathered with it.

Furthermore, this section describes how GPS data can be processed to be meaningful for answering research questions. The third section describes how GPS can be applied to study the interaction between neighbourhood characteristics and health. At the end of this chapter, a conclusion will be drawn, and strengths and weaknesses of using GPS devices will be described.

Theoretical Background and Practical Information on How to Use GPS

This section describes what a GPS is and describes how GPS data can be handled to be meaningful for answering research questions. The section is structured in three parts: (1) a description of what GPS is, (2) a description of what kind of information can be gathered with GPS, (3) some background information on how accurate a GPS device is, (4) an overview of existing types of GPS devices and (v) a manual of how GPS data can be handled.

What Is GPS?

The global positioning system (GPS) is a system that makes it possible to determine positions of objects and persons on the Earth's surface. The system, which is officially called NAVSTAR, was built in the 1970s and 1980s for use by US military forces. For various reasons, the USA has lifted the restrictions for civilian use, and it has now become ubiquitous in civilian navigation products and applications. The most important 'hardware' that makes the GPS system work is the 24–32 satellites that orbit the Earth at an altitude of 20,200 km and send out radio signals. From almost every location on the Earth's surface, the signals from at least 6 up to about 10 satellites can be received.

The determination of positions of GPS receivers is based on measuring the transmission times of signals from the satellites to the receivers. The transmission times are used to calculate distances to the satellites. Using the positions of the satellites, which are known very accurately, and some complicated geometrical calculations, the position of a receiver is calculated.

What Kind of Information Can Be Gathered with GPS?

The main output information of GPS receivers are (1) the x and y coordinates, (2) the altitude relative to (standardised) sea level and usually also (3) the exact time. See Table 9.1 for an example of data that is obtained from a GPS recorder. In this example, there is a fixed time period (*epoch*) of 5 s between two data points. GPS devices may have different or adjustable epochs, or they may have varying time intervals depending on the speed or on the curvature of the track. For example,

Table 9.1 Raw GPS data

Index	Date	Time	Latitude	N/S	Longitude	E/W	Altitude
1	11-09-2010	19:15:53	52.47757	N	4.819151	E	48.6567
2	11-09-2010	19:16:48	52.47767	N	4.819817	E	107.2862
3	11-09-2010	19:16:53	52.47751	N	4.819658	E	76.51211
4	11-09-2010	19:16:58	52.47755	N	4.819583	E	76.10406
5	11-09-2010	19:17:03	52.47752	N	4.819275	E	54.46672
..	..	..	..	..	..	..	..
5000	14-09-2010	13:18:23	52.47745	N	4.819642	E	48.13932
5001	14-09-2010	13:18:28	52.47745	N	4.819646	E	48.08909
5002	14-09-2010	13:18:33	52.47745	N	4.819651	E	48.00119
5003	14-09-2010	13:18:38	52.47744	N	4.819643	E	48.40571
5004	14-09-2010	13:18:43	52.47743	N	4.819611	E	48.26397
5005	14-09-2010	13:18:48	52.47744	N	4.819546	E	48.68541

in curves, it may record points every 3 s, while on straight ends when travelling at higher speeds, it may record points every 10 s.

When interpreting raw GPS data, one must be careful about which geographical coordinate system is used and which time zone the times refer to. More information about geographical coordinate systems can be found in Chap. 8 of this book.

GPS devices usually record position data in internal memory, e.g. on an SD card. Recorded data can then be transferred to computers for post-processing and presentation. The frequency at which the position is updated internally can be up to many times per second, but in commonly used devices, data points are stored not more than once every second up to a few times per minute. In Fig. 9.1, an example is given of GPS tracks with different position update frequencies of someone who was driving a car. The green tracks have a frequency of once per 5 s, whereas the red ones have a frequency of once per 15 s. The figure shows that an update frequency of 15 s is not enough to accurately record travel through sharp curves.

Most receivers also provide derived information from the position and time like speed, bearing (direction), acceleration and distance travelled. Some receivers also gather 'internal' information like signal quality, number of satellites in sight and calculated location error. That kind of information may be useful when the data is filtered or smoothed; for more information see the section on GPS data handling below.

Accuracy

The position measurement accuracy of GPS receivers is variable. Even in good circumstances, the position error[1] of GPS devices for consumer use is usually around 10–15 m

[1] Position error is often expressed as the "circular error probable" (CEP). A CEP of 5 m means that 50 % of the position measurements are within a circle with a radius of 5 m around the actual location and that the other 50 % of measurements are outside of that circle.

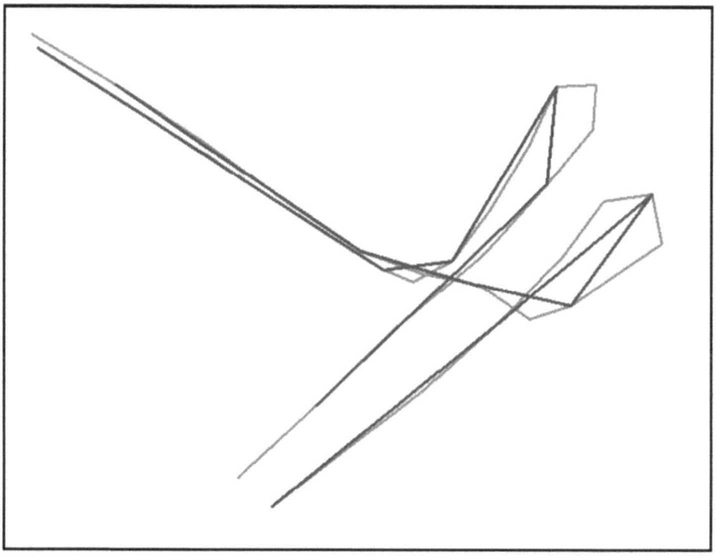

Fig. 9.1 Comparison of GPS tracks from a subject driving a car with different position update frequencies. The *dark line* indicates a lower position update frequency than the *light line*

(Kerr et al. 2011). The reception of satellite signals can be disturbed by surrounding obstacles like buildings, thick trees or steep mountainsides. Reflections of signals against walls or complete loss of signal from some of the satellites often results in a deterioration of the accuracy of position determination or complete inability to establish a position. Unfortunately, in most practical cases where GPS devices are used to study neighbourhood interaction, situations where the satellite 'fix' is lost occur regularly.

It is possible to enhance the accuracy of GPS receivers by using augmentation systems such as DGPS (differential GPS), WAAS (wide area augmentation system), EGNOS (European geostationary overlay service), INS (inertial navigation system) or A-GPS (assisted GPS). Most of these augmentation systems are already integrated into consumer GPS devices, smartphones and GPS data loggers. Such devices have higher accuracies and less frequent loss of ability to determine a position than devices without augmentation. Another means to enhance the accuracy of position measurements, used mostly in navigation applications, is to use geographical information to 'snap' the calculated position to the most likely nearby location (e.g. a road or parking place).

Types of GPS Devices

There are various types of devices available which contain GPS receivers. In health and environment-related research, where subjects carry devices for one or more whole days, GPS data loggers and GPS transmitters are most often used. The main difference between GPS data loggers or GPS transmitters and handheld GPS devices

Table 9.2 Examples of types of GPS devices and their advantages and disadvantages

Type of device	Advantages	Disadvantages
GPS data logger	Subjects cannot manipulate settings of the device	
GPS transmitter	Transmission of data in real time (no need to transfer data at the end of a recording period)	Battery power consumption
Handheld GPS device	Suitable for outdoor use (more or less shock and water proof)	Memory may not be sufficient to record for several days
		Subjects may manipulate settings of the device
GPS navigation system (for car or motor bike)	Easy to operate	Does not operate (or only for a short time) without power supply
	Large display	Relatively large and heavy
Smart phone with GPS	Possibility to transmit data in real time (no need to transfer data at the end of a recording period)	Expensive
	Possibility for feedback to subjects	Subjects may manipulate settings of the device

is that they do not have a display on which the current position is shown. For outdoor use like hiking and mountain biking, small and lightweight handheld GPS devices are used that are more weather resistant. For use as navigation systems in cars and on motorbikes, larger devices with touch screens that are easy to operate while driving are available. Last but not least, smartphones with GPS functionality are becoming more and more ubiquitous. Table 9.2 from the article of Kerr et al. (2011) describes examples of types of GPS devices and their advantages and disadvantages.

For more detailed information concerning several technical as well as practical aspects that are important when using GPS devices in health research, the reader is advised to read the excellent article by Kerr and others (Kerr et al. 2011) that was published in the American Journal of Preventive Medicine. They also provide a description of features to consider in GPS purchasing decision.

Device Selection

For most health and environment-related studies, a GPS logger (see Table 9.2) is the most suitable device type. There are many manufacturers and very many different models on the market. The most suitable device for a specific study depends on aspects like accuracy, memory size, battery life, fix time and other factors, which are described in detail in the article by Kerr and others (2011). It is advised to verify whether the relevant performance factors as specified by the manufacturer are achieved in realistic circumstances, either by conducting your own performance tests or by finding test results or reviews done by others.

Proper Usage by Participants

The GPS signal reception and therefore the accuracy of the recorded locations may be affected by how the GPS device is worn or carried by the participants. Carrying the device inside pockets, bags or backpacks is not recommended. Attaching the device to a belt usually works well because it does not hinder normal transportation behaviour. However, when the subjects wear long coats, GPS signal reception might be affected. As an alternative wearing location, one can use a small backpack with the GPS device attached to the outside of it.

When subjects are to carry the GPS devices for longer periods (whole days or even multiple days), one must make sure that the participants do not forget to wear the device and also remind them to recharge the batteries regularly. If possible, one should send reminder messages to the participants every day. Asking the participants to write down (log) when the device was worn and when it was charged also helps to avoid that they forget to wear or charge it. More tips concerning participant compliance can be found in (Kerr et al. 2011).

GPS Data Handling

In its raw form, recorded GPS data consists of a table with data points that list a time and a location, as illustrated in Table 9.1. In Fig. 9.2, consecutive locations are plotted on a map and connected with lines. Such a group of consecutive locations is called a *track*. A device may record multiple tracks, separated by time gaps when it has been turned off or unable to determine locations. The raw track data need to be processed to obtain information that is meaningful for the study that is being carried out.

The following processing steps are often necessary:

- Elimination of 'bad data' (in other words: filtering out noise)
- Calculating derived variables like speed, bearing, acceleration, climb rate, etc.
- Determination of trips (also called journeys)
- Determination of mode of transport
- Association with neighbourhood characteristics (using GIS information)
- Aggregation of results

In the next sections, examples are given of (1) how 'bad data' can be eliminated, (2) how trips/journey can be detected and (3) how the mode of transport can be determined.

Elimination of 'Bad Data'

It has already been mentioned that GPS tracks often contain groups of data points that are recorded during periods with bad satellite signal reception resulting in poor position accuracy. An example of a track that contains such periods of bad signal reception is shown in Fig. 9.2.

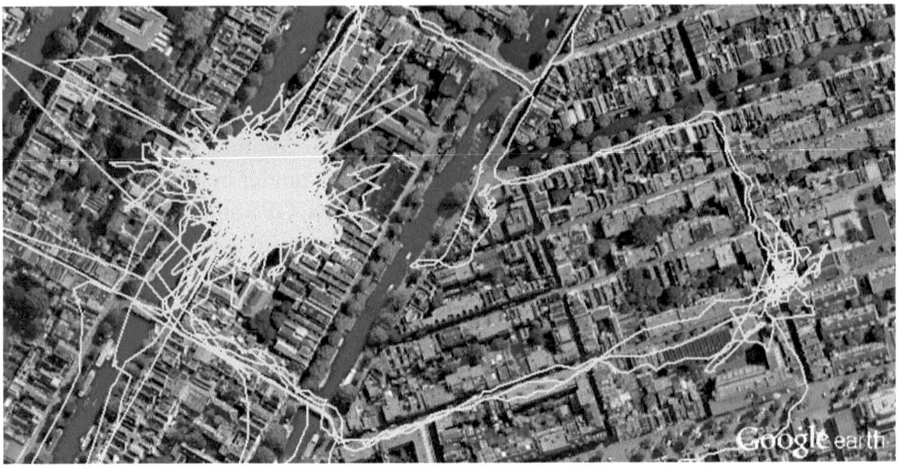

Fig. 9.2 Raw GPS track data, shown on a map. This example shows two typical clusters of "bad data" as recorded while the receiver is inside a building

Before further data processing takes place, data points that contain this type of noise should be identified and, in most cases, eliminated. In Textbox 9.1, such a method is described.

Other indications of inaccurate data that results from bad signal reception are unrealistic values of speed, bearing, acceleration or altitude. The exact threshold values above which speed, altitude, etc. are considered to be unrealistic depend on the type of GPS device, on the environment and on the transportation behaviour of the person that carried the device.

Trip/Journey Detection

A trip or journey is usually defined as a part of a track that begins when movement starts away from a fixed position and ends when the movement reaches (approaches) another fixed position. When the GPS device has been turned on long before the journey begins and is kept on after the destination is reached, establishing the start and end points (in time) of the journey from the recorded data may be complicated. This is especially the case when there is no a priori knowledge about the positions of the start and end points of the journey. Also, if the GPS device had to make a cold start when leaving the start location, which means the device has not been used before and therefore it takes a while before the GPS device can find the satellites. This makes it possible that the start of the journey may have been recorded with only bad accuracy or not at all. For the detection of journey end points, the 'dwell time' is often used. Dwell time is the length of time when there is no movement (Kerr et al. 2011). More or less equivalent is the possibility to use cluster detection to identify locations where much time is spent while hardly moving. The moment of reaching a cluster location is then the end point of a trip.

Textbox 9.1. Identification of Indoor/Outdoor Using Cluster Detection

The procedure for indoor/outdoor discrimination consists of the following steps:

First, the GPS data points are projected onto a raster of grid cells of 25 m.

Then, the grid cell that contains the highest number of GPS locations is selected. The process is illustrated in Fig. 9.3.

If it contains less than 100 locations, the procedure stops (there is no cluster).

A list is made that contains all GPS data points in the selected grid cell, plus all data points in its 8 neighbour grid cells. The centre of gravity (COG_k) of these data points is calculated, and then the root mean square of the distances (d_{RMS}) of the data points to the COG. Data points that lie more than three times d_{RMS} away from the COG are labelled as outliers and eliminated from the list of GPS data points.

The COG is calculated again (COG_{k+1}), and if the COG is more than 5 m from its previous location, the outlier removal procedure is repeated.

The data points that lie less than 2 d_{RMS} away from the COG are labelled as belonging to the cluster.

Extra processing steps can be added here to make sure that the 'spikes' are also labelled as 'indoors' and eliminated. This can be done by taking the temporal relations between those data points and the cluster points into account.

The whole procedure is repeated, without the already found cluster points, to find new clusters, until no new clusters are found.

Determination of Mode of Transport

Many studies try to gather information on the times, distances and locations spent walking, cycling, running or using motorised transportation like cars, buses or trains. The most straightforward approach to do this using GPS data is to define upper an. lower bounds for the speed for each mode of transportation and use the average speed during the trip as classifying variable. Unfortunately, we have found that this approach does not work very well, because trips through cities and towns often involve periods with low speeds, which cause the average speed to drop below the threshold value that belongs to the actually used mode of transportation.

Also, multimodal trips like walking-vehicle-walking may be wrongly classified in this way. If mode changes during a trip can be identified, e.g. by identifying dwell times when mounting a vehicle or by using GIS information about the location of parking places or bus stops, trips can be separated into trip segments and these segments can be classified more reliably.

Instead of using the average speed to determine the mode of transportation, using the maximum speed as the classifying variable is likely to be more reliable. Especially if high-frequency noise ('spikes') is filtered out, the maximum speed

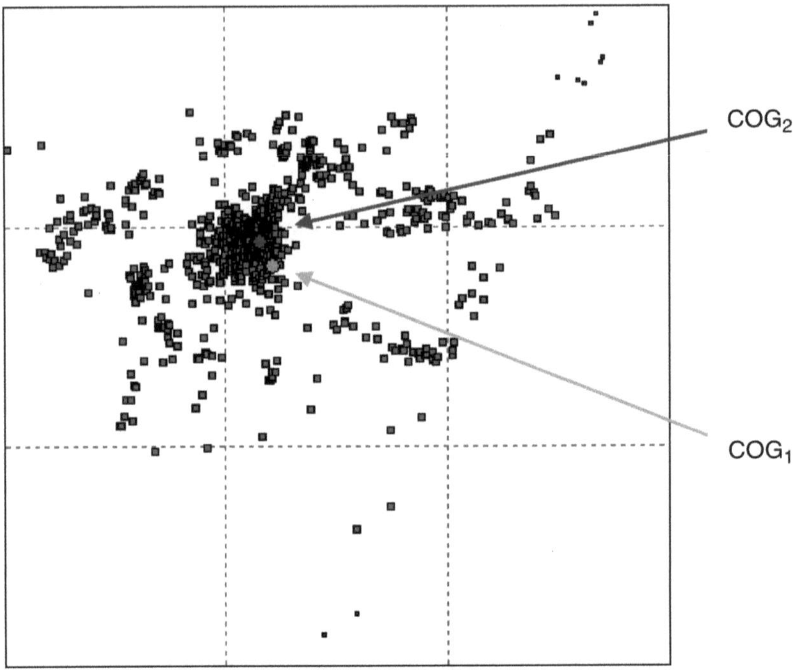

Fig. 9.3 Cluster detection, showing two iterations of finding the center of gravity (COG)

over the whole trip is a good indicator of whether the trip was made walking, cycling or using motorised transportation. In the 'Park or Flowerbed' study (see Textbox 9.2 below), using a maximum of 9 km/h for walking and 25 km/h for cycling provided satisfactory results.

Application of GPS in Neighbourhood and Health Research

This section describes how GPS can be applied to study the interaction between neighbourhood characteristics and health. The section is structured in three parts: (1) how to link GPS data to neighbourhood characteristics, (2) some examples from studies on the relationship between neighbourhood and physical activity using GPS and (3) some other examples of studies on personal exposure linked to GPS.

How to Link GPS Data to Neighbourhood Characteristics?

As described in the previous section, GPS registers time and position in *x* and *y* coordinates. These *x* and *y* coordinates can be linked to neighbourhood characteristics which have a spatial component that can be expressed in x and y coordinates. This is in essence how in a GIS it is possible to assign personal exposure to neighbourhood characteristics along a person's tracks. In reality, the collection and analysis of GIS data require substantial GIS expertise for linkage of GPS tracks with neighbourhood characteristics. This is because the data in GIS information layers is not as detailed as the GPS data. An understanding of the origin of GIS methods is also essential to determine the optimal choice of statistical analysis methods to analyse the impact of neighbourhood on PA and health. Most GIS software packages can easily export data in a format that is compatible with statistics software.

Neighbourhood Characteristics That Can Be Linked to GPS

A wide scope of neighbourhood characteristics can be linked to GPS, including physical and social items, quantitative and qualitative data. Not only the typical information that we find in topographical maps (e.g. roads, water, buildings, vegetation, recreational areas) is an important source. Also, population statistics and results of interviews and neighbourhood observations can be input for GIS, on the condition that a value can be assigned for different geographic units (e.g. per house, street, block). The input can, e.g. be based on questionnaires on proximity of facilities, interviews on perceived traffic safety, observations of pavement quality, satellite images of urban heat islands or fully automated counts of the volume of road traffic.

Examples of Neighbourhood and Physical Activity Research Using GPS

The neighbourhood environment is related to physical activity levels, and therefore the way we design and build our environment can affect healthy physical activity behaviour. In other words, spatial planning is relevant as a means of health promotion. In research on environment and physical activity, more objective and quantitative insights into persons' activities and exposures are needed. Such information can be added by application of GPS.

This section provides examples from two Dutch studies which applied GPS to investigate the relationship between neighbourhood characteristics and physical activity, i.e. the 'Spatial Planning and Children's Exercise (SPACE) study' and the 'Park or Flowerbed study' (see Textbox 9.2). The examples are presented in 3 subsections that illustrate that GPS can be used to assess (1) whether the respondent is indoors or outdoors, (2) whether respondents were using inactive or active transportation and (3) environmental exposure to neighbourhood characteristics by combining GPS, GIS data and data gathered via interviews.

Textbox 9.2. Overview of the SPACE and Park or Flowerbed Study

SPACE Study

Purpose: To identify neighbourhood characteristics that determine physical activity behaviour and to develop recommendations for a activity-friendly neighbourhood

Setting: Longitudinal study in 5 Dutch city neighbourhoods, both in 2004 and 2008

Sample: About 1,000 children of primary school age (6–11 years of age)

Methods: Anthropometry, neighbourhood observation, 7-day activity diary, GPS and accelerometry

Reference: de Vries et al. (2010)

Park or Flowerbed

Purpose: To identify neighbourhood characteristics that determine physical activity behaviour and develop recommendations for a activity-friendly neighbourhood

Setting: Qualitative study in 4 deprived neighbourhoods in Amsterdam (The Netherlands)

Sample: 111 respondents from three age groups (youth (age 13–17), adults (30–50) and elderly adults (60–80) living in one of the four selected deprived

Methods: Neighbourhood observation, 5-day activity diary, GPS, semi-structured interviews

More information: j.maas@vumc.nl

Examples of Using GPS to Classify Whether People Are Indoors or Outdoors

Figure 9.4 shows a section of a Park or Flowerbed participant's GPS track, where segments of the tracks are categorised as either indoors or outdoors. The section above on how to use GPS describes how the track segments were classified, which is partially automated by software. By classification of all trips in a study population, for example, the time spent outdoors and indoors can be quantified and can be analysed for personal and environmental determinants. This information can be relevant for research questions such as '*how much time is spent outdoors, what is the physical activity level outdoors and what are the determinants of being outdoors*'. Such questions are relevant as to inform decision makers on how to design a neighbourhood that attract people to engage in outdoor activities, which may be relevant for, e.g. physical activity and social interaction.

Examples of Using GPS to Classify Whether People Are Using Active Transportation

GPS data can be processed in such a way that the mode of transport of people can be determined. Figure 9.5 provides an example of how GPS tracks were classified as inactive (motorised) or active transportation in the Park or Flowerbed study. Figure 9.4 depicts segments within a GPS track of a Park or Flowerbed participant that were classified as walking, cycling and motorised transport.

The classification of the mode of transport can and has been used to address research questions like '*What percentage of subject's trips is by motorised or active means of transportation?*' (illustrated by Fig. 9.6), or '*What distance do people travel by bike, or on foot?*' or '*For which destinations do people favour active transportation?*' or '*Is traffic safety a determinant of the choice for cycling to school?*' The latter two questions require additional information on neighbourhood characteristics (exposure), as illustrated later in this chapter.

Figure 9.7 shows the frequency distribution of the distance travelled from home to their elementary school for a group of 88 children in the SPACE study. This data illustrates the distance to school that can be bridged by active transportation to school for this study sample. This data was used to assess the willingness of subjects to use active transportation from home to school as a function of the distance from home to school.

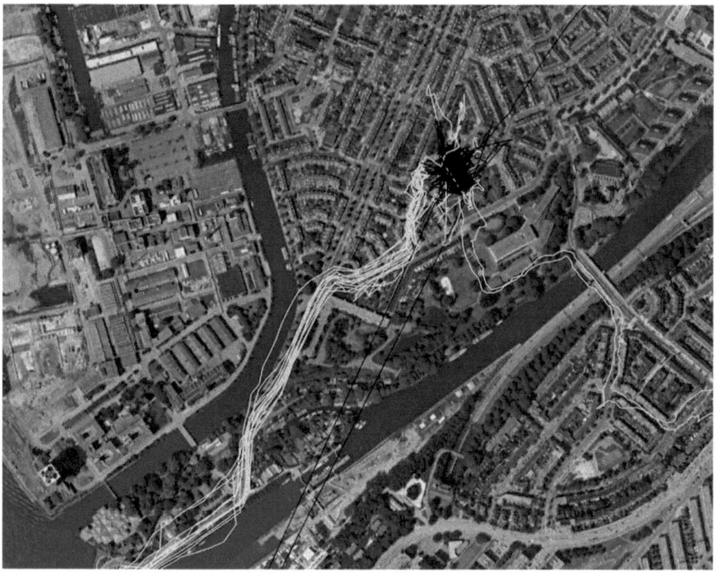

Fig. 9.4 GPS track where indoor (*black*) and outdoor (*light*) segments are differentiated, based on a filter (see Textbox 9.1)

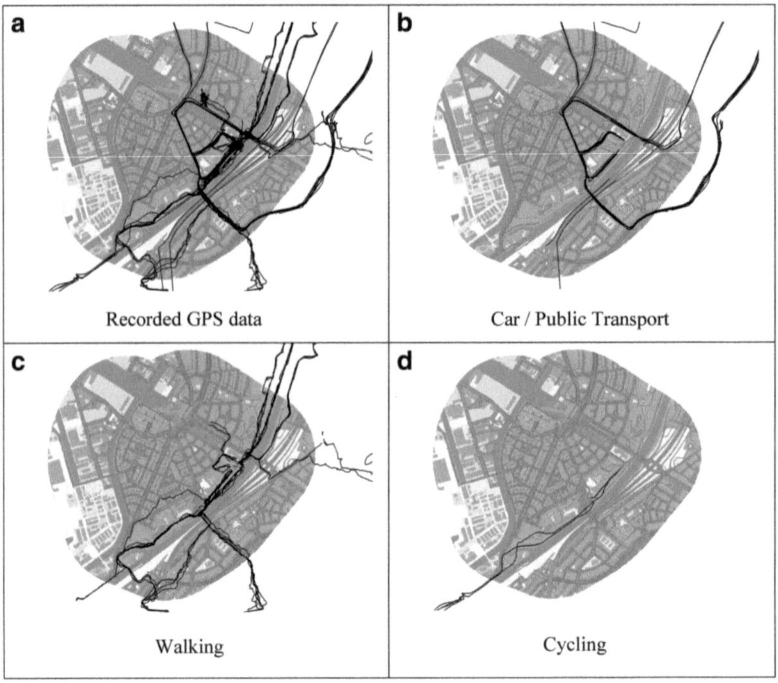

Fig. 9.5 Example of which modes of transport a respondent from the Park or Flowerbed study took during 5 days. Figures **b**, **c** and **d** show which routes were taken with the different modes of transport that were used by this respondent

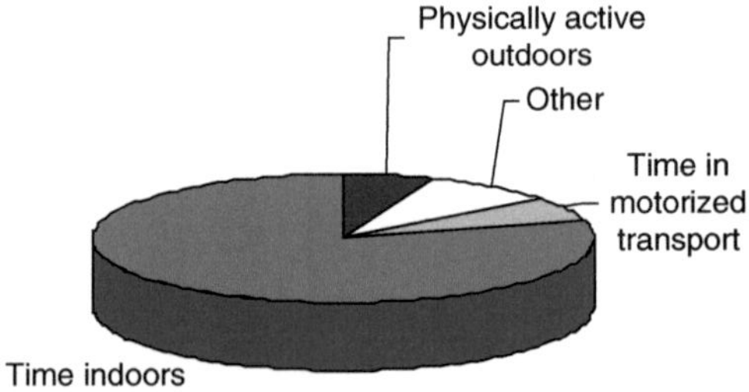

Fig. 9.6 Example for a distribution of the percentage of GPS track-time spent indoors, outdoors and with different activities, for a group of participants

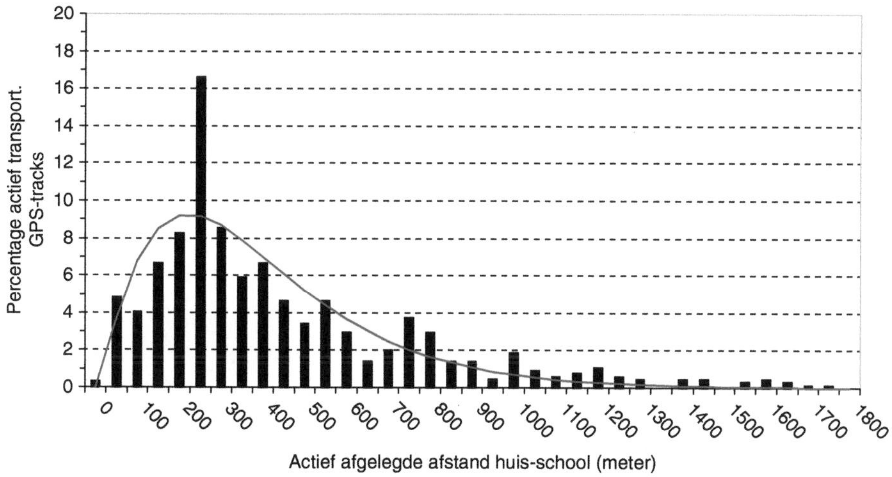

Fig. 9.7 Distribution of the percentage of active transportation measured by GPS tracks (*y*-axis) by distance between home and elementary school in meters on the *x* axis travelled by active transportation

Examples of Using GPS to Assess Exposure to Neighbourhood Characteristics

Where the sections above illustrated how GPS tracks can be classified as outdoors or indoors, and respectively per mode of transportation, the figures in this section show how further context can be added to GPS tracks to study neighbourhood characteristics of physical activity behaviour.

Figure 9.8 is a schematic example of a GPS track plotted over different layers of GIS information, in this case the percentage of green surface and the height of buildings. In this example, the coloured GPS track overlaps a 500×500 m grid where the colour of the grid cell expresses the percentage of green surface area. Another information layer is 'building height', represented by the numbers printed inside the grey squares (buildings). There are many GIS methods to assist data linkage. In the example above, the overlap of GPS track with 'green surface' can be used, and for building height, the proximity of high-rise buildings was assigned to the recorded GPS locations.

By linking the percentage of green surface per cell to the overlapping GPS track segment, we can analyse, among others, the availability of green surface along a person's route through the neighbourhood. The 'exposure' to green space can be analysed, for example, to answer the question '*Are green environments visited more frequent by foot or by bike than less green parts of the neighbourhood?*'

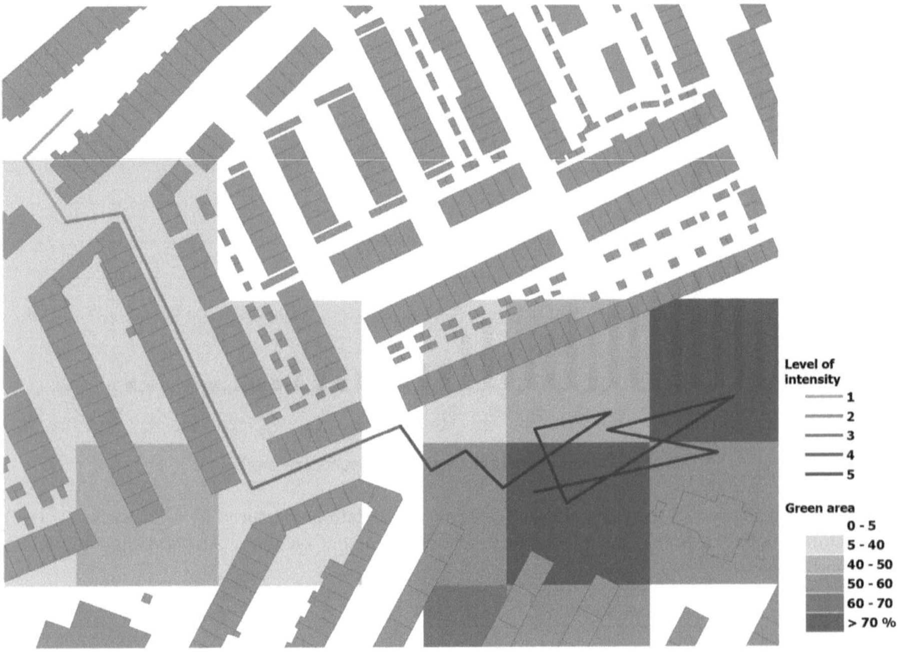

Fig. 9.8 GPS track linked to neighbourhood exposure to green space

Figure 9.9 is an example of Park or Flowerbed where GPS tracks were linked to geoinformation of the road network. The GPS data of all respondents of one neighbourhood was aggregated to illustrate how intensively certain roads were used, by means of transportation by foot. Subsequently, the figure can be used to analyse research questions like '*What were the motives and destinations for these trips?*' and '*What additional characteristics of the street determined the choice for this route* (e.g. *safety, green space)?*' by adding additional geoinformation. Such analyses in Park of Flowerbed showed, for instance, that especially older people walk to places were shops are located. Furthermore, the analyses showed that some neighbourhood residents chose for a route along green vegetation, which the residents also confirmed in the interviews when asked what the motive was for taking a certain route.

Figure 9.10 shows the result of adding perceived attractiveness data to the same area as in Fig. 9.9. In interviews, Park or Flowerbed participants answered how they experienced and appreciated their neighbourhood. They were also asked to name positive and negative places in their neighbourhood. The figure gives an overview of the spaces in one of the four neighbourhoods which were experienced as positive and negative. When the perceived attractiveness was overlaid with aggregated GPS data, it shows that certain places that are regarded as unsafe are avoided by people. For instance, at the border of

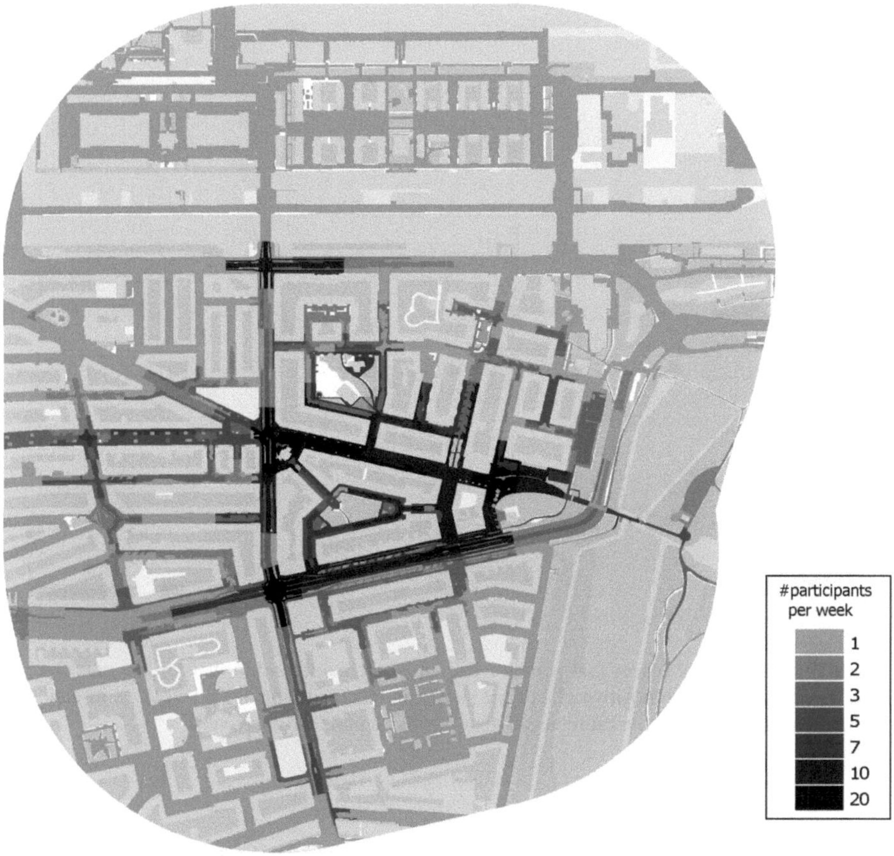

Fig. 9.9 Number of participants (from *light to dark*) that used a specific street segment by foot during 1 week of observation

the neighbourhood, there is a park (lower right part of Figs. 9.9–9.10). This park can be reached via two different ways, and only one of these ways was used. The tunnel which is perceived as unsafe is not used by the neighbourhood residents.

Another example of a research question could be: 'Are there differences in how different age groups use their neighbourhood?' Figure 9.11 shows the frequency of use of parts of the neighbourhood while walking for children, adults and elderly. The comparison shows that certain areas are more intensively used by a specific age group.

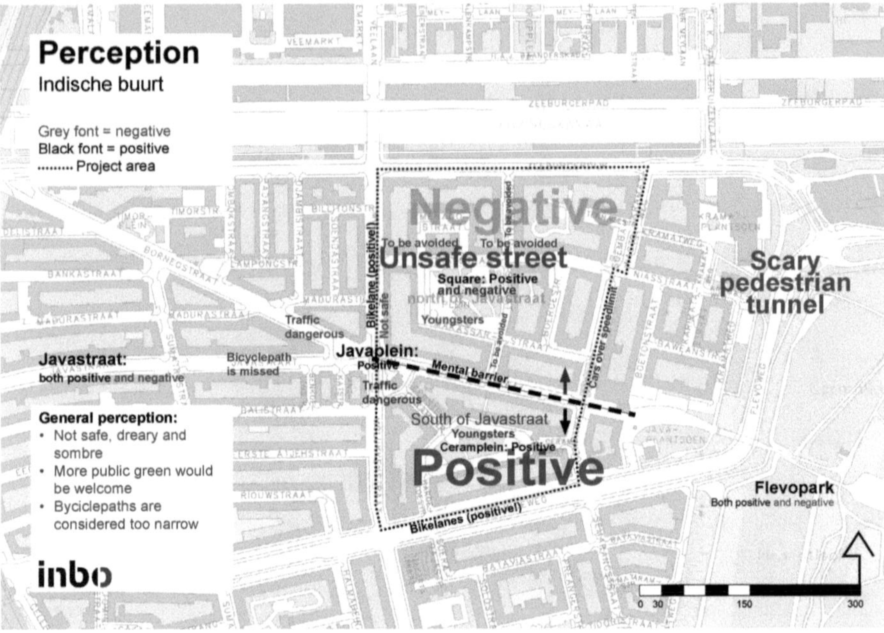

Fig. 9.10 Overview of places that people living in a neighbourhood in Amsterdam perceived as positive or negative. The positive places are shown in black and the negative places in *grey*. The larger the word is written, the more negative or positive a place was perceived

Examples of Using GPS to Assess Environmental Exposure on Other Outcomes

Although the focus of this chapter is on application of GPS in neighbourhood and physical activity behaviour, there are many other fields in which GPS enables a better understanding of the relationship between environmental exposure and health. Air pollution and noise are important contributors to the environmental burden of disease (WHO 2008). Figure 9.12 shows the noise exposure during a bicycle ride through a neighbourhood in the city of Rotterdam. The noise level was assessed by a portable meter, and the sound level averaged over 30 s is shown by the colour of the GPS track. Peaks in sound level were, e.g. observed near major roads. The effect of ambient noise levels on cardiovascular and stress effects by additional echocardiography (ECG) registrations is subject of research in ongoing studies.

Figure 9.13 is a similar figure, but showing ambient exposure to particulate. A mobile particle counter assessed the exposure during a car drive through the Netherlands. Peak levels of particulate matter were observed when in situation of busy traffic, and particularly when driving closely behind a heavy truck.

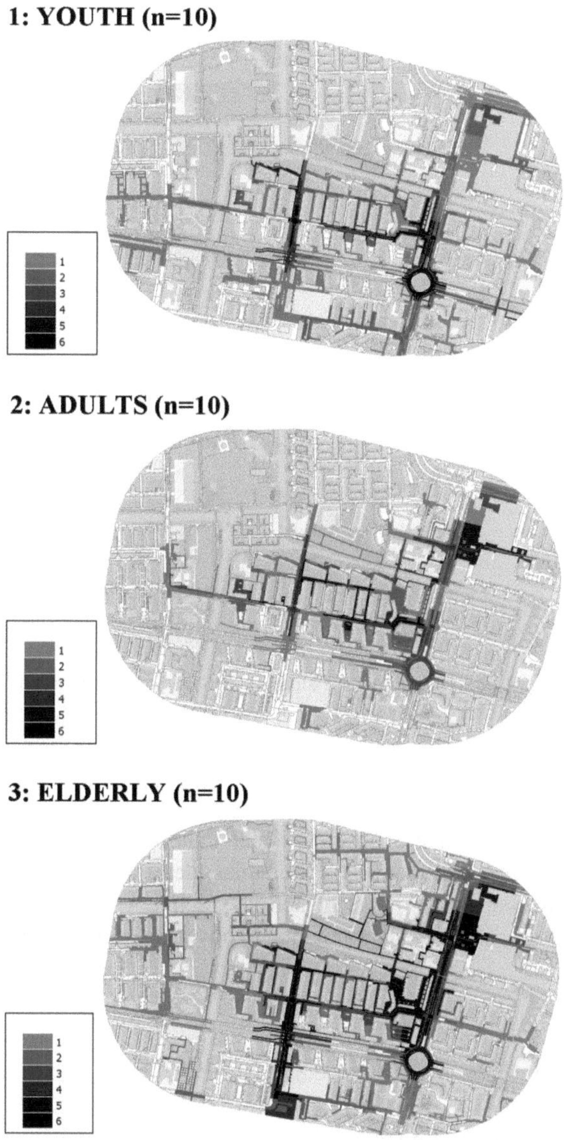

Fig. 9.11 Example of where youth (1), adults (2) and elderly (3) walked in their neighbourhood during 1 week. For instance the roundabout in the lower *right* part is in relatively frequently used by youth, but not by adults, whereas adults and the elderly are observed relatively frequently near the shopping *center* in the *upper right* corner

Discussion

This chapter illustrates the added value of GPS applications for gaining insight into the role of neighbourhood characteristics on physical activity and health in general, and in health promotion. GPS provides exact and objective insight into personal activities and

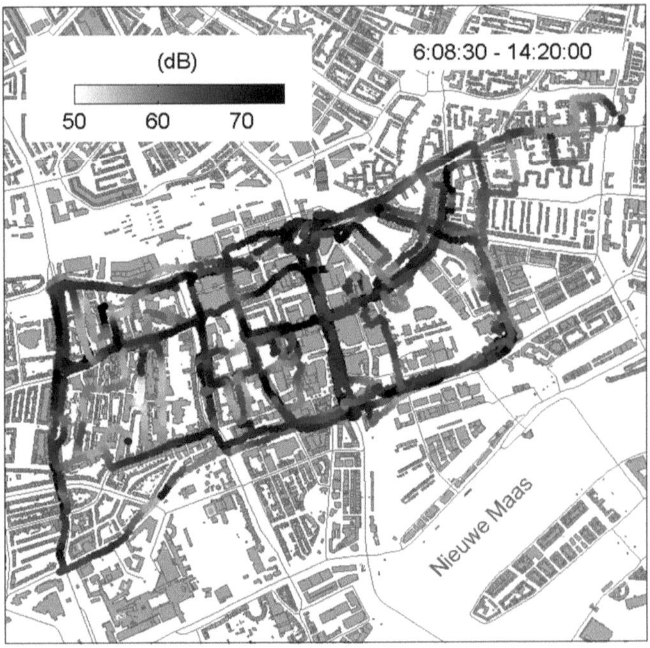

Fig. 9.12 Noise exposure along a GPS track on a topography layer

environmental exposures, which cannot be achieved by 'traditional' methods. Several examples show that GPS enables identification of location (indoors versus outdoors), assessment of physical activity (active versus motorised transportation, speed) and assessment of environmental exposure (e.g., green areas, air pollution).

Advantages and Considerations

Textbox 9.3 gives an overview of the advantages and considerations of using GPS in research. The textbox is based on the experience of the authors of this chapter during the past 5 years. Further applications and advantages will undoubtedly arise from additional experience. In our experience, acceptance of GPS by study respondents is relatively high. However, the privacy aspect is an important issue for respondents and should receive appropriate attention when recruiting and informing subjects.

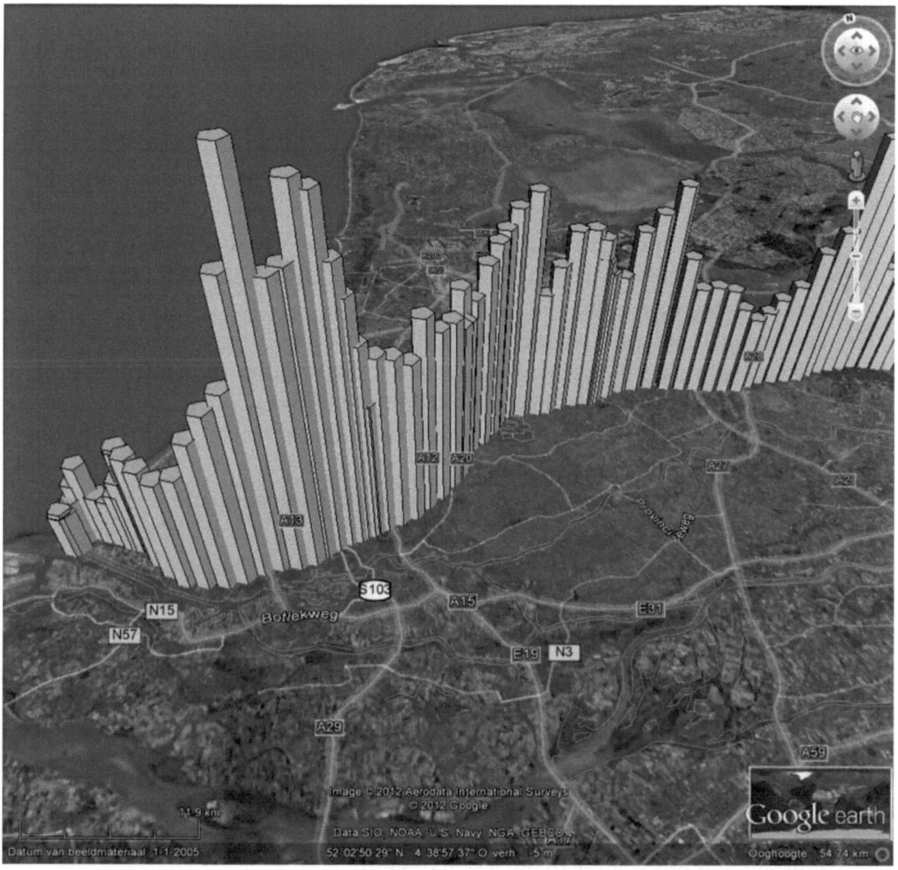

Fig. 9.13 Air pollution exposure along a GPS track. The height of the columns indicates the air pollution concentration

Several limitations and considerations need to be taken into account when designing a study employing GPS. For example, an active role of study participants is required; thus ample information and assistance on usage should be provided. The variety of specifications of the GPS devices can accommodate diverse research questions and designs. Per research question, it is advisable to choose the most appropriate device based on the requirements for accuracy, size, battery life, sample frequency and study duration. Besides the most appropriate hardware, it is also advisable to gather complementary data from the respondents besides the GPS data depending on the research question. For instance, it can be wise to complement the data with diaries or via an interview to ask people about their motives to be at certain places.

Textbox 9.3. Summary of Advantages and Considerations for Using GPS

Advantages

- Small, light, unobtrusive and affordable devices are now available.
- The variety in GPS devices allows usage for many different study designs (e.g. from memory equipped GPS loggers that operate for 2–3 days without charging, to smart phones that send GPS tracks to a central server).
- The position error is generally 10–15 m, and GPS is more accurate than self-reported travel surveys.
- Indoor and outdoor positions can be differentiated.
- GPS aids in identifying trips and active transportation and differentiating the mode of transport (motorised, walking, cycling).
- GPS allows quantification of environmental exposures (e.g. noise, air pollution, built environment).
- GPS provides insight in the intensity level of physical activity.

Considerations

- The precision of GPS position assessment can be hampered by shedding of radio signals (e.g. by high-rise buildings, leafy trees, indoors), which should be considered, e.g. by filtering of data.
- A good manual, preferably with pictures, can help respondents to wear and handle GPS devices in order to collect as much valid data as possible.
- Technical expertise is required to operate GPS devices, and GIS skills are essential for acquiring environmental exposures linked to GPS.
- Privacy issues should be taken into account, e.g. by IRB approval, informed consent and procedures to ensure anonymity.
- GPS data can be complemented with diaries, interviews or other sensor data (e.g. accelerometer, heart rate monitor).

References

Adams, C., Riggs, P., & Volckens, J. (2009). Development of a method for personal, spatiotemporal exposure assessment. *Journal of Environmental Monitoring, 11*(7), 1331–1339.

American Journal of Preventive Medicine. (1998). Physical activity interventions. *American Journal of Preventive Medicine, 15*, 255–432.

Badland, H. M., Duncan, M. J., Oliver, M., Duncan, J. S., & Mavoa, S. (2010). Examining commute routes: applications of GIS and GPS technology. *Environmental Health and Preventive Medicine, 15*(5), 327–330.

Brownson, R. C., Hoehner, C. M., Day, K., Forsyth, A., & Sallis, J. F. (2009). Measuring the built environment for physical activity: state of the science. *American Journal of Preventive Medicine, 36*(4S), 99–123.

Burton, L. M. M., Matthews, S. A. P., Leung, M., Kemp, S. P. A., & Takeuchi, D. T. T. (2011). *Communities, neighborhoods, and health: expanding the boundaries of place*. New York: Springer.

Clark, M. I., Berry, T. R., Spence, J. C., Nykiforuk, C., Carlson, M., & Blanchard, C. (2010). Key stakeholder perspectives on the development of walkable neighbourhoods. *Health & Place, 16*(1), 43–50.

de Vries, S. I., Hopman-Rock, M., Bakker, I., Hirasing, R. A., & van Mecheeln, W. (2010). Built environmental correlates of walking and cycling in Dutch urban children: Results from the SPACE study. *International Journal of Environmental Research and Public Health, 7*(5), 2309–2324.

Dishman, R. K., & Buckworth, J. (1996). Increasing physical activity: a quantitative synthesis. *Medicine and Science in Sports and Exercise, 28*, 706–709.

Dollman, J., Norton, K., & Norton, L. (2005). Evidence for secular trends in children's physical activity behaviour. *British Journal of Sports Medicine, 39*(12), 892–897.

Duncan, M. J., & Mummery, W. K. (2007). GIS or GPS? A comparison of two methods for assessing route taken during active transport. *American Journal of Preventive Medicine, 33*(1), 51–53.

Giles-Corti, B., & King, A. C. (2009). Creating active environments across the life course: thinking outside the square. *British Journal of Sports Medicine, 43*(2), 109–113.

Giles-Corti, B., Timperio, A., Bull, F., & Pikora, T. (2005). Understanding physical activity environmental correlates: increased specificity for ecological models. *Exercise and Sport Sciences Reviews, 33*(4), 175–181.

Kawachi, I., & Berkman, L. F. (2003). *Neighbourhoods and health*. Oxford: Oxford University Press.

Kerr, J., Duncan, S., & Schipperijn, J. (2011). Using global positioning systems in health research: A practical approach to data collection and processing. *American Journal of Preventive Medicine, 41*(5), 532–540.

Krenn, P. J., Mag, D. I., Titze, S., Oja, P., Jones, A., & Ogilvie, D. (2011). Use of global positioning systems to study physical activity and the environment. *American Journal of Preventive Medicine, 41*(5), 508–515.

Lauretani, F., Maggio, M., Valenti, G., Dall'Aglio, E., & Ceda, G. P. (2010). Vitamin D in older population: new roles for this "classic actor"? *The Aging Male, 13*(4), 215–232.

Marcus, B. H., Dubbert, P. M., Forsyth, L. H., McKenzie, T. L., Stone, E. J., et al. (2000). Physical activity behavior change: issues in adoption and maintenance. *Health Psychology, 19*, 17–32.

McDonald, N. C. (2007). Active transportation to school: trends among U.S. schoolchildren, 1969–2001. *American Journal of Preventive Medicine, 32*(6), 509–516.

Morabia, A., Mirer, F. E., Amstislavski, T. M., et al. (2010). Potential health impact of switching from car to public transportation when commuting to work. *American Journal of Public Health, 100*(12), 2388–2391.

Ooijendijk, W. T. M., Hildebrandt, V. H., & Chorus, A. M. J. (2008). Physical activity in the Netherlands 2000–2007 [In Dutch]. In V. H. Hildebrandt, W. T. M. Ooijendijk, & M. Hopman-Rock (Eds.), *Trend report physical activity and health [In Dutch]* (pp. 9–42). Leiden: De Bink.

Saelens, B. E., & Handy, S. L. (2008). Built environment correlates of walking: A review. *Medicine and Science in Sports and Exercise, 40*(7 Suppl), S550–S566.

Saelens, B. E., Sallis, J. F., & Frank, L. D. (2003). Environmental correlates of walking and cycling: findings from the transportation, urban design, and planning literatures. *Annals of Behavioral Medicine, 25*(2), 80–91.

Sallis, J. F., Cervero, R., Ascher, W., Henderson, K. A., Kraft, M. K., & Kerr, J. (2006). An ecological approach to creating active living communities. *Annual Review of Public Health, 27*, 297–322.

Stopher, P., Fitzgerald, C., & Xu, M. (2007). Assessing the accuracy of the Sydney Household Travel Survey with GPS. *Transportation, 34*(6), 723–741.

Swinburn, B., Egger, G., & Raza, F. (1999). Dissecting obesogenic environments: the development and application of a framework for identifying and prioritizing environmental interventions for obesity. *Preventive Medicine*, Part 1 *29*(6), 563–570.

WHO. (2008). *The global burden of disease: 2004 update*. Geneva: World Health Organization.

Chapter 10
Mathematical Approaches to Analysing Area-Level Effects on Health

Ulrike Grittner and Kim Bloomfield

Introduction

In social research, studies that investigate the relationship between individuals and the society they live in are very common. Individuals interact within the social context of their group; i.e. they are influenced by group and contextual characteristics and, in turn, group characteristics are influenced by the individuals who constitute the group. As a result of group clustering, data from individuals of a group are often more similar to each other (i.e. correlated) in contrast to data from individuals from different groups.

Such clustered or hierarchical data can be analysed at different hierarchical levels, while variables at each level may be incorporated. This leads to research that identifies the variance in the outcome that is related to the different levels of. Additionally it evaluates the association of individual or group characteristics at the appropriate levels with the outcome. This kind of analysis is referred to as 'multilevel analysis' (Snijders and Bosker 1999). The method has been described under various names such as hierarchical models (Raudenbush and Bryk 2002), random effects models (Dunson 2008) and mixed models (Verbeke and Molenberghs 2000; Zuur et al. 2009).

With respect to social epidemiology, most studies of neighbourhood effects on health aim at controlling individual factors (such as age, sex, educational achievement, income) in the analysis. This requires multilevel modelling due to the fact that

U. Grittner (✉)
Department for Biostatistics and Clinical Epidemiology,
Charité-University Medicine, Charitéplatz 1, 10117 Berlin, Germany
e-mail: ulrike.grittner@charite.de

K. Bloomfield
Center for Alcohol and Drug Research, School of Business and Social Science,
Aarhus University, Artillerivej 90, 2300 Copenhagen S, Denmark
e-mail: kb@crf.au.dk

C. Stock and A. Ellaway (eds.), *Neighbourhood Structure and Health Promotion*,
DOI 10.1007/978-1-4614-6672-7_10,

data nested at different levels of sampling are combined into one analysis. Some examples of hierarchical data include pupils who are nested in classes or in schools, residents who live in neighbourhoods, employees who are nested in firms, teeth that are nested in patients and municipalities that are nested in regions and a prominent example: repeated measurements are nested in subjects. Here, we name the lower level units (individuals, pupils, employees, teeth, municipalities, repeated measurements) as level 1 units and the higher level units (neighbourhoods, schools, firms, regions, subjects) as level 2 units.

In all these cases, there might be dependence or correlation between the level 1 units that cannot be ignored with regard to the analysed outcome. It makes a difference if analysing, for example, data on 300 pupils from 300 different classes (no hierarchical data structure) in contrast to an analysis of data on 300 pupils from 15 different classes (20 pupils per class, nested data structure). Pupils in one class tend to be more similar to each other than to pupils in different classes with regard to an outcome variable such as results of a math test. To ignore this dependency may yield misleading results.

We assume that the reader is familiar with linear and logistic regression. If needing additional reading about linear or logistic regression, we recommend, for example, Montgomery and Peck (1992) or Kleinbaum and Klein (2010). We will not explain here the more technical details or the mathematical background of the models used. For further reading, we recommend, for example, Verbeke and Molenberghs (2000), Zuur et al. (2009) or Raudenbush and Bryk (2002). We also recommend the webpage of the Centre for Multilevel Modelling at the University of Bristol which contains helpful material (http://www.bristol.ac.uk/cmm/).

Using a small data example, we will first demonstrate how traditional techniques fail to model the data in an appropriate way and will then show how a linear multilevel model could be applied. We will then analyse the whole data set and also demonstrate how to apply a logistic multilevel model for dichotomous outcomes. We will provide software commands in different software languages.

The Data Example

As an illustrative example, we use data from the 'Danish Youth Cohort' from 2005 (Stock et al. 2011). The data set consists of information from 10,380 seventh-grade Danish pupils from 407 schools. Stock et al. (2011) analysed how individual and school district characteristics are related to active transportation to school.

In our example, we focus on the relationship between individual (level 1) and school district characteristics (level 2) on one hand and the academic performance of the pupils (the outcome variable) on the other hand. The information about the pupils' academic performance comes from the following question: 'How well do you think you are doing at school academically?' with response categories: 'not good' (1), 'average' (2), 'good' (3) and 'very good' (4). For illustrative reasons, we treat academic performance here as a metric variable even if it is an ordinal variable and assume a linear relationship between academic performance and several individual- or school-level characteristics.

Information about academic performance was available for 10,272 pupils in the sample [percentages in the different categories were as follows: 'not good' (3.1 %), 'average' (20.6 %), 'good' (56.3 %) and 'very good' (20.1 %)].

For the following examples, let us take a subsample of 10 selected school districts containing information on 162 pupils from this larger Danish pupil data set. We wish to examine if there is any relationship between academic performance and daily physical activity [physical activity of less than 1 h a day (0) or 1 h or more (1)].

Traditional Techniques

Ordinary Linear Regression at Pupil Level: Ignoring Nested Data Structure and Dependence

Let us first analyse these data using traditional statistical techniques such as ordinary least-squares regression (Kreft and De Leeuw 1998). Linear regression models have some assumptions. These are: normally distributed residuals after applying the model, homogeneity in the variance of the outcome over all covariates, fixed covariate matrix, independence among the analysed units (individuals) and correct model specification.

We now perform a simple linear regression to examine the relationship between physical activity and academic performance, assuming that there are no substantial differences *between the schools* regarding average academic performance of the pupils. Such a model takes the form of

$$y_i = \beta_0 + \beta_1 x_{1i} + \varepsilon_i, \tag{10.1}$$

where y_i is the academic performance value of the *i*th pupil (range 1–4),
β_0 is the intercept,
β_1 is the slope which is related to the physical activity of the pupil,
x_{1i} is the value for the physical activity (0: <1 h a day, 1: 1 h or more) of the *i*th pupil and ε_i is the residual for the *i*th pupil (mean 0, constant variance σ_ε^2).

For completeness and for later comparisons, we also calculate a *null model* without covariates and obtain the coefficients that are reported in Table 10.2.

Let us interpret the model (Table 10.2) with the covariate for physical activity. The intercept (beta = 2.93) can be interpreted as the mean academic performance for those pupils who are physically active <1 h a day. Those who are physically active 1 h or more a day have an average performance value that is 0.04 points higher as indicated by the slope coefficient. But the standard error (se) for the slope

Table 10.1 Descriptive data for ten selected schools, (size, mean of academic performance, % of pupils who are more than 1 h a day physically active)

School	Number of pupils	Mean of academic performance[a]	% of pupils who are physically active for more than 1 h per day
1	29	2.93	79.3
2	10	2.30	30.0
3	13	2.77	84.6
4	30	3.30	80.6
5	16	3.25	75.0
6	11	2.73	72.7
7	10	2.70	50.0
8	15	3.07	86.7
9	11	2.82	72.7
10	17	2.94	82.4

[a]Range: 1–4; 1: not good; 4: very good

Table 10.2 Linear regression models for academic performance (significant coefficients in bold), $N=162$ pupils in ten schools

	Null model		With physical activity	
	Beta	se	Beta	se
Intercept β_0	**2.96**	**0.06**	**2.93**	**0.12**
Slope β_1 (1 h or more physical activity per day)	–		0.04	0.14
R^2	0		0.001	
σ_ε^2	0.60		0.60	

coefficient is relatively high (i.e., 0.14, greater than twice the coefficient), meaning that the slope coefficient is not significant. Therefore, we would conclude that physical activity is not significantly related to the academic performance of the pupils.

With such a simple regression, we would ignore the fact that pupils are nested in schools. But pupils in one school might be more similar with regard to their academic performance than pupils in another school, and the relationship between academic performance and physical activity might also differ between schools. In fact, the range between the ten schools with regard to the mean academic performance of the pupils of a school is between 2.3 and 3.3 (Table 10.1), and with a Kruskal–Wallis test, we would conclude that there are significant differences with regard to academic performance between the ten schools ($p=0.024$). Further, in five of the schools (schools 2, 4, 5, 6, 7), the mean performance of pupils who are more active is higher, while in the remaining five schools (schools 1, 3, 8, 9, 10), the opposite is true. Therefore, we cannot assume that the nested structure of the data is unimportant. Taking this into consideration would be a better use of all the information that the data set provides and would offer more explanatory power regarding academic performance (Table 10.2).

Table 10.3 Linear regression models for academic performance with aggregated data, $N=10$ schools (significant effects in bold)

	Null model		With physical activity	
	Beta	se	Beta	se
Intercept β_0	**2.96**	**0.09**	**2.00**	**0.37**
Slope β_1 (fraction of physical active pupils)	–		**1.28**	**0.49**
R^2	0		0.47	
σ_ε^2	0.008		0.005	

Regression with Aggregated Data on School Level: Ignoring Within-School Variance

However, if we are more interested in the differences between *schools* with regard to academic performance than in the differences between *individual pupils*, we could simply use aggregated data from the 10 schools. Here, we use the mean performance and the percentage of pupils who are more active (1 or more hour per day) at each school to fit the following model:

$$y_j = \beta_0 + \beta_1 x_{1j} + \varepsilon_j, \tag{10.2}$$

where y_j is the mean performance value of the jth school,
β_0 is the intercept,
β_1 is the slope which is related to the percentage of pupils per school who are more physically active,
x_{1j} is the fraction of pupils who more active per school at the jth school (range 0–1) and ε_j is the residual (mean 0, constant variance σ_ε^2).

Additionally, the regression is weighted by the number of pupils for the particular school divided by the total number to account for different sample sizes in schools.

We also calculate a null model without covariates to obtain the coefficients that are reported in Table 10.3.

We would conclude that the mean self-rated academic performance of pupils in a school is significantly related to the fraction of physically active pupils insofar as those schools where more pupils are physically active also have a better mean academic performance (higher value).

With such an aggregated regression, however, we ignore variability within the schools (i.e. among the pupils). This regression is based only on 10 units of observation (schools). The results must be interpreted cautiously because we cannot say anything about the individuals (i.e. if individual physical activity would be related to individual academic performance). This problem is known as the ecological fallacy (Freedman 2004).

Analysis on Pupil Level Accounting for Different Schools: Analysis of Covariance

With an analysis of covariance (ANCOVA), we can test the relationship between physical activity and academic performance while accounting for differences between schools with regard to average academic performance. If we additionally include an interaction term for schools and physical activity, we can test if the relationship between physical activity and academic performance differs between schools. If the interaction term is significant, it is more appropriate to calculate 10 individual regressions with ordinary least-square estimation instead of ANCOVA analysis as stated in many textbooks; otherwise the F-tests are biased (see, e.g. Kreft and De Leeuw 1998; Bijleveld and van der Kamp 1998).

In our example the interaction term is significant and we obtain 10 single regressions of the type:

$$y_{ij} = \beta_{0j} + \beta_{1j}x_{1ij} + \varepsilon_{ij}, \tag{10.3}$$

where y_{ij} is the academic performance value of pupil i in school j,
β_{0j} is the mean value of academic performance at school j for pupils who are not physically active,
β_{1j} is the slope of school j for physical activity,
x_{1ij} is the physical activity (0 or 1) value of pupil i at school j and
ε_{ij} is the error term at the pupils' level (mean 0, variance $\sigma^2_{\varepsilon j}$),

where each school has three coefficients for extra regression equations (intercept β_{0j}, slope β_{1j}, error variance $\sigma^2_{\varepsilon j}$) which results for the 10 schools in a total of 30 regression parameters (Table 10.4, error variance not shown).

As a result of the ANCOVA in our example, we can conclude that there are significant differences between the schools with regard to average academic performance ($F=77.12$, $df=10$, $p<0.001$) and that there are significant differences between the schools with regard to the relationship between physical activity and academic performance ($F=3.59$, $df=10$, $p<0.001$). The latter finding is also illustrated in (Fig. 10.1) where we see that in some schools pupils who are more active have a better academic performance (schools 2, 4, 5, 6, 7), while in other schools the opposite is true (schools 1, 3, 8, 9, 10).[1]

The advantage of ANCOVA or separate regressions for every school is that we model more adequately the differences between schools with regard to mean academic performance as well as the relationship of pupils' physical activity and academic performance. This is in contrast to a total or aggregated regression where

[1]Note that every regression line is defined by only two points.

Table 10.4 ANCOVA and single regressions for academic performance in ten schools, $n = 162$ pupils (significant effects in bold)

School	Null model (ANCOVA)		With physical activity (10 single regressions)			
	Beta	se	Intercept	se	Slope for physical activity (β_{1j})	se
1	**2.93**	**0.14**	**3.50**	**0.31**	**−0.72**	**0.35**
2	**2.30**	**0.24**	**2.00**	**0.27**	1.00	0.49
3	**2.77**	**0.21**	**4.00**	**0.46**	**−1.46**	**0.50**
4	**3.30**	**0.14**	**3.00**	**0.26**	0.38	0.21
5	**3.25**	**0.19**	**3.00**	**0.22**	0.33	0.25
6	**2.73**	**0.23**	**2.00**	**0.54**	1.00	0.64
7	**2.70**	**0.24**	**2.40**	**0.28**	0.60	0.40
8	**3.07**	**0.19**	**4.00**	**0.59**	−1.08	0.63
9	**2.82**	**0.23**	**3.33**	**0.31**	−0.71	0.36
10	**2.94**	**0.18**	**3.67**	**0.40**	−0.88	0.44
R^2	0.89					

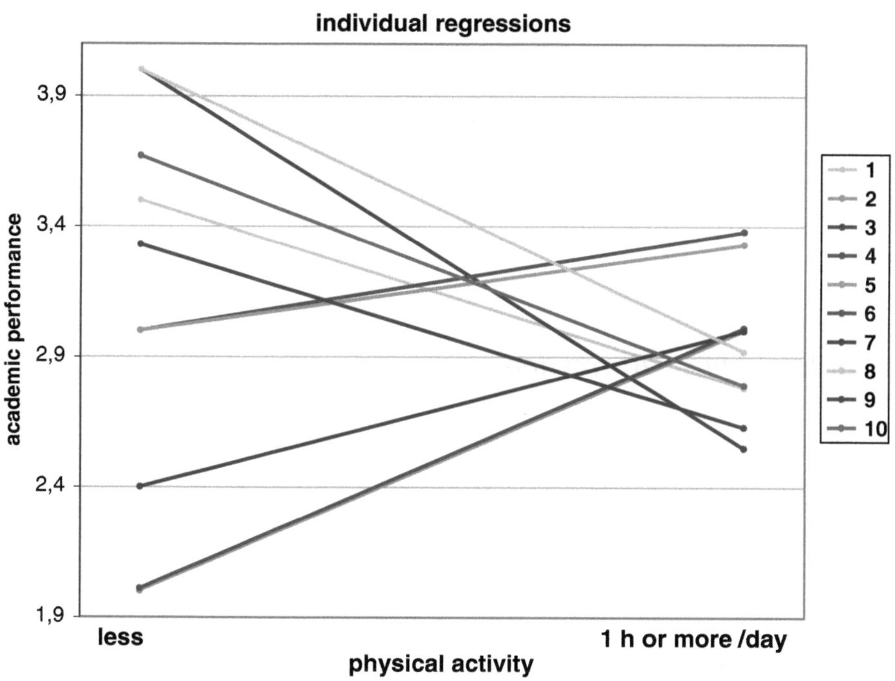

Fig. 10.1 Regression *lines* for each school for the relation between physical activity and academic performance

we have only one overall (for all pupils from all schools) slope coefficient for the relationship between physical activity and academic performance.

However, there are some drawbacks to ANCOVA or separate regressions including that ANCOVA indicates that differences exist between schools, but we cannot test or further explain why differences between schools exist. It is not possible to incorporate school-level characteristics as covariates in the model. Another disadvantage is the large number of parameter estimates. Even if there would not be significant interaction, we would still obtain 11 regression parameters (10 intercepts for the districts and a slope parameter for physical activity), and this number increases with every additional level 2 unit. That means that ANCOVA or separate regressions are only reasonable if the number of level 2 units is small (<20).

Multilevel Modelling

The main idea of multilevel modelling is to integrate the regression at level 1 (e.g. individuals) with level 2 (e.g. schools) or higher levels into one regression equation and also to incorporate covariates at appropriate levels. In addition, it is possible to adjust for correlation between level 1 units, i.e. similarity of the level 1 units that belong to the same level 2 unit. In other words, we account for heterogeneity between higher level units, i.e. differences between the groups of level 1 units. Alternatively, if a clustered data structure is present, we could simply conduct extra regressions for each cluster. But if we also want to make overall inferences about relationships between lower level as well as higher level characteristics and the outcome, we can combine these regressions into one regression model with multilevel techniques.

Multilevel Linear Regression

The assumptions underlying the multilevel linear regression model are similar to those for ordinary multiple regression analysis: linear relationships, homoscedasticity and normal distribution of the residuals (Hox and Maas 2004). But now, dependence of lower level units is also accounted for.

For a multilevel analysis, most software packages require that the data be arranged in the following way (Fig. 10.2): one line for every level 1 unit (e.g. pupils: 'pupil_id'), a variable for identification of higher level units (e.g. schools: here 'school' with a school id number), covariates that contain information about level 1 or higher level characteristics as variables with entries in every line (here academic performance: 'perform' range: 1–4, physical activity: 'activ': 0 or 1).

The following section demonstrates how multilevel linear regression modelling works step by step.

Fig. 10.2 Example of multilevel data structure

school	pupil_id	perform	activ
1	1	1	1
1	2	4	0
1	3	3	0
1	4	1	1
2	5	2	0
2	6	3	1
2	7	1	0
2	8	4	1
3	9	4	1
3	10	2	1
3	11	1	1
…	…	…	…

Step 1: The Random Intercept Model Without Covariates

In the first step, we analyse a model with no explanatory variables. This model is similar to the null model which we calculated with traditional regression techniques and is called the intercept-only model.

The equation is

$$y_{ij} = \beta_0 + u_{0j} + \varepsilon_{ij}, \tag{10.4}$$

where y_{ij} is the academic performance value of pupil i in school j,
β_0 is the intercept,
u_{0j} is the residual or random effect for school j (mean 0, variance σ^2_{u0}) and
ε_{ij} is the error term for pupil i at school j (mean 0, variance σ^2_{ε}).

This model does not explain factors that are related to the academic performance of pupils. It only decomposes the variance of academic performance into a component that is related to school differences (σ^2_{u0}) and a component that is related to differences between pupils (σ^2_{ε}).

The SAS (SAS institute Inc., 2008) syntax to run this model is:

```
proc mixed data=walk covtest ;
     class school ;
     model perform= /Solution cl ;
     random intercept / subject=school;
run;
```

Table 10.5 Multilevel linear model for academic performance, random intercept model without covariates (10 schools, 162 pupils) (significant effects in bold)

Fixed effects	Beta	se
Intercept β_0	**2.91**	**0.09**
Variance estimates for random effects		
Variance between schools σ^2_{u0}	0.04	0.04
Variance between pupils σ^2_{ε}	**0.56**	**0.06**

where *walk* is the name of our data set, *school* is a variable that contains one specific numeric value for every school and *perform* is the variable that contains the values for academic performance of the pupils.

In the Appendix, we list the corresponding commands in STATA (StataCorp. 2007), R (R Development Core Team 2011; Pinheiro et al. 2011) and SPSS (SPSS for Windows 2011). We will not explain in detail here what the commands stand for. For further details, see Zuur et al. (2009), Venables and Ripley (2002) or Verbeke and Molenberghs (2000).[2]

With Equation 10.4 for the intercept-only model, we are interested in the intercept β_0 and the two variance estimates σ^2_{u0} for the variance between schools and σ^2_{ε} for the variance between pupils. From the output, we obtain the values depicted in Table 10.5.

'Fixed effects' are the overall effects across all schools and can be interpreted in the same way as in non-hierarchical linear regression. Here, the fixed effect is the parameter for the intercept (β_0). But we know already that the schools differ with regard to the academic performance of the pupils. Especially when we analyse a sample with many schools, we are not interested in the particular intercepts and effects from each school, but more in the *distribution* of intercepts across schools, because then we see if pupils in different schools are more or less similar with regard to the outcome. Thus, we examine the variance estimate for the school intercepts (σ^2_{u0}). It is not significant here, meaning that the 10 schools do not differ significantly from each other with regard to the mean academic performance of their pupils. However, this may be because our sample is small; significance could be present if we had included many more schools in the analysis.

The value for σ^2_{ε} is a measure for the residual variance on the pupil level and is significant, meaning that there are significant differences with regard to academic performance among the individual pupils after taking into account differences in mean performance between schools.

We can now calculate the intra-class correlation (ICC) which is a measure of the average degree of dependence of level 1 units (pupils) within a school. Here, we obtain an estimate for the average similarity or dependence of pupils within a school with regard to academic performance.

[2]Note: for the random effects in STATA and R, the standard deviation is given, while in SAS and SPSS, the variance (the square of the standard deviation) is given in the output.

The equation for calculation of the ICC is

$$\rho = \frac{\sigma_{u0}^2}{\sigma_{u0}^2 + \sigma_\varepsilon^2}.$$

It is the proportion of variance that is accounted for by the schools.

In our example, the ICC is $\rho = \frac{0.04}{0.04 + 0.56} = 0.07$.

That means that 7 % of the variance between the pupils' academic performance is explained by school differences. We conclude that differences of academic performance between pupils are present but are only explained to a small degree by school differences.

Step 2: Integrating Covariates on the Individual Level as Fixed Effects

Now we want to extend our model to see how physical activity is related to academic performance.

Our model can be described by the following equation:

$$y_{ij} = \beta_0 + \beta_1 x_{1ij} + u_{0j} + \varepsilon_{ij}, \tag{10.5}$$

where y_{ij} is the academic performance value of pupil i in school j,
β_0 is the fixed effect intercept,
β_1 is the fixed effect slope for physical activity,
x_{1ij} is the value for physical activity (0 or 1) of pupil i in school j,
u_{0j} is the residual or random effect for the intercept for school j (mean 0, variance σ_{u0}^2) and
ε_{ij} is the error term for pupil i at school j (mean 0, variance σ_ε^2).

To run this model, we modify the previous syntax by adding to the command line '*activ*' which is a dichotomous variable describing the physical activity of each pupil as 1 h per day physical active (1) or not (0).

In SAS:

```
proc mixed data=walk covtest ;
     class school ;
     model perform= activ /Solution cl ;
     random intercept / subject=school;
run;
```

As the results of the analysis show (Table 10.6) the slope coefficient for physical activity (β_1) is not significant, meaning that there is no significant relationship overall between physical activity and academic performance of pupils.

However, the regression-related graph (Fig. 10.3) looks very different compared to Fig. 10.1. The separate regressions (Fig. 10.1) describe our data more exactly

Table 10.6 Multilevel linear model for academic performance, random intercept model with individual level covariate (10 schools, 162 pupils) (significant effects in bold)

Fixed effects	Beta	se
Intercept β_0	**2.93**	**0.14**
Slope for physical activity β_1	−0.03	0.14
Variance estimates for random effects		
Variance between school intercepts σ_{u0}^2	0.05	0.04
Variance between pupils σ_ε^2	**0.56**	**0.07**

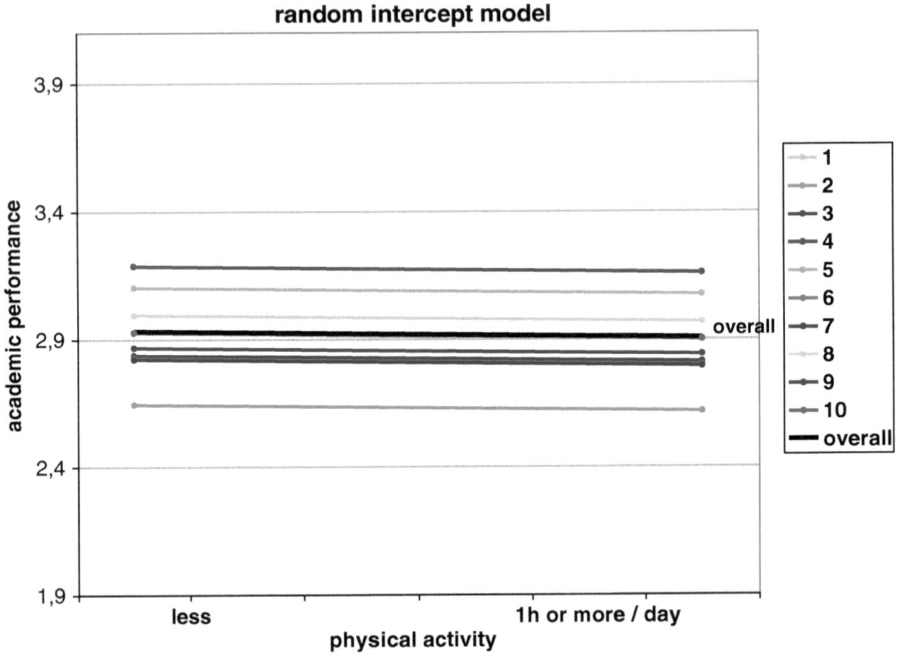

Fig. 10.3 Regression-based *lines* for every school for the random intercept model with regard to the relationship between physical activity and academic performance

because in the random intercept model, we have assumed that the relationship between physical activity and academic performance (the slope) is the same in each school, which is clearly not the case. We conclude that the random intercept model is not a very good model for our data because so far we have not allowed the slope to vary between schools.

It should be noted that other covariates on the individual level could also be integrated in the model. When analysing data sets with more units on the higher level, additional covariates on that level could also be tested, for example, different school characteristics.

Table 10.7 Multilevel linear model for academic performance, random intercept and slope model with individual level covariate (10 schools, 162 pupils) (significant effects in bold)

Fixed effects	Beta	se
Intercept β_0	**2.95**	**0.14**
Slope for physical activity β_1	−0.04	0.16
Variance estimates for random effects		
Variance between school intercepts σ^2_{u0}	0.06	0.08
Variance between school slopes σ^2_{u1}	0.07	0.10
Variance between pupils σ^2_{ε}	**0.53**	**0.07**

Step 3: Adding a Random Slope

We will now add a random slope for physical activity to the model. That means we allow not only for the intercepts to vary between schools but also the slopes.

The equation is now extended by $u_{1j}x_{ij}$:

$$y_{ij} = \beta_0 + \beta_1 x_{1ij} + u_{0j} + u_{1j}x_{1ij} + \varepsilon_{ij}. \tag{10.6}$$

Here, $\beta_1 + u_{1j}$ is the slope for physical activity in school *j*, where β_1 is the fixed part and u_{1j} is the random part with mean 0 and variance σ^2_{u1}.

In SAS:

```
proc mixed data=walk covtest ;
     class school ;
     model perform= activ /Solution cl ;
     random intercept activ / subject=school;
run;
```

As indicated by the fixed effect for the slope (β_1), physical activity is not significantly related to academic performance (Table 10.7). The variance coefficients for the random effects (σ^2_{u0}, σ^2_{u1}) now show that there are no significant differences between schools with regard to the intercepts or slopes. But again, this is not to be expected with only 10 schools in the analysis. Figure 10.4 shows the regression-based lines for the 10 schools. When comparing Figs. 10.1 and 10.4, it is obvious that the real slopes are much steeper and that the intercepts and slopes from the separate regressions differ more than those from the multilevel model.

The reason for this is due to the weighting of the regression coefficients of the 10 schools which is called 'shrinkage'. The 'shrinkage' method, which is present in every multilevel regression, is a method that 'borrows strength' for the estimates of a particular school from the overall estimates (Kreft and De Leeuw 1998). This prevents our variance estimate on the second level to be affected by outliers and produces more precise estimates. Thus, individual estimates of single schools are 'shrunken' in the direction toward the overall estimate. The 'shrinkage estimates' (so-called Empirical Bayes estimates) are weighted averages of the specific ordinary least squares estimate in each school and the overall regression coefficient

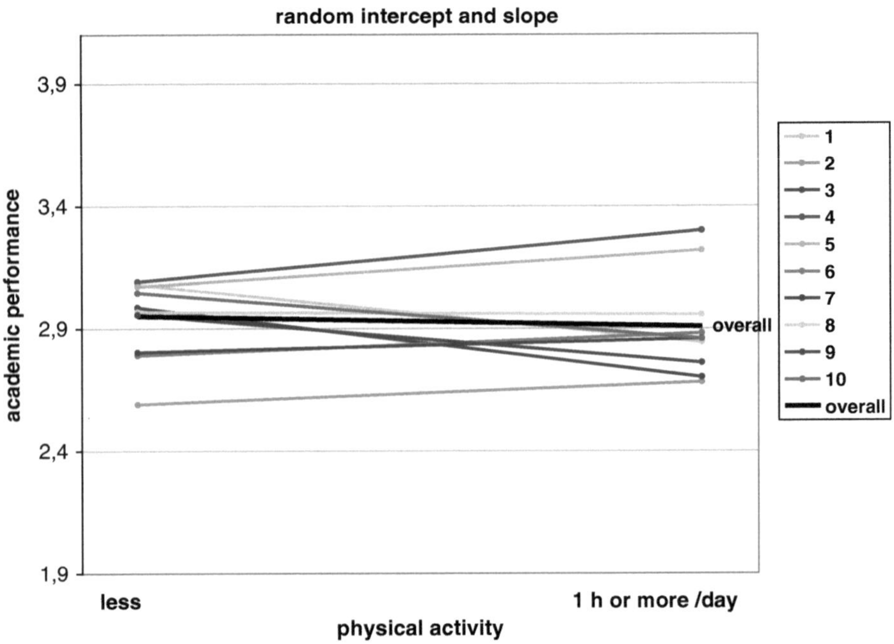

Fig. 10.4 Regression-based *lines* for every school for the random intercept and slope model with regard to the relationship between physical activity and academic performance

(Hox 2002). The extent of shrinkage depends on the group size and the difference between school-specific estimates and overall estimates. If the group size is relatively small and the distance between school-based estimates to the overall estimate is relatively high, the shrinkage will be larger than for larger group sizes and lower distance of school-specific estimates to overall estimates. The underlying assumption is that the school-specific estimates constitute a random sample from a normal distribution of such estimates. If particular group values are based on only a small number of pupils, these will most likely be biased and lead to extreme values, leading to poor representation of the distribution of such estimates.

Calculations with the Whole Data Set

So far we have worked with a small data subsample. We now calculate the model for the whole example data set. We incorporate the results from the different models (all steps) into one table. Note that for our smaller example, we intentionally selected schools with different slopes. When analysing the whole data set, the picture looks different.

In the final model (Table 10.8, right column), we have included additional covariates for sex, school enjoyment and parents' socio-economic position. School

Table 10.8 Multilevel linear model for academic performance, random intercept and slope model with individual level covariate (406 schools, 10,214 pupils) (significant effects in bold)

	Intercept only model	+ Covariate	+ Random slope	Random intercept model and more covariates
	Model 0	Model 1	Model 2	Model 3
Fixed effects	Beta (se)	Beta (se)	Beta (se)	Beta (se)
Intercept β_0	**2.93 (0.01)**	**2.76 (0.02)**	**2.76 (0.02)**	**2.56 (0.02)**
Physical activity, β_1	–	**0.21 (0.02)**	**0.21 (0.02)**	**0.14 (0.02)**
Enjoyment β_2				**0.33 (0.01)**
Sex (boys; ref: girls) β_3				**0.07 (0.01)**
FAS (ref: low)				
Middle β_4				**0.15 (0.02)**
High β_5				**0.17 (0.02)**
Variance estimates for random effects				
Variance between school intercepts σ^2_{u0}	**0.007 (0.002)**	**0.007 (0.002)**	**0.007 (0.002)**	**0.002 (0.001)**
Variance between school slopes σ^2_{u1}	–	–	0	–
Variance between pupils σ^2_{ε}	**0.515 (0.007)**	**0.508 (0.007)**	**0.508 (0.007)**	**0.434 (0.006)**
ICC	**0.014**			
Likelihood-ratio-test for comparing model 1 and 3				**1667.3 (df: 10, $p<0.001$)**

enjoyment was assessed with the question 'How much do you like going to school?' and response categories 'not much' (1), 'average' (2), 'much' (3) and 'very much' (4). The parents' socio-economic position was assessed with a three-item Family Affluence Scale (FAS) (Torsheim et al. 2004). The FAS asks about the number of cars owned by the household, whether the child has his/her own bedroom and the number of family holidays in the past year. A FAS score is calculated by summing the responses of these three items. The scale ranges from 0 to 6 points and was further categorised into low (0–2), medium (3–4) and high levels (5–6).

Variable selection methods which are used to find a final model can be done by using the likelihood-ratio test that compares the model fit and improvement of the model when adding covariates (Lehmann 1986). In the example the test statistic shows that the final model is significantly better than the model with only one covariate (Table 10.8).

In the third column we tested a random slope for physical activity (σ^2_{u1}), but because in the majority of schools pupils who are more active have higher academic performance, the slopes were similar and there was no significant variation between the slopes of the schools. Therefore, we continue with the random intercept model and columns 2 and 3 describe the same model.

The equation for the final model in the last column is

$$y_{ij} = \beta_0 + \beta_1 x_{1ij} + \beta_2 x_{2ij} + \beta_3 x_{3ij} + \beta_4 x_{4ij} + \beta_5 x_{5ij} + u_{0j} + \varepsilon_{ij}, \qquad (10.7)$$

where y_{ij} is the academic performance value of pupil i in school j,
β_0 is the fixed effect intercept,
β_1 is the fixed effect for physical activity, x_{1ij} is the value for physical activity of pupil i in school j (0 or 1),
β_2 is the fixed effect for school enjoyment, x_{2ij} is the value for school enjoyment of pupil i in school j (range −1.5 to 1.5 after centring),
β_3 is the fixed effect for sex, x_{3ij} is the value for sex of pupil i in school j (0 for girls, 1 for boys),
β_4 is the fixed effect for middle FAS, x_{4ij} is 1 for pupils with middle FAS, 0 for others,
β_5 is the fixed effect for high FAS, x_{5ij} is 1 for pupils with high FAS, 0 for others,
u_{0j} is the residual or random effect for the intercept for school j (mean 0, variance σ_{u0}^2) and
ε_{ij} is the error term for pupil i at school j (mean 0, variance σ_ε^2).

Interpretation of the Final Model

In addition to physical activity, school enjoyment was positively related to the academic performance of pupils (as indicated by significant coefficients β_1 and β_2). Pupils who were more active and who enjoyed school more had also a better academic performance. Boys reported better performance than girls (as indicated by the coefficient β_3), and those pupils from middle or higher socio-economic households performed better than those of lower socio-economic background (indicated by β_4 and β_5).

After adjusting for more individual characteristics, the variance between intercepts of schools and the residual variance of pupils in the model were reduced. There were no significant random slope variables, indicating that the relationship between a covariate and the outcome (academic performance) did not differ significantly between schools (e.g. positive association in some schools, negative association in other schools). Further, we could not find significant school-level variables which were related to the academic performance of the pupils. Therefore, we might conclude that the self-reported academic performance of pupils is related to their individual characteristics, not to the school characteristics which were analysed here (compare Stock et al. 2011), and that the relationship between the individual characteristics and the academic performance is similar in different schools (e.g. higher school enjoyment is related to higher academic performance). However, as indicated by the significant variance coefficient for the random intercept, there are significant differences between schools with regard to the mean performance of the pupils, although we do not know what these differences are related to because we did not find significant school-level characteristics.

Multilevel Logistic Models for Dichotomous Data

We will also discuss the case of a dichotomous outcome where a logistic model is appropriate. As an example, we refer to the study of Stock et al. (2011), who analysed which individual- and school district-level characteristics were associated with daily active transportation to school.

Active transportation to school was assessed by the question: 'How do you usually get to and from school?' and was dichotomised into daily active transportation for those who answered 'Every day I walk or use a bicycle, roller skates or the like' and less than daily active transportation for those who answered 'On some days I am taken by car or bus, on other days by foot, bicycle, roller skates or the like' or 'I am always taken by bus or car'.

We consider the equation for multilevel logistic null model (without covariates), and therefore, we denote $E(y_{ij}) = \pi_{ij} = \Pr(y_{ij} = 1)$ as the expectation of our outcome or the probability of pupil *i* in school *j* to use daily active transport to school.

Now the equation is

$$\log(\frac{\pi_{ij}}{1-\pi_{ij}})=\beta_0+u_{0j}, \quad \text{where } \pi \sim \text{Binomial}(n_{ij},\mu), \tag{10.8}$$

β_0 is the log-odds that $y = 1$ (daily active transport to school) when $u = 0$,
u_{0j} is the effect of being in group *j* (school *j*) on the log-odds that $y = 1$, or the level 2 residual (mean 0, variance σ^2_{u0}),
n_{ij} is the sample size and
μ is the expected value of π_{ij}.

As in the linear case, we would like to know how much variation is on the school level and how much is on the individual level. But as stated by Larsen and Merlo (2005), components of the variance are not as straightforward to investigate and to interpret when analysing dichotomous outcome variables. Classical interpretative schemes such as the ICC may be inappropriate. Larsen and Merlo therefore suggest calculating median odds ratios (MOR) instead (Merlo et al. 2006).

For illustrative reasons, we will describe a model with one individual-level covariate, one school district-level covariate and a cross-level interaction. The full regression model is described in Stock et al. (2011). Stock et al. report that academic performance of the pupils is related to active school transportation: 69.4 % of those with very good performance are active on their way to school in contrast to only 53.3 % of those with bad performance. In addition to other individual and school district characteristics, the differentiation between more urban school districts and more rural districts (as measured by the area size of farming land use of the district) is also related to active transportation. In districts with less farming land use (more urban areas) 72.9 % of the pupils use active daily transportation in contrast to only 52.3 % in districts with more farming land use (for the exact definition of the farming land use variable, see Stock et al. 2011). One reason could be that in more rural areas, car use is more common and walking or going by bicycle is less supported by the infrastructure (Stock et al. 2011).

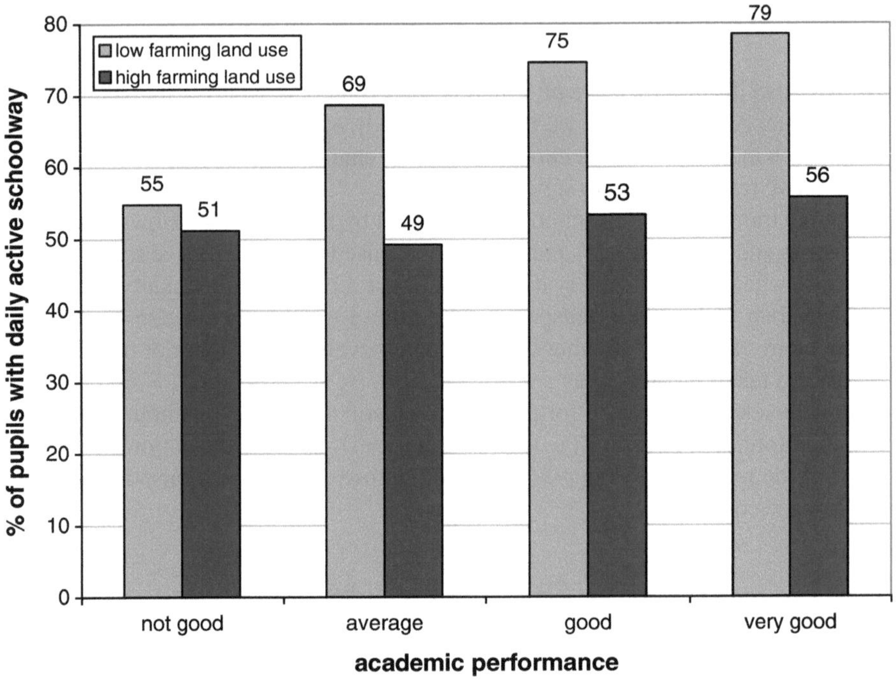

Fig. 10.5 Prevalence of daily active school transportation in relation to academic performance of pupils and type of school district

Figure 10.5 shows how individual academic performance and the proportion of farming land use in the school district interact with regard to daily active school transportation. In districts with less farming land use, the relationship between academic performance and active transportation is much stronger than in districts with more farming land use.

The command in SAS for the null model is:

```
proc glimmix data=walk method=quad(qpoints=10) oddsratios ;
     class school ;
     model walkschool (event="1")= /Solution dist=binary ;
     random intercept / subject=school type=un ;
     ods output oddsratios=o2;
run;
```

where *walk* is our data set, *school* is the variable that contains the school id numbers and *walkschool* is the dichotomous variable that indicates if a pupil is active daily on his or her way to school (1) or not (0).

The SAS-command for the model with covariates is:

```
proc glimmix data=walk method=quad(qpoints=10) oddsratios ;
     class school ;
     model walkschool (event="1")= perform less_farm
```

Table 10.9 Multilevel logistic model for active daily transport to school, random intercept model without covariates (406 schools, 10,380 pupils) (significant effects in bold)

	Null model	Model with 2 covariates and cross-level interaction
Fixed effects	Beta (se)	Beta (se)
Intercept β_0	**0.63 (0.05)**	0.06 (0.06)
At individual level		**Odds ratios (95 %CI)**
Academic performance (range: 1–4, higher values: better performance)		**1.11 (1.02–1.21)**
At school district level		
Areas with less farming land use (ref: areas with more farming land use)		**2.54 (2.15–2.99)**
Cross-level interaction		
Academic performance × low farming land use		**1.24 (1.09–1.39)**
Variance estimates for random effects		
Variance between school intercepts σ^2_{u0}	**0.67 (0.07)**	**0.39 (0.05)**

```
        perform_less_farm/Solution dist=binary ;
        random intercept / subject=district type=un ;
        ods output oddsratios=o2;
run;
```

where *perform* is the variable for academic performance of the pupil (centred), *less_farm* is the variable for the school district type (lower farming land use: 1, higher farming land use: 0) and *perform_less_farm* is a dummy variable constructed as an interaction term by multiplying *perform* and *less_farm.*

Table 10.9 shows results of the null model and the model with covariates. In the null model, the significant term for σ^2_{u0} shows that there are significant differences between school districts with regard to the proportion of pupils who use active daily transportation.

The model with covariates shows that pupils with higher academic performance and pupils in areas with less farming land use are more often walking or cycling to school daily than pupils with lower academic performance or pupils in areas with more farming land use. The significant coefficient for the interaction between academic performance and proportion of farming land use shows that the association between academic performance and active transportation is much stronger in more urban areas than in more rural areas.

Conclusion

This chapter is an application-oriented introduction into both linear and logistic multilevel modelling. It has explained the main idea of multilevel modelling and described the procedures for a multilevel analysis as well as how to interpret the results. It has shown how multilevel modelling allows for differentiation between relationships of individual characteristics (lower level characteristics) or group characteristics (higher level characteristics) and the outcome of interest in a single analysis. It has demonstrated how it is possible to make inferences regarding the impact of individual characteristics after controlling for group characteristics or vice versa. The chapter has also shown how multilevel modelling can assess whether the relationship between individual characteristics and the outcome differs in different groups.

Multilevel modelling has become an increasingly useful analytic tool not only in the social sciences and medicine but also within epidemiological, public health and health promotion research (e.g. Kothari and Birch 2004; Diez-Roux and Aiello 2005; Diez-Roux 2000). This technique has expanded the range and depth of analyses such that researchers may now take into account more than one level of data. This is, for example, relevant for research in health promotion which is often based on a socio-ecological theoretical framework (Kothari and Birch 2004). Influencing the health of individuals may occur not only directly but also via the families, neighbourhoods and communities in which they live, the places at which they work and the schools that they attend. Recent research has employed multilevel modelling to examine a variety of subjects including the effect of the community on the rate of unplanned pregnancies (Koren and Mawn 2010), the effects of the social and built environment on stress and health (Matthews and Yang 2010) and the effects of fast-food outlet density and car ownership on body mass (Inagami et al. 2009).

The technique has also found wide use in intervention research including such recent studies as one of blood pressure reduction among African-American men visiting barber shops (Victor et al. 2009), an evaluation of a web-based anti-smoking campaign in Toronto secondary schools (Norman et al. 2008) and a trial to reduce stress among young restaurant workers (Petree et al. 2012).

It is thus clear that multilevel approaches have become well accepted in the health research field. They add an extra 'dimension' of analysis to produce results that more fully take into account additional avenues of influence upon human health and behaviour.

For further reading, we recommend Verbeke and Molenberghs (2000), Zuur et al. (2009) or Raudenbush and Bryk (2002) and the webpage of the Centre for Multilevel Modelling at the University of Bristol which contains helpful material (http://www.bristol.ac.uk/cmm/). Graduate School of Education, Bristol Institute of Public Affairs (2012).

Appendix

Syntax commands for the examples in STATA, R and SPSS. In R, we used the following libraries: *nlme* (Pinheiro et al. 2011), *MASS* (Venables and Ripley 2002) and *lme4* (Bates et al. 2011).

Multilevel Linear Regression: The Intercept-Only Model

In STATA:

```
xtmixed perform || school:, var
```

In R:

```
library (nlme)
L1 <- lme (fixed=perform~1, random= ~1 | school, data=walk)
summary (L1)
```

In SPSS:

```
MIXED perform
/PRINT = SOLUTION TESTCOV
/FIXED = INTERCEPT
/RANDOM = INTERCEPT | SUBJECT (school) .
```

Multilevel Linear Regression: Random Intercept Model with One Individual-Level Covariate

In STATA:

```
xtmixed perform activ|| school:, var
```

In R:

```
library (nlme)
L2 <- lme (fixed=perform ~ 1+activ , random = ~1 | school,
data=walk)summary (L2)
```

In SPSS:

```
MIXED perform WITH activ
/PRINT = SOLUTION TESTCOV
/FIXED = INTERCEPT activ
/RANDOM = INTERCEPT | SUBJECT (school).
```

Multilevel Linear Regression: Random Intercept and Slope Model with One Individual-Level Covariate

In STATA:

```
xtmixed perform activ|| school: activ, var
```

In R:

```
library (nlme)
L3 <- lme (fixed=perform ~ 1+active, random=~activ|school,
data=walk)
Summary (L3)
```

In SPSS:

```
MIXED perform WITH activ
/PRINT = SOLUTION TESTCOV
/FIXED = INTERCEPT activ
/RANDOM = INTERCEPT activ| SUBJECT (school).
```

Multilevel Logistic Model for Binary Outcome: Intercept-Only Model

In STATA:

```
xtset school
xtlogit walkschool
```

In R:

```
library (MASS)
library (lme4)
L4<-glmer (walkschool~1+(1|school),family=binomial,
data=walk)
summary (L5)
```

In SPSS:

```
GENLINMIXED
/DATA_STRUCTURE SUBJECTS=school
/FIELDS TARGET=walkschool
/TARGET_OPTIONS DISTRIBUTION=BINOMIAL LINK=LOGIT
/FIXED USE_INTERCEPT=TRUE
/random use_intercept=true subjects=school.
```

Multilevel Logistic Model for Binary Outcome: Random Intercept Model with Individual-Level and School District-Level Covariates and Cross-Level Interaction

In STATA:

```
xtlogit walkschool perform less_farm perform_less_farm, or
```

In R:

```
library (MASS)
library (lme4)
L5<-glmer (walkschool~1+perform+less_farm+perform_less_
farm+ (1|school),family=binomial, data=walk)
summary (L5)
```

In SPSS:

```
GENLINMIXED
/DATA_STRUCTURE SUBJECTS=school
```

```
/FIELDS TARGET=walkschool
/TARGET_OPTIONS reference=0 DISTRIBUTION=BINOMIAL
LINK=LOGIT
/FIXED effects= perform less_farm perform_less_farm
USE_INTERCEPT=TRUE
/random use_intercept=true subjects=school
COVARIANCE_TYPE =UNSTRUCTURED.
```

References

Bates, D., Maechler, M., & Bolker, B. (2011). lme4: Linear mixed-effects models using S4 classes. 0.999375-42 ed. p. R package. Accessed February 11, 2013, from http://CRAN.R-project.org/package=lme4.

Bijleveld, C. C. J. H., & van der Kamp, L. J. T. (Eds.). (1998). *Longitudinal data analysis. Designs, models and methods*. London: Sage.

Diez-Roux, A. V. (2000). Multilevel analysis in public health research. *Annual Review of Public Health, 21*, 171–192.

Diez-Roux, A. V., & Aiello, A. E. (2005). Multilevel analysis of infectious diseases. *The Journal of Infectious Diseases, 191*(suppl 1), 25–33.

Dunson, D. (Ed.). (2008). *Random effect and latent variable model selection* (1st ed.). New York: Springer.

Freedman, D. A. (2004). The ecological fallacy. In M. Lewis-Beck, A. Bryman, & T. F. Liao (Eds.), *Encyclopedia of social science research methods*. London: Sage.

Graduate School of Education, Bristol Institute of Public Affairs. (2012). Centre for multilevel modelling. University-of-Bristol. Accessed February 24, 2012, from http://www.bristol.ac.uk/cmm/.

Hox, J. (2002). *Multilevel analysis. Techniques and applications*. Mahwah, NJ: Lawrence Erlbaum Associates, Inc.

Hox, J., & Maas, C. J. M. (2004). The influence of violations of assumptions on multilevel parameter estimates and their standard errors. *Computational Statistics & Data Analysis, 46*, 427–440.

Inagami, S., Cohen, D. A., Brown, A. F., & Asch, S. M. (2009). Body mass index, neighborhood fast food and restaurant concentration and car ownership. *Journal of Urban Health, 86*(5), 683–695.

Kleinbaum, D. G., & Klein, M. (2010). *Logistic regression. A self-learning text* (3rd ed.). New York: Springer.

Koren, A., & Mawn, B. (2010). The context of unintended pregnancy among married women in the USA. *Journal of Family Planning and Reproductive Health Care, 36*(3), 150–158.

Kothari, A. R., & Birch, S. (2004). Multilevel health promotion research: conceptual and analytical considerations. *The Canadian Journal of Nursing Research, 36*(1), 56–75.

Kreft, I., & De Leeuw, J. (1998). *Introducing multilevel modeling*. London: Sage.

Larsen, K., & Merlo, J. (2005). Appropriate assessment of neighbourhood effects on individual health: Integrating random and fixed effects in multilevel logistic regression. *American Journal of Epidemiology, 161*, 81–88.

Lehmann, E. L. (1986). *Testing statistical hypotheses* (2nd ed.). New York: Wiley.

Matthews, S. A., & Yang, T.-C. (2010). Exploring the role of the built and social neighborhood environment in moderating stress and health. *Annals of Behavioral Medicine, 39*, 170–183.

Merlo, J., Chaix, B., Ohlsson, H., Beckman, A., Johnell, K., Hjerpe, P., et al. (2006). A brief conceptual tutorial of multilevel analysis in social epidemiology: Using measures of clustering in multilevel logistic regression to investigate contextual phenomena. *Journal of Epidemiology and Community Health, 60*, 290–297.

Montgomery, D. C., & Peck, E. A. (1992). *Introduction to linear regression analysis*. New York: Wiley.

Norman, C. D., Maley, O., Li, X., & Skinner, H. A. (2008). Using the internet to assist smoking prevention and cessation in schools: A randomized, controlled trial. *Health Psychology, 27*(6), 799–810.

Petree, R. D., Broome, K. M., & Bennett, J. B. (2012). Exploring and reducing stress in young restaurant workers: Results of a randomized field trial. *American Journal of Health Promotion, 26*(4), 217–224.

Pinheiro, J., Bates, D., DebRoy, S., & Sarkar, D., R-Development-Core-Team. (2011). nlme: Linear and nonlinear mixed effects models. R package version 3.1-102.

R Development Core Team. (2011). R: A language and environment for statistical computing. http://www.R-project.org, Vienna.

Raudenbush, S. W., & Bryk, A. S. (2002). *Hierarchical linear models. Applications and data analysis methods* (2nd ed.). London: Sage.

SAS System for Windows. (2008). (9.2 ed.). Cary, NC: SAS Institute Inc.

Snijders, T. A. B., & Bosker, R. J. (1999). *Multilevel analysis. An introduction to basic and advanced multilevel modeling*. London: Sage.

SPSS for Windows. (2011). (20.0.0 ed.). Chicago: SPSS Inc.

StataCorp. (2007). *Stata statistical software, Stata/IC* (101st ed.). College Station, TX: StataCorp LP.

Stock, C., Bloomfield, K., Ejstrud, B., Vinther-Larsen, M., Meijer, M., Grønbæk, M., et al. (2011). Are characteristics of the school district associated with active transportation to school in Danish adolescents? *European Journal of Public Health, 22*(3), 398–404.

Torsheim, T., Currie, C., Boyce, W., Kalnins, I., Overpeck, M., & Haugland, S. (2004). Material deprivation and self-rated health: A multilevel study of adolescents from 22 European and North American countries. *Social Science & Medicine, 59*, 1–12.

Venables, W. N., & Ripley, B. D. (2002). *Modern applied statistics with S*. New York: Springer.

Verbeke, G., & Molenberghs, G. (2000). *Linear mixed models for longitudinal data*. New York: Springer.

Victor, R. G., Ravenell, J. E., Freeman, A., Bhat, D. G., Storm, J. S., Shafig, M., et al. (2009). A barber-based intervention for hypertension in African-American men: Design of a group randomized trial. *American Heart Journal, 157*(1), 30–36.

Zuur, A. F., Ieno, E. N., Walker, N. J., Saveliev, A. A., & Smith, G. M. (Eds.). (2009). *Mixed effects models and extensions in ecology with R*. New York: Springer.

Part III
Neighbourhood and Lifestyle

Chapter 11
Vitamin G (Green Spaces and Health): Potential Mechanisms, Policy Implications and Ideas for Further Research

Jolanda Maas

Introduction

In our society, which is becoming increasingly densely populated and in which large numbers of people live in urban areas, green space is no longer an obvious component of the direct living environment. According to a United Nations report, the urban population now amounts to 50 % of the world population, and this figure will have risen to about 70 % by 2030 (Vlahov and Galea 2002). At the same time, urban green space is under pressure because of shortage of land on which to build housing (De Vries 2001). The quality and quantity of green in and around cities has diminished noticeably. Due to increasing urbanisation, combined with a spatial planning policy of densification, more people are facing the prospect of living in less green residential environments. If the availability of green space positively influences health, living in less green residential environments could have negative health consequences. People with a low socio-economic status, who do not have the resources to move to greener (often more expensive) areas outside cities, will be particularly affected by these developments, which may lead to environmental injustice with regard to the distribution of (access to) public green spaces.

Notions about the beneficial effects of green space have persisted throughout history (Van den Berg and Van den Berg 2001). However, scientific evidence of a direct relationship between the amount of green space in the living environment and health has been limited until fairly recently. The first part of this chapter provides an overview of (the results) from studies on the direct relationship between green space and health.

J. Maas (✉)
Department of Public and Occupational Health, EMGO + Institute,
VU Medical Center, Postbus 7057, 1007 MB, Amsterdam, The Netherlands
e-mail: j.maas@vumc.nl

C. Stock and A. Ellaway (eds.), *Neighbourhood Structure and Health Promotion*,
DOI 10.1007/978-1-4614-6672-7_11, © Springer Science+Business Media New York 2013

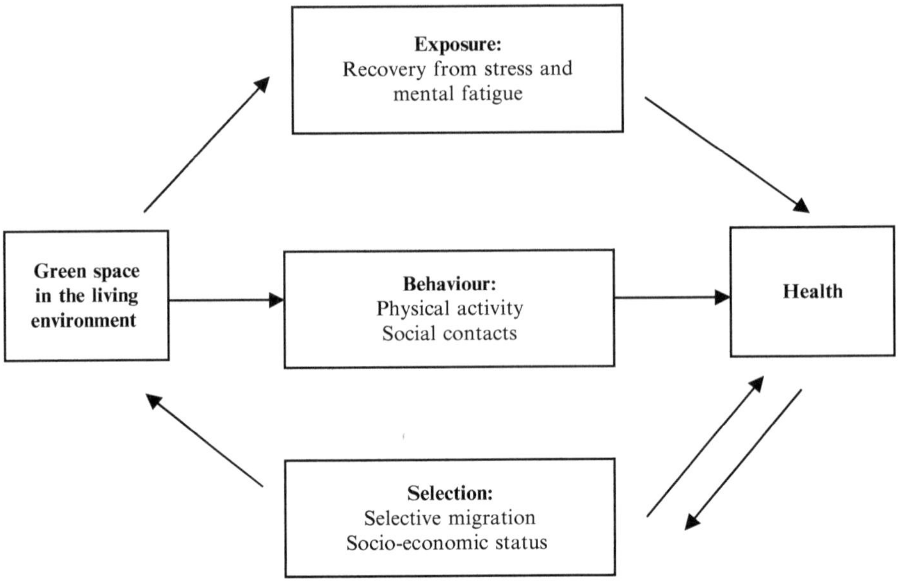

Fig. 11.1 Conceptual model for the relationships between green space, health and the explanatory mechanisms

Once a link between green space and health can be established, the next question is to examine the mechanisms through which green space might exert a beneficial effect on health. In the second part of this chapter, we will give an overview on the literature, investigating mechanisms related to exposure and behaviour, e.g. restoration from stress, stimulating physical activity and encouraging social contacts.

There are other factors which might also play an important role in explaining the relationship between green space and health, for example, children's physical and social development (Health Council of the Netherlands 2004). However, this chapter focuses on the mechanisms related to exposure and behaviour because of their relevance to contemporary health problems, such as chronic stress, burnout, depression, lack of physical activity and obesity. Figure 11.1 summarises the relationships between green space, health and the explanatory mechanisms in a conceptual model.

Green Space and Health

Studies investigating the direct relationship between green space and health can be divided into studies focussing on (i) investigating the relationship between green space and perceived (mental and physical) health and (ii) studies focussing on mortality or morbidity. The main results of these studies will be described in the following two sections.

Associations with Perceived Mental and Physical Health

There are several studies which investigate the relationship between green space and health. In 2003, the first study on the direct relationship between green space and perceived health was published by De Vries et al. (2003). This study showed that residents of neighbourhoods with abundant green space tend, on average, to enjoy better general health and a better mental health and reported fewer symptoms. This positive link was found to be most apparent among the elderly, among housewives and among people from lower socio-economic groups (De Vries et al. 2003). In 2006, this study was replicated by Maas et al. (2006), using larger ($n = 250{,}000$ as opposed to $n = 10{,}000$), more recent (2001 as opposed to 1989) and more comprehensive datasets that are better attuned to each other (both green space and health data are from the same year). The findings of this study corresponded with the findings of De Vries et al. (2003). In their study, Maas et al. (2006) showed that the amount of green space in people's living environment is positively associated with perceived general health. This relationship was apparent in both urban and rural areas and is considerable; the chance that residents would describe their health as less than good was 1.5 times as large in living environments with little green space than it was in living environments with very much green space. Moreover, the results of this study suggest that the availability of green space might be an important factor in explaining urban/rural health differences. A previous study has shown that the association between level of urbanity and people's self-reported health cannot be explained by demographic, socio-economic and behavioural factors or by selective migration (Verheij et al. 2008). The results of the study by Maas et al. (2006) indicated that the availability of green space is more strongly associated with people's perceived general health than with level of urbanity, controlling for age, gender, socio-economic status, job status and ethnicity. As in the study of De Vries et al. (2003), in the study of Maas et al. (2006), the relationship between green space and health was stronger for people with a lower socio-economic status as opposed to people with a high socio-economic status and was stronger for young people and the elderly compared to adults aged between 25 and 64 years. A study from van Dillen et al. (2011) also performed in the Netherlands showed that besides the quantity of green space, the quality of green space is also important for health. The study also showed that streetscape greenery is at least as strongly related to self-reported health as green areas.

The described studies have all been performed in the Netherlands, but indications of a positive relationship between green space and health have also been found in other countries. In England, Mitchell and Popham (2007) found that a higher proportion of green space in an area is generally associated with better self-reported health, although the association depended on the degree of urbanity and level of income deprivation. There was no significant association between green space and health in higher income suburban and rural areas, which the authors believed might be explained by the quality of green space, a factor that had not been taken into account in the study. In Sweden, Nielsen and Hansen (2007) found that people who had access to a garden or had green areas a short distance away from their houses were less stressed and had a lower likelihood of obesity. Also in Sweden, Björk et al. (2008) found no relationship between self-perceived health and the amount of green space within a 100-m and a 300-m radius around the house. Ellaway et al. (2005) investigated the relationship between individuals' obesity and the amount of vegetation and greenery visible in their residential environment (as assessed by trained surveyors). They used a European cross-sectional survey and found that respondents whose residential environment contained high levels of greenery had about a 40 % lower likelihood of being overweight and obese.

The results of a study by Sugiyama et al. (2008) performed in Australia showed that people who perceived their neighbourhood as 'very green' had respectively 1.37 and 1.60 times higher odds of having better physical and mental health. Perceived neighbourhood greenness appeared to be more strongly associated with mental health than it was with physical health. People living in neighbourhoods that were perceived as 'medium green' did not have higher odds of better physical or mental health, which indicates that only very green neighbourhoods have a particularly beneficial effect on health. In 2010, Stigsdotter et al. (2010) showed that Danes living more than 1 km away from the nearest green space report poorer health and health-related quality of life than respondents living closer.

In conclusion, a positive association between neighbourhood green space and several self-reported general indicators of physical and mental health has been found in a number of countries that differ in population density and the availability (and quality) of green space.

Associations with Mortality and Morbidity

Relatively few studies on the relation between green space and health have gone beyond examining the relationship with self-reported health measures. They have investigated whether morbidity and mortality were related to the amount of green space in people's living environment. In this section, the results of these studies will be described.

Takano et al. (2002) were among the first to study the relationship between the amount of green space and mortality risk. In their Japanese longitudinal study among citizens in Tokyo, they showed that living in a neighbourhood with relatively plentiful walkable green space correlated with a lower mortality risk (Takano et al. 2002). Mitchell and Popham (2008) showed that the association between income deprivation and mortality differed significantly across population groups in the UK with varying amount of exposure to green space and that the strength of the association was dependent on the health measures used. Only mortality from all causes and circulatory disease were related to exposure to green space. Mortality from lung cancer or intentional self-harm was not (Mitchell and Popham 2008). In a study conducted in New Zealand, Richardson et al. (2010) found no association between green space and cardiovascular disease mortality. According to the authors, the fact that no association was found might be explained with the inability to adjust for individual-level factors with a significant influence on cardiovascular disease mortality risk (e.g. diet and alcohol consumption). Another study from Richardson et al. (2011) performed in the largest US cities also found no relation between greenness and mortality from heart disease, diabetes, lung cancer or automobile accidents. On the other hand, a study form Coutts et al. (2010) performed in Florida (USA) found that, after controlling for some of the leading influences of mortality—including the levels of obesity, smoking, old age and education—the amount of green space within defined distances of census tracts in each county was associated with both all cause and cardiovascular mortality.

Only one study to date has investigated the relationship between the *amount* of green space in the living environment and morbidity. In a study performed in the Netherlands, Maas et al. 2009b investigated whether several clusters of physician-assessed diseases were related to the amount of green space in people's living environment. They used large-scale representative medical record data on morbidity to show that the annual prevalence rates for 15 of 24 selected disease clusters were lower in living environments with more green space within a 1 km radius around people's homes, controlling for demographic and socio-economic characteristics and level of urbanicity. No significant relationships were found for the amount of green space within a 3 km radius around people's homes. Green space close to home appeared to be more important where the prevalence of disease is concerned. Where the disease clusters were concerned, the relationship was strongest for anxiety disorder and depression. The chance of depression was 1.33 times higher in living environments with little green space than in living environments with very much green space. The relationship appeared to be particularly strong in children and people with a low socio-economic status.

Green Space and Health in Summary

A number of studies performed in different countries show that green space is positively related to, for example, perceived health, specific diseases, stress, number of health complaints and mental health (De Vries et al. 2003; Mitchell and Popham 2007; Takano et al. 2002; Nielsen and Hansen 2007; Sugiyama et al. 2008). For mortality, the results are inconclusive. Some studies find a relation while others do not.

With regard to the strength of the relationship, self-reported health seems to be more strongly related to the amount of green space in the living environment than the prevalence of specific diseases. The chance of feeling unhealthy is 1.5 times larger in living environments with little green space than it is in living environments with very many green areas (Maas et al. 2006). This relationship is weaker for the prevalence of specific diseases. In the case of depression, which is one of the disease clusters strongly related to the amount of green space in the living environment, the chance of this disorder is 1.33 times greater in areas with little green space (Maas et al. 2009b).

The relation between green space and health appears to be stronger for people with a lower socio-economic status (De Vries et al. 2003; Maas et al. 2006, 2009b; Mitchell and Popham 2007, 2008). Furthermore, three studies performed in the Netherlands showed that the relationship between green space and health was stronger for younger people and the elderly. This might be explained by the fact that these population groups spend more time in the vicinity of their homes as a result of lower mobility (Schwanen et al. 2002; Harms 2006). Another explanatory factor could be that the health situation of people with lower socio-economic status is worse on average, which leaves more room for health improvement. As a result, they might be more susceptible to the amount of green space in their living environment.

Mechanisms Linked to the Relationship Between Green Space and Health

The previous section showed that the amount of green space in the living environment is related to health. But these studies provide little insight into the mechanisms behind this relationship. In this section, we will discuss the plausibility of various mechanisms which might be related to exposure to green space and behaviour, e.g. restoration from stress, stimulating physical activity and encouraging social contacts.

Exposure: Restoration from Stress and Mental Fatigue

A small but growing body of well-controlled empirical research deals directly with the restorative effects of green space (Health Council of the Netherlands and RMNO 2004; Van den Berg et al. 2007). In general, these studies have shown more positive affective, cognitive and physiological responses to natural settings as compared to built environment settings city centres. These positive responses have been observed in diverse settings including remote wilderness areas (Hartig et al. 1991, 2003) as well as nearby green space such as gardens (Ottosson and Grahn 2005; Rodiek 2002). Notably, people need not go outdoors to profit from nature's restorative functions. Merely viewing green space through a window can already have positive effects. Several studies have shown that residents of apartments with views of green space, in particular women and children who presumably spend much time at home, tend to report less stress and perform better on tests for cognitive functioning than their counterparts in apartments with barren views (Faber Taylor et al. 2002; Kaplan 2001; Kuo and Sullivan 2001; Tennessen and Cimprich 1995; Wells 2000).

Laboratory experiments have shown that viewing slides or videos of natural environments leads to a faster and more complete affective, cognitive and psychophysiological stress recovery than viewing built environments (e.g. Berto 2005; Hartig et al. 1996; Ulrich et al. 1991; Van den Berg et al. 2003). In sum, there is convergent evidence from different lines of research that contact with real or simulated natural environments can provide restoration from stress and mental fatigue (Van den Berg et al. 2010).

The restorative effects of green space have generally been explained from an evolutionary perspective. What most of these explanations have in common is the argument that, as a result of two or three million years of evolution in natural environments, modern humans have developed a partly genetic readiness to respond positively to habitable settings that were favourable to well-being and survival for premodern people (Van den Berg et al. 2010; Appleton 1975; Orians 1986; Kaplan and Kaplan 1989; Ulrich 1993). Notably, this readiness to respond positively to habitable settings is assumed to be triggered by natural environments alone; humans do not possess such a disposition for most built environments and materials (Ulrich 1993). An important implication of people's readiness to respond positively to nature is that their attention is easily and almost effortlessly held by natural scenes. This attention-drawing quality of natural settings is referred to as 'soft fascination' (Kaplan and Kaplan 1989), which is assumed to play an important role in the restorative quality of nature. When nature captures people's attention, executive systems that regulate directed attention are allowed to rest, pessimistic thoughts are blocked, and negative emotions are replaced by positive ones (Hartig et al. 1996; Parsons 1991; Van den Berg et al. 2010).

Behaviour: Physical Activity and Social Contacts

The second mechanism behind the relationship between green space and health that is discussed is that of behaviour modification. The general idea behind this potential mechanism is that green space may promote two forms of behaviour which positively influence health, viz. physical activity and social contacts. These two forms of behaviour and the evidence for a relationship with green space are discussed in the following two sections.

Physical Activity

Green space can have beneficial effects on health because green space promotes physical activity. The relationship between physical activity and health has received increased attention in recent years as it is seen to play a key role in the promotion of good health and the prevention of diseases, such as Type II diabetes, obesity, cardiovascular diseases and hypertension (US Department of HHS 1996; Booth et al. 2000; Pate et al. 1995; NIH Consensus Development Panel on Physical Activity and Cardiovascular Health 1996; Paffenbarger et al. 1993). According to the social ecological model (Sallis and Owen 1996; Giles-Corti and Donovan 2002), the physical and social environment determines physical activity beyond biological characteristics (i.e. age, gender) and psychological characteristics (Sallis et al. 1998; King et al. 2002; Giles-Corti and Donovan 2002, 2003). One characteristic of the physical environment that might influence physical activity is the amount of green space in the living environment. Green environments are perceived as more attractive than built environments (Van den Berg et al. 2003), and because some bodily movement (e.g. walking or cycling) is often necessary to experience them, it may be that they do inherently promote physical activity. Furthermore, green environments are multifunctional and can be used for different kinds of physical activity.

Several studies have investigated whether the amount of green space in the living environment stimulates physical activity. The results differ for children, adolescents and adults. Most of the studies which focus on the relationship between neighbourhood green space and physical activity for children or adolescents find positive relationships (e.g. Mota et al. 2005; De Vries et al. 2007; Roemmich et al. 2006). Some studies were interested in differences between boys and girls or focussed only on boys or girls. Two studies have shown that accessibility to a park was stronger (Epstein et al. 2006) or even exclusively (Roemmich et al. 2007) associated to physical activity behaviour in boys only. Jago et al. (2005) also found a relationship between green space and physical activity for male adolescents in two studies which only followed male adolescents. Jago et al. (2005, 2006) also found positive relations between the number and height of trees in a 400-m radius around adolescents houses (Jago et al. 2005) as well as the number of parks in the environment (Jago et al. 2006) and the level of physical activity of male adolescents. Two studies which followed only girls found a positive association between green space and physical activity for girls (Cohen et al. 2006; Timperio et al. 2004).

The scientific evidence on the relationship between green space and physical activity for adults is ambiguous. Several studies have found that aesthetics of the environment and the availability and accessibility of parks stimulate certain types of physical activity (e.g. Pikora et al. 2003; McGinn et al. 2007). On the other hand, there are also studies that did not find a relationship between green space and physical activity (e.g. Hillsdon et al. 2006; Kaczynski and Henderson 2007). A study from Maas et al. (2008) found that people with more green space in their living environment spent more time on gardening and on commuting to work.

Aside from the issue that a green environment might offer an opportunity for individuals to be physically active, it might also encourage people to exercise for longer periods of time. Research by Pennebaker and Lightner (1980) showed that joggers who jogged in a green stimulating environment ran faster then joggers jogging on a lap track. At the same time, no differences were found in heart rate or blood pressure between the two run courses. Furthermore, research by Pretty et al. (2007) showed that people who participated in outdoor exercise programmes were more likely to complete the programme compared to people who participated in indoor exercise programmes. These two studies imply that people engage in physical activity for longer periods in a green environment than in an indoor environment, and this has the potential to offer positive health benefits. A systematic review from Bowler et al. (2010) concluded that there is some evidence that activity in a natural environment compared to a different environment can have a positive impact on mental well-being. These results are drawn from short-term tests on self-reported feelings such as ‘anger/aggression’, ‘sadness/depression’ and ‘fatigue/tiredness’. There are only a limited number of studies which also indicate there might be an impact on physiological outcomes.

Branas et al. (2011) performed an interesting implementation study where they conducted a decade-long difference-indifferences analysis of the impact of a vacant lot greening programme in Philadelphia, Pennsylvania, on health and safety outcomes. Regarding safety, the study showed that vacant lot greening was associated with consistent reductions in gun assaults and some consistent reductions in vandalism. Regarding health, the study showed that vacant lot greening was associated with residents' reporting less stress and more exercise in select sections of the city.

Social Contacts

Besides influencing physical activity, green space might also stimulate social contacts. Social contacts can take many forms, including having a conversation, undertaking joint activities and paying visits. It is widely recognised that social relationships can influence a variety of health outcomes (e.g. Berkman et al. 2000; Hawe and Shiell 2000). Persons actively involved in communities or socially engaged with others tend to live longer (Kawachi et al. 1997) and are healthier both physically and mentally (e.g. Kawachi and Berkman 2000; Leyden 2003).

Attractive green areas in the neighbourhood may serve as a focal point of tacit coordination for positive informal social interaction, strengthening social ties and social cohesion by extension (Kweon et al. 1998). Furthermore, natural settings in common spaces can attract neighbourhood inhabitants as they can provide shelter, privacy and sound buffering from surrounding environments and they could have restorative effects (Coley et al. 1997; Hartig et al. 2003; Kaplan and Kaplan 1989). Besides offering opportunities for meeting, green spaces can also promote a general sense of community by increasing feelings of emotional attachment to a neighbourhood and people's identification with a place, which could in turn decrease feelings of loneliness and increase social support (Prezza et al. 2001; Pretty et al. 1994).

Three closely related studies, performed by the same research group in an underprivileged area of Chicago, provided the first indications of a positive relationship between the presence of green public facilities and social ties (Coley et al. 1997; Kuo et al. 1998; Kweon et al. 1998). These studies showed that the presence of trees predicted greater use of outdoor space (Coley et al. 1997) and increased neighbourhood social ties (Kuo et al. 1998) and that use of nearby green common spaces predicted stronger social ties and a better sense of community for older adults (Kweon et al. 1998). All these studies were conducted in highly deprived urban areas where green elements were very scarce. The question is whether these relationships will also be found in other, richer and greener areas.

Only a few studies have addressed the relation between green space and social contacts. A study by Ewert and Heywood (1991) conducted in the United States of America showed that undertaking activities in natural environments appeared to have stimulating effects on social contacts and social cohesion. The results of a study by Leyden (2003) show that people in Ireland in walkable neighbourhoods, characterised by the availability of local parks, for example, are 'more likely to know their neighbours, to participate politically, to trust others, and to be involved socially'. Flap and Völker (2005) showed that Dutch neighbourhoods with more open green space and recreational facilities promote a sense of community. Another study performed in the Netherlands found that residents of neighbourhoods with a higher quantity of green space felt less lonely and less often experienced a shortage of social support than residents in neighbourhood with a lower quantity of green space (Maas et al. 2009a). This study also showed that loneliness and perceived shortage of social support partly mediated the relation between green space and health. On the other hand, in Western Australia, Wood et al. (2007) did not find a relationship between distance to park from the respondents' home and social capital.

Overall, the available studies indicate that there is a relationship between neighbourhood green space and social contacts. One study even showed that form and degree of social interaction (loneliness and social support) mediated the relation between green space and health. Although it must be emphasised that there are only a few studies which investigate this relationship, these studies give positive indications for the existence of social contacts as a possible mechanism explaining the link between green space and health.

Selection Effects

Apart from these causal mechanisms, the relationship may partly be the result of direct or indirect selection. Direct selection occurs when people's health influences their chances of living in a favourable environment. The neighbourhood in which people live may not only influence their health, but the health of individuals may also influence the area where they will live. Several studies have observed that residential mobility is associated with individual health. Positive health is correlated with greater residential mobility among younger adults in particular (Bentham 1998; Boyle et al. 2004; Van Hooijdonk et al. 2007). On the other hand, longitudinal studies of health-related migration show that direct selection cannot be held responsible for geographical differences that remain if socio-economic and demographic factors are taken into account (Verheij et al. 1998; Van Lenthe et al. 2007). The current available studies on the relation between green space and health were all unable to control for direct selection, as they all used a cross-sectional study design. Longitudinal studies should be performed to find out whether direct selection plays a role in explaining the relation.

Indirect selection takes place when people with certain characteristics that are related to health, such as income, can afford to live in a favourable environment (Verheij 1999). Migration flows are related to such socio-demographic characteristics as age, income and education (Heins 2002). Most available studies on the relation between green space and health have controlled statistically for the possibility of indirect selection by taking socio-demographic and socio-economic characteristics of people into account. This helps to reduce the role of indirect selection.

Conclusions on Possible Mechanisms

Taking all scientific evidence into account, it can be concluded that restoration from stress and mental fatigue might be the most likely mechanism behind the relationship between green space and health This is the only mechanism for which there is convergent evidence from different lines of research which shows that contact with real or simulated natural environments, including nearby green space, can provide restoration from stress and mental fatigue. Scientific evidence on the influence of the other mechanisms is scarce. The studies from Maas et al. (2008, 2009a) were among the first to investigate the triad of a mechanism, green space and health. Sugiyama et al. (2008) also examined whether mechanisms of physical activity and social contacts might explain the relationship between green space and health. More specifically, they examined whether walking, social coherence of the neighbourhood (measured with questions like it is easy to make friends in my neighbourhood) and local social interaction mediated the relationship between greenness and physical and mental health. Their results showed that recreational walking mediated the relationship between greenness and physical health, whereas the relationship between greenness and mental health was partly accounted for by recreational walking and social coherence. Where physical activity is concerned, the available studies indicate that physical activity might be an underlying mechanism for children and adolescents but that the relation might be less important for adults.

Policy Implications

Although notions of the beneficial effects of green space have existed throughout history (Van den Berg and Van den Berg 2001) and people generally believe that green space is good for their health (Frerichs 2004), until a few years ago, there was hardly any scientific evidence for a direct relationship between green space and health. However, in the past few years, several studies performed in different countries show that green space is positively related to, for example, perceived health, specific diseases, stress, number of complaints and mental health.

These studies provided evidence for the proposition that green space is more than just a luxury since the availability of green space is positively related to perceived and objective health. The development of green space should thus be allocated a more central position in policy related to health, nature and spatial planning. The studies also provide arguments that are needed to place the topic of green space and health on the political agenda and to legitimise policy in this field.

Vulnerable Population Groups

Several studies have shown that vulnerable population groups, such as the elderly, children and adolescents and people with a low socio-economic status may benefit more from neighbourhood green spaces. This suggests that policymakers should take the amount and quality of green space in the living environment into account when endeavouring to improve the health situation of the elderly, young people and groups with lower socio-economic status, especially in urban environments where there is little green space.

Urban Planning

The findings of studies on green space and health could be seen as extra arguments for preserving or—if possible—enlarging the amount of green space in urban living environments for health reasons, especially in the urban environment where space is under pressure because of shortage of land on which to build housing. The greatest opportunities for including green space in neighbourhoods can be found in those areas where radical changes are planned. Urban planners should take green space into account when redesigning existing neighbourhoods or when new neighbourhoods are being developed.

Indication for Designing Green Spaces

The available studies provide little insight on how green space should be designed for optimal health benefits. The studies on the mechanisms behind the relationship between green space and health could provide information on the kind and amount of necessary green space because the ideal design of green spaces differs per mechanism. Walking and cycle paths would be convenient for physical activity, benches for social contacts and quietness is important for recovery from stress. In view of the degree of uncertainty about the exact mechanism behind the relationship, it seems wise to design green spaces that provide a combination of quietness and opportunities for physical activity and social contacts.

Recommendations for Further Research

As has been mentioned before, research on the relation between green space and health is still in its infancy. The available studies have shown that green space might play a role in stimulating health. But a lot of questions remain unanswered. This section raises some important issues which need further investigation.

Type and Amount of Green Space

The available studies on the relation between green space and health provide little insight into the type of green space which optimally influences health. Will tree-lined streets suffice? Or does nature need to be more like a park or wooded area? And is the same type of green space equally useful for health benefits for different population groups?

In order to be able to translate the findings of research on the relationship between green space and health into more specific policy implications, research is needed on how much green space is needed to improve people's health. For example, in the Netherlands, is the norm of 75 m^2 per dwelling imposed by the Ministry of Housing, Spatial Planning and the Environment of the Netherlands (Ministerie van VROM 2004) sufficient, or should there be more green space?

Studies on the relation between green space and health give little insight into the importance of the proximity, quality and accessibility of green space for people's health. Is a large green area within 3 km radius from the residential area sufficient, or should green spaces be closer by? And is proximity of green space for all population groups equally important, or is proximity for elderly and children more important than for adults?

Mechanisms Linked to Green Space and Health

No clear conclusions could be drawn concerning the influence of the behavioural mechanisms. Future research should, therefore, focus on whether mechanisms related to physical activity and social contacts might explain the relationship between green space and health. Apart from the mechanisms discussed here, other mechanisms such as microclimate and the development of children should also be taken into account in future research.

Cost and Benefit Analyses

Urban planning is often supported by analyses of the cost and benefit of building plans. It would be useful to examine the way in which possible reductions in health care costs related to the amount of green space in the living environment can be added to the cost and benefit analyses.

Causality of the Relationship Between Green Space and Health

Most of the studies on the relation between green space and health are cross-sectional, which means that part of any relationship found might be due to direct or indirect selection. Most studies have tried to rule out indirect selection as much as possible by controlling statistically for demographic and socio-economic characteristics of the individual. Apart from individual characteristics, neighbourhood characteristics like neighbourhood socio-economic status, which could differ from individual socio-economic status when most neighbourhood residents have a low socio-economic status but the individual does not, might also be responsible for the relationship found between green space and health. Future research should also take neighbourhood characteristics into account. Furthermore, longitudinal studies are needed to control for direct selection.

Research Aimed at Specific Population Groups

Most studies on the relation between green space and health focus on assessing the relation for large population groups. More knowledge is needed on what kind of green space influences the health of these population groups beneficially. Do neighbourhoods with a high child population need the same amount and type of green space as neighbourhoods with mainly elderly people?

Use of Green Space in Health Care Settings

This chapter shows that green space in the residential area has the potential to influence health. There exist, however, only a few studies which focus on health benefits of green space in health care settings (Ulrich 1984; Lechtzin et al. 2010). This could be due to the lack of scientific evidence conclusively showing that people's health benefits from green space in health care settings. Several initiatives of using green space in health care settings taken by health care providers could possibly be improved, if they were accompanied by good research. Initiatives for using green space in the health care sector should be evaluated in order to increase insight into their effectiveness. Future research should focus on evaluating examples of good practices that aim to increase the amount of green space in health care settings.

Individual Interaction with Green Space

Few studies have investigated how use of and exposure to green spaces influences health. Questions that need to be answered are for instance: Are people who use green spaces more often healthier? This kind of information could be gathered using a GPS device, a device which measures where someone is at a certain time (see Chap. 9 in this book).

Most studies on the relationship between green space and health have used objective measures of green space, which reduced the risks of respondent bias.

Subjective measures of green space, however, can also provide important information. People's perception of green spaces may, in fact, affect their behaviour more than the actual amount of green space available. Green spaces that are considered unsafe or of poor quality tend to be avoided, which means that supplementing objective measures of green space with measures of people's perception of green space will improve our understanding of how the green environment affects health, behaviour and feelings of social safety (Coley et al. 1997; Kuo et al. 1998; Kweon et al. 1998).

References

Appleton, J. (1975). *The experience of landscape*. London: Wiley.

Bentham, G. (1998). Migration and morbidity: Implications for geographical studies of disease. *Social Science & Medicine, 26*(1), 49–54.

Berkman, L. F., Glass, T., Brisette, I., & Seeman, T. E. (2000). From social integration to health. Durkheim in the new millennium. *Social Science & Medicine, 51*, 843–857.

Berto, R. (2005). Exposure to restorative environments helps restore attentional capacity. *Journal of Environmental Psychology, 25*, 249–259.

Björk, J., Albin, M., Grahn, P., Jacobson, H., Ardö, J., Wadbro, J., et al. (2008). Recreational values of the natural environment in relation to neighbourhood satisfaction, physical activity, obesity and wellbeing. *Journal of Epidemiology and Community Health, 62*(e2).

Booth, M. L., Owen, N., Nauman, A., Clavisi, O., & Leslie, E. (2000). Social-cognitive and perceived environment influences associated with physical activity in older Australians. *Preventive Medicine, 31*, 15–22.

Bowler, D. E., Buyung-Ali, L. M., Knight, T. M., & Pullin, A. S. (2010). A systematic review of evidence for the added benefits to health of exposure to natural environments. *BMC Public Health, 10*, 456. doi:10. 1186/1471-2458-10-456.

Boyle, P., Norman, P., & Rees, P. (2004). Changing places: Do changes in the relative deprivation of areas influence limiting long-term illness and mortality among non-migrant people living in non-deprived households? *Social Science & Medicine, 58*, 2459–2471.

Branas, C. C., Cheney, R. A., MacDonald, J. M., Tam, V. W., Jackson, T. D., & Ten Have, T. R. (2011). A difference-in-differences analysis of health, safety, and greening vacant urban space. *American Journal of Epidemiology, 174*(11), 1296–1306.

Cohen, D. A., Ashwood, J. S., Scott, M. M., Overton, A., Evenson, K. R., Staten, L. K., et al. (2006). Public parks and physical activity among adolescent girls. *Pediatrics, 118*, e1381–e1389.

Coley, R. L., Kuo, F. E., & Sullivan, W. C. (1997). Where does community grow? The social context created by nature in Urban Public Housing. *Environment and Behavior, 29*(4), 468–494.

Coutts, C., Horner, M., & Chapin, T. (2010). Using geographical information system to model the effects of green space accessibility on mortality in Florida. *Geocarto International, 25*(6), 471–484.

De Vries, S. (2001). *Nature and Health: The importance of green space in the urban living environment*. Proceedings of the symposium Open space functions under urban pressure, September 19–21, 2001, Ghent.

De Vries, S. I., Bakker, I., Van Mechelen, W., & Hopman-Rock, M. (2007). Determinants of activity friendly neighborhoods for children: Results from the SPACE Study. *American Journal of Health Promotion, 21*(14 Suppl), 312–316.

De Vries, S., Verheij, R. A., Groenewegen, P. P., & Spreeuwenberg, P. (2003). Natural environments – healthy environments? An exploratory analysis of the relationship between green space and health. *Environment and Planning A, 35*, 1717–1731.

Ellaway, A., Macintyre, S., & Bonnefoy, X. (2005). Graffiti, greenery, and obesity in adults: Secondary analysis of European cross sectional survey. *BMJ, 331*, 611–612.

Epstein, L. H., Raja, S., Gold, S. S., Paluch, R. A., Pak, Y., & Roemmich, J. N. (2006). Reducing sedentary behavior: The relationship between park area and the physical activity of youth. *Psychological Science, 17*, 654–659.

Ewert, A., & Heywood, J. (1991). Group development in the Natural Environment. Expectations, outcomes and techniques. *Environment and Behavior, 23*(5), 592–615.

Faber Taylor, A., Kuo, F. E., & Sullivan, W. C. (2002). Views of nature and self-discipline. Evidence from inner city children. *Journal of Environmental Psychology, 22*, 49–63.

Flap, H., & Völker, B. (2005). Gemeenschap, informele controle en collectieve kwaden. In B. Völker (Ed.), *Burgers in de buurt: samen leven in school, wijk en vereniging* (pp. 41–70). Amsterdam: Amsterdam University Press.

Frerichs, R. (2004). *Gezondheid en natuur: een onderzoek naar de relatie tussen gezondheid en natuur*. Amsterdam: TNS-NIPO.

Giles-Corti, B., & Donovan, R. J. (2002). The relative influence of individual, social and physical environment determinants of physical activity. *Social Science & Medicine, 54*, 1793–1812.

Giles-Corti, B., & Donovan, R. J. (2003). Relative influences of individual, social environmental, and physical environmental correlates of walking. *American Journal of Public Health, 93*, 1583–1589.

Harms, L. (2006). *Op weg in de vrije tijd: context, kenmerken en dynamiek van vrijetijdsmobiliteit*. Den Haag: Sociaal Cultureel Planbureau.

Hartig, T., Böök, A., Garville, J., Olssen, T., & Gärling, T. (1996). Environmental influences on psychological restoration. *Scandinavian Journal of Psychology, 37*, 378–393.

Hartig, T., Evans, G. W., Jamner, L. D., Dows, D. S., & Gärling, T. (2003). Tracking restoration in natural and urban field settings. *Journal of Environmental Psychology, 23*, 109–123.

Hartig, T., Mang, M., & Evans, G. W. (1991). Restorative effects of natural environment experiences. *Environment and Behavior, 23*, 3–27.

Hawe, P., & Shiell, A. (2000). Social capital and health promotion: A review. *Social Science & Medicine, 51*, 871–885.

Health Council of the Netherlands, Dutch Advisory Council for research on Spatial Planning, Nature and the Environment (2004). *Nature and health: The influence of nature on social, psychological and physical well-being*. The Hague: Health Council of the Netherlands/RMNO. http://www.gezondheidsraad.nl/sites/default/files/Nature %20and %20health.pdf. Accessed 23 Dec 2011.

Heins, S. (2002). *Rurale woonmilieus in stad en land. Plattelandsbeelden, vraag naar en aanbod van rurale woonmilieus*. Delft: Eburon.

Hillsdon, M., Panter, J., Foster, C., & Jones, A. (2006). The relationship between access and quality of urban green space with population physical activity. *J R Institute of Public Health, 120*, 1127–1132.

Jago, R., Baranowski, T., & Harris, M. (2006). Relationships between GIS environmental features and adolescent male physical activity: GIS coding differences. *Journal of Physical Activity and Health, 3*, 230–242.

Jago, R., Baranowski, T., Zakeri, I., & Harris, M. (2005). Observed environmental features and the physical activity of adolescent males. *American Journal of Preventive Medicine, 29*, 98–104.

Kaczynski, A. T., & Henderson, K. A. (2007). Environmental correlates of physical activity: A review of evidence about parks and recreation. *Leisure Sciences, 39*, 315–354.

Kaplan, R. (2001). The nature of the view from home: Psychological benefits. *Environment and Behavior, 33*, 507–542.

Kaplan, R., & Kaplan, S. (1989). *The experience of nature: A psychological perspective*. Cambridge: Cambridge University Press.

Kawachi, I., & Berkman, L. (2000). Social cohesion, social capital, and health. In L. Berkman & I. Kawachi (Eds.), *Social epidemiology*. New York: Oxford University Press.

Kawachi, I., Kennedy, B. P., Lochner, K., & Prothrow-Stith, D. (1997). Social capital, income inequality, and mortality. *American Journal of Public Health, 87*(9), 1491–1498.

King, A. C., Stokols, D., Talen, E., Brassington, G. S., & Killingsworth, R. (2002). Theoretical approaches to the promotion of physical activity: Forging a transdisciplinary paradigm. *American Journal of Preventive Medicine, 23*, 15–25.
Kuo, F. E., Sullivan, W. C., & Wiley, A. (1998). Fertile ground for community: Inner-city neighborhood common spaces. *American Journal of Community Psychology, 26*, 823–851.
Kuo, F. E., & Sullivan, W. C. (2001). Aggression and violence in the inner-city. Effects of environment via mental fatigue. *Environ Beh, 33*(4):543–571.
Kweon, B. S., Sullivan, W. C., & Wiley, A. (1998). Green common spaces and the social integration of inner-city older adults. *Environment and Behavior, 30*, 823–858.
Lechtzin, N., Busse, A. M., Smith, M. T., Grossman, S., Nesbit, S., & Diette, G. B. (2010). A randomized trial of nature scenery and sounds versus urban scenery and sounds to reduce pain in adults undergoing bone marrow aspirate and biopsy. *Journal of Alternative and Complementary Medicine, 16*(9), 965–972.
Leyden, K. M. (2003). Social capital and the built environment: The importance of walkable neighborhoods. *American Journal of Public Health, 93*, 1546–1551.
Maas, J., Van Dillen, S., Verheij, R. A., & Groenewegen, P. P. (2009a). Social contacts as a possible mechanism behind the relation between green space and health. *Health & Place, 15*(2), 586–595.
Maas, J., Verheij, R. A., de Vries, S., Spreeuwenberg, P., Schellevis, F. G., & Groenewegen, P. P. (2009a). Morbidity is related to a green living environment. *Journal of Epidemiology and Community Health, 63*, 967–973.
Maas, J., Verheij, R. A., Groenewegen, P. P., De Vries, S., & Spreeuwenberg, P. (2006). Green space, urbanity and health: How strong is the relation? *Journal of Epidemiology and Community Health, 60*, 587–592.
Maas, J., Verheij, R. A., Spreeuwenberg, P., & Groenewegen, P. P. (2008). Physical activity as a possible mechanism behind the relation between green space and health: A multilevel analysis. *BMC Public Health, 8*(206), 1–13.
McGinn, A. P., Evenson, K. R., Herring, A. H., & Huston, S. L. (2007). The relationship between leisure, walking and transportation activity with the natural environment. *Health & Place, 13*, 588–602.
Ministerie van Volkshuisvesting, Ruimtelijke Ordening en Milieubeheer. (2004). *Kamerbrief: Nationale aanpak Milieu en Gezondheid 2008–2012*. Den Haag: Ministerie van VROM.
Mitchell, R., & Popham, F. (2007). Green space, urbanity and health: Relationships in England. *Journal of Epidemiology and Community Health, 61*, 681–683.
Mitchell, R., & Popham, F. (2008). Effects of exposure to natural environments on health inequalities: An observational population study. *The Lancet, 372*, 1655–1660.
Mota, J., Almeida, M., Santos, P., & Ribeiro, J. C. (2005). Perceived neighborhood environments and physical activity in adolescents. *Preventive Medicine, 41*, 834–836.
Nielsen, T. S., & Hansen, K. B. (2007). Do green areas affect health? Results from a Danish survey on the use of green areas and health indicators. *Health Place, 13*, 839–850.
NIH. (1996). Consensus development panel on physical activity and cardiovascular health: Physical activity and cardiovascular health. *Journal of the American Medical Association, 276*, 241–246.
Orians, G. H. (1986). An ecological and evolutionary approach to landscape aesthetics. In E. C. Penning-Rowsell & D. Lowenthal (Eds.), *Landscape meanings and values* (pp. 3–22). London: Allen and Unwin.
Ottosson, J., & Grahn, P. (2005). A comparison of leisure time spent in a garden with leisure time spent indoors: On measures of restoration in residents in geriatric care. *Landscape Research, 30*(1), 23–55.
Paffenbarger, R. S., Hyde, R. T., Win, A. L., Lee, I., Jong, D. L., & Kampert, J. B. (1993). The association of changes in physical-activity level and other lifestyle characteristics with mortality among men. *New England Journal of Medicine, 328*, 538–545.
Parsons, R. (1991). The potential influences of environmental perception on human health. *Journal of Environmental Psychology, 11*, 1–23.

Pate, R., Pratt, M., Blair, S. N., Haskell, W. L., Macere, C. A., Bouchard, C., et al. (1995). Physical activity and public health: A recommendation from the Centers for Disease Control and Prevention and the American College of Sports Medicine. *Journal of the American Medical Association, 273*, 402–407.

Pennebaker, J. W., & Lightner, J. M. (1980). Competition of internal and external information in an exercise setting. *Journal of Personality and Social Psychology, 39*, 165–174.

Pikora, T., Giles-Corti, B., Bull, F., Jamrozik, K., & Donovan, R. (2003). Developing a framework for assessment of the environmental determinants of walking and cycling. *Social Science & Medicine, 56*, 1693–1703.

Pretty, G. M. H., Andrews, L., & Collett, C. (1994). Exploring adolescents' sense of community and its relationship to loneliness. *Journal of Community Psychology, 22*, 346–358.

Pretty, J., Peacock, J., Hine, R., Sellens, M., South, N., & Griffin, M. (2007). Green exercise in the UK countryside: Effects on health and psychological well-being, and implications for policy and planning. *Journal of Environmental Planning and Management, 50*, 211–231.

Prezza, M., Amici, M., Roberti, T., & Tedeschi, G. (2001). Sense of community referred to the whole town: It's relations with neighboring, loneliness, life satisfaction, and area of residence. *Journal of Community Psychology, 29*(1), 29–52.

Richardson, E. A., Mitchell, R., Hartig, T., de Vries, S., Astell-Burt, T., & Frumkin, H. (2011). Green cities and health: A question of scale? *Journal of Epidemiology and Community Health*. doi:10.1136/jech.2011.137240.

Richardson, E., Pearce, J., Mitchell, R., Day, P., & Kingham, S. (2010). The association between green space and cause-specific mortality in urban New Zealand: An ecological analysis of green space utility. *BMC Public Health, 10*, 240. doi:10.1136/jech.2011.137240.

Rodiek, S. D. (2002). Influence of an outdoor garden on mood and stress in older persons. *Journal of Therapeutic Horticulture, 13*, 13–21.

Roemmich, J. N., Epstein, L. H., Raja, S., & Yin, L. (2007). The neighborhood and home environments: Disparate relationships with physical activity and sedentary behaviors in youth. *Annals of Behavioral Medicine, 33*, 29–38.

Roemmich, J. N., Epstein, L. H., Raja, S., Yin, L., Robinson, J., & Winiewicz, D. (2006). Association of access to parks and recreational facilities with the physical activity of young children. *Preventive Medicine, 43*, 437–441.

Sallis, J. F., Bauman, A., & Pratt, M. (1998). Environmental and policy: Interventions to promote physical activity. *American Journal of Preventive Medicine, 15*, 379–397.

Sallis, J. F., & Owen, N. (1996). Ecological models. In K. Glanz, B. K. Rimer, & F. M. Lewis (Eds.), *Health behavior and health education: Theory, research and practice* (pp. 403–424). San Francisco: Jossey-Bass.

Schwanen, T., Dijst, M., & Dieleman, F. M. (2002). A microlevel analysis of residential context and travel time. *Environment and Planning A, 34*, 1487–1507.

Stigsdotter, U. K., Ekholm, O., Schipperijn, J., Toftager, M., Kamper-Jørgensen, F., & Randrup, T. B. (2010). Health promoting outdoor environments—associations between green space, and health, health-related quality of life and stress based on a Danish national representative survey. *Scandinavian Journal of Public Health, 38*(4), 411–417.

Sugiyama, T., Leslie, E., Giles-Corti, B., & Owen, N. (2008). Associations of neighbourhood greenness with physical and mental health: Do walking, social coherence and local social interaction explain the relationships? *Journal of Epidemiology and Community Health, 62*, e9.

Takano, T., Nakamura, K., & Watanabe, M. (2002). Urban residential environments and senior citizens' longevity in megacity areas. The importance of walkable green spaces. *Journal of Epidemiology and Community Health, 56*, 913–918.

Tennessen, C. M., & Cimprich, B. (1995). Views to nature: Effects on attention. *Journal of Environmental Psychology, 15*, 77–85.

Timperio, A., Crawford, D., Telford, A., & Salmon, J. (2004). Perceptions about the local neighborhood and walking and cycling among children. *Preventive Medicine, 38*, 39–47.

Ulrich, R. (1984). View through a window may influence recovery from surgery. *Science, 224*, 420–421.

Ulrich, R. S. (1993). Biophilia, biophobia and natural landscapes. In S. R. Kellert & E. O. Wilson (Eds.), *The Biophilia hypothesis* (pp. 85–137). Washington, DC: Island Press.
Ulrich, R. S., Simons, R. F., Losito, B. D., Fiorito, E., Miles, M. A., & Zelson, M. (1991). Stress recovery during exposure to natural and urban environments. *Journal of Environmental Psychology, 11*, 201–203.
US Department of Health and Human Services (1996). *Physical activity and health: A report of the Surgeon General*. US Department of HHS, Centers for Disease Control and Prevention, National Center for Chronic Disease Prevention and Health Promotion, Atlanta.
Van den Berg, A. E., Hartig, T., & Staats, H. (2007). Preference for nature in urbanized societies: Stress, restoration, and the pursuit of sustainability. *Journal of Social Issues, 63*, 79–96.
Van den Berg, A. E., Koole, S. L., & Van der Wulp, N. Y. (2003). Environmental preference and restoration: How are they related? *Journal of Environmental Psychology, 23*, 2135–2146.
Van den Berg, A. E., Maas, J., Verheij, R. A., & Groenewegen, P. P. (2010). Green space as a buffer between negative life events and health. *Soc sci med, 70*(8), 1203–1210. http://dx.doi.org/10.1016/j.socscimed.2010.01.002.
Van den Berg, A. E., & Van den Berg, M. M. H. E. (2001). *Van buiten word je beter*. Alterra: Wageningen.
Van Dillen, S. M. E., De Vries, S., Groenewegen, P. P., & Spreeuwenberg, P. (2011). Greenspace in urban neighbourhoods and residents' health: Adding quality to quantity. *Journal of Epidemiology and Community Health*. doi:10.1136/jech.2009.104695.
Van Hooijdonk, C., Droomers, M., Van Loon, J. A. M., Van der Lucht, F., & Kunst, A. E. (2007). Exceptions to the rule: Healthy deprived areas and unhealthy wealthy areas. *Social Science & Medicine, 64*, 1326–1342.
Van Lenthe, F. J., Martikainen, P., & Mackenbach, J. P. (2007). Neighbourhood inequalities in health and health-related behaviour: Results of selective migration? *Health & Place, 13*, 123–137.
Verheij, R. A., Maas, J., Groenewegen, P. P. (2008). Urban-rural health differences and the availability of green space. *Eur Urban Regional Studies, 15*(4):307–316.
Verheij, R. A. (1999). *Urban–rural variations in health care*. Dissertation NIVEL, Utrecht.
Verheij, R. A., Van de Mheen, H. D., De Bakker, D. H., Groenewegen, P. P., & Mackenbach, J. P. (1998). Urban–rural variations in health in the Netherlands: Does selective migration play a part? *Journal of Epidemiology and Community Health, 52*, 487–493.
Vlahov, D., & Galea, S. (2002). Urbanization, urbanicity, and health. *Journal of Urban Health, 79*(4 Suppl 1), 1–12.
Wells, N. M. (2000). At home with nature. Effects of "greenness" on children's cognitive functioning. *Environment and Behavior, 32*, 775–795.
Wood, L., Shannon, T., Bulsara, M., Pikora, T., McCormack, G., & Giles-Corti, B. (2007). The anatomy of the safe and social suburb: An explanatory study of the built environment, social capital and residents' perceptions of safety. *Health & Place, 14*(1), 15–31.

Chapter 12
Socioeconomic Differences in Physical Activity: The Role of Neighbourhood Factors

Carlijn Kamphuis and Frank van Lenthe

Introduction

Physical activity is an important determinant of health; however, many people do not meet recommendations for sufficient physical activity. Also, studies have shown large socioeconomic inequalities in physical activity, with those with a lower socioeconomic position (SEP) less likely to participate in recreational and vigorous activities than high SEP groups. From this respect, it is important to investigate to what extent physical activity and inequalities in physical activity are associated with environmental factors, such as physical and social neighbourhood characteristics. Certain characteristics of neighbourhoods, like aesthetics and social cohesion, may have a positive association with residents' physical activity levels, but lower exposures among low socioeconomic groups. These characteristics may then serve as entry points for interventions to increase physical activity levels and reduce inequalities in physical activity. Also, to achieve environmental justice (with all people having equal access to health-enhancing environments), it is important to improve neighbourhood conditions for low socioeconomic groups.

In this chapter, we start with explaining socioeconomic health inequalities and how health behaviours, like physical activity, may contribute to these inequalities. Subsequently, we will introduce theoretical models (i.e. the Theory of Planned Behaviour and social ecological models of health behaviour) that formed the theoretical basis for a series of studies on inequalities in physical activity and neighbourhood characteristics. Then, the results of two empirical studies are presented, namely, regarding inequalities in sports participation and recreational walking. Subsequently, we discuss to what extent socioeconomic inequalities in

C. Kamphuis (✉) • F. van Lenthe
Department of Public Health, Erasmus University Medical Centre, P.O. Box 2040, 3000 CA Rotterdam, The Netherlands
e-mail: c.kamphuis@erasmusmc.nl; f.vanlenthe@erasmusmc.nl

C. Stock and A. Ellaway (eds.), *Neighbourhood Structure and Health Promotion*, DOI 10.1007/978-1-4614-6672-7_12,

neighbourhood perceptions are due to differences in objective neighbourhood characteristics or subject to other influences. We end this chapter with a discussion of challenges for future research into neighbourhood influences on health behaviours.

Socioeconomic Inequalities in Health and Health Behaviours

Socioeconomic inequalities in health have existed for centuries and are observed in many countries in Europe (Antonovsky 1967; Mackenbach et al. 2008). Despite increased attention in research and policy for health inequalities over the last decades, the health gap between higher and lower socioeconomic groups has not declined. In fact, socioeconomic health inequalities have even widened over recent decades (Mackenbach et al. 2003). In the Netherlands, people with a low SEP live about 7 years shorter than their higher status counterparts. Moreover, they spend about 18 *more* years in poorer health (Lucht and Polder 2010). The reduction of these health inequalities is a major priority for public health from a scientific and societal perspective, both at the international and national level. The potential gain in healthy life years resulting from a reduction of health inequalities—and its related societal and economic impact—could be enormous. However, current approaches to tackle health inequalities have been far from successful.

An important mechanism behind the association between SEP and health is that of the behavioural explanation. Low socioeconomic groups have a less healthy lifestyle, as characterised by physical inactivity, poorer eating habits and more smoking, which leads to their poorer health status. Recent research suggests that the importance of health behaviours as contributors to socioeconomic inequalities in mortality is even higher than previously thought (Stringhini et al. 2010). There is a clear need to promote healthy behaviours in lower socioeconomic groups and to reduce socioeconomic inequalities in health behaviours. To achieve this, interventions and policies should match with the most important determinants of socioeconomic inequalities in health behaviours. However, what are those determinants, or in other words, why do poor people behave poorly? (Lynch et al. 1997) Obviously, relevant determinants of health behaviours differ greatly for different behaviours. Access to healthy foods in supermarkets may be important for fruit intake, but obviously not for sport participation. Therefore, it is important to study specific determinants for specific behavioural outcomes. In this chapter, we focus on several specific outcomes of one particular health behaviour, namely, physical activity.

The protective effects of physical activity for total mortality, cardiovascular disease and diabetes are widely known and supported by a large amount of evidence (Batty 2002; Schnohr et al. 2006, 2003). Physical activity also increases chances for longevity: life expectancy for sedentary people at age 50 years is 1.5 years shorter than for people engaging in moderate daily physical activity and more than 3.5 years shorter than for people with high physical activity levels (Franco et al. 2005). How much activity is required to achieve health benefits is still a topic of debate. While many studies show that moderate intensity exercise, like walking, is sufficient to reduce the risk of cardiovascular disease (Wannamethee and Shaper 2001; Wannamethee et al. 1998), others conclude that only heavy or vigorous activity, like sports, confers benefit (Rothenbacher et al. 2006; Swain and Franklin 2006).

Over time, the prevalence of individuals not meeting recommendations for sufficient physical activity has increased to more than 50 % of the population (Lucht and Polder 2010), and many studies have shown large educational inequalities in physical activity (Dowler 2001). Compared to people from high socioeconomic groups, people from lower socioeconomic groups are more likely to be physically inactive (Crespo et al. 1999; Droomers et al. 1998; Marshall et al. 2007), to have lower levels of leisure time physical activity (Lindstrom et al. 2001; Lynch et al. 1997) and walking for recreation (Ball et al. 2007) and to show decreases in leisure physical activity over time (Droomers et al. 2001). To be able to reduce socioeconomic differences in physical activity, it is important therefore to understand which factors may offer good entry points for interventions, i.e. factors that are related to physical activity *and* are patterned by SEP. To ascertain the relevant determinants, theoretical models that try to explain and predict variations in health behaviours were consulted.

Theoretical Guidance: Theory of Planned Behaviour and Ecological Models

Following a long tradition in health promotion and health education (Baranowski et al. 2003; Weinstein 1993), individual differences in health behaviours can be explained by socio-cognitive factors as part of planned, cognitive appraisal processes. Among the most commonly employed theoretical models to predict health behaviours is Fishbein and Ajzen's Theory of Planned Behaviour (TPB) (Ajzen 1991). The TPB assumes that one's intention to change his/her behaviour (e.g. I want to become physically activity on a daily basis) is determined by attitudes towards the behaviour (e.g. daily physical activity is fun, daily physical activity is healthy), subjective norms that are associated with the behaviour (e.g. family and friends think that I should be physically active on a daily base) and perceived behavioural control to perform the behaviour (e.g. I'm sure I could be physically active daily).

Attitudes, subjective norms and perceived behavioural control predict general variations in health behaviours, accounting for 27 % and 39 % of the variance in behaviour and intention, respectively (Armitage and Conner 2001). Especially perceived behavioural control—very similar to the concept of self-efficacy—is known as a particularly strong correlate of health behaviours (Trost et al. 2002). These individual cognitions have been utilised less frequently for understanding *socioeconomic* variations in health behaviours. However, lower socioeconomic groups have shown to be less health consciousness and to have stronger beliefs about effects of destiny on health, which were associated with less healthy behavioural choices (Wardle and Steptoe 2003). Self-efficacy, enjoyment of physical activity and intentions were found to contribute to the explanation of socioeconomic differences in walking (Ball et al. 2007).

Although some of the variations in health behaviours can be accounted for by individual cognitions, social-cognitive theories have been criticised for their focus on such motivational factors only, paying little attention to environmental, nonvoluntary factors which are beyond the individual's control. To better understand why people behave as they do and to increase the likelihood of behaviour change, it is important to put behaviour into context. This renewed interest in environmental factors for health and health behaviours has shifted the focus from social-cognitive towards ecological models of health behaviours.

Ecological models emphasise that besides intrapersonal and interpersonal factors, the environment also has an important effect on health behaviours (Sallis and Owen 2002). All these factors together function to promote or hinder an individual's engagement in health behaviours (Sallis et al. 2006). Many different environmental settings may impact on behaviours, e.g. factors from the neighbourhood, work or household environment, but also city- and country-level variables (e.g. policies, regulations, media) (Swinburn et al. 1999). Environments can restrict people acting in a healthy way by promoting (and sometimes demanding) other actions and by discouraging or prohibiting health behaviours. Empirical studies have shown that neighbourhood aesthetics, connectivity of streets and the availability and accessibility of facilities may have a positive association with physical activity (McCormack et al. 2004; Wendel-Vos et al. 2007).

Also from the perspective of socioeconomic inequalities in health behaviours, it is important to consider environmental influences. Given that most unhealthy behaviours systematically cluster within the low socioeconomic groups, the core underlying determinants are most likely to be found in factors to which socioeconomic groups are differentially exposed, e.g. environmental factors. The growing body of evidence for place effects on health supports this hypothesis (Macintyre et al. 2002). Even after adjustment for individual-level variables such as age, gender and individual SES, residents of disadvantaged neighbourhoods were found to be in poorer health (Bosma et al. 2001; Pickett and Pearl 2001) and have higher rates of unhealthy behaviours, i.e. smoking, physical inactivity and poor diet (Diez-Roux et al. 2000; Ecob and Macintyre 2000; Sundquist et al. 1999; Van Lenthe et al. 2005). This means that the higher prevalence of unhealthy behaviours among people of low SEP may be partly due to either direct or indirect adverse effects of their neighbourhood of residence. We have investigated the contribution of specific neighbourhood characteristics to socioeconomic differences for two specific physical activity outcomes: sports participation and recreational walking.

Socioeconomic Inequalities in Sports Participation: The Role of Environmental Factors

Participation in vigorous activities like sports is low among the socioeconomically disadvantaged groups; however, regular vigorous activity can have an important positive health effect (Andersen et al. 2000; Franco et al. 2005). For a better understanding of the determinants of socioeconomic inequalities in sports participation, we examined the contribution of neighbourhood, household and individual factors to these inequalities (Kamphuis et al. 2008b).

Data were obtained by a large-scale postal survey among a stratified sample of the adult population (age 25–75 years) of Eindhoven (which is the fifth largest city of the Netherlands) and surrounding cities ($N=4{,}785$; response rate 64.4 %). Participants reported on their highest attained educational level and household income level (as indicators of their socioeconomic position (SEP)) and several level neighbourhood, household and individual factors, as described in Table 12.1. Also, they reported on their physical activity behaviour in the SQUASH questionnaire—a validated Dutch questionnaire to measure various types of physical activity among an adult population: commuting, leisure time, sports, occupational and housekeeping activities (Wendel-Vos et al. 2003). Participants wrote down up to four sports they did on a weekly basis during previous month (open question). For these sports they reported frequency (times per week), average duration (minutes per day) and intensity (low, average, high). Self-reported intensity, in combination with participant's age, and activity-specific MET values were used to calculate intensity scores. As almost half of the sample did not do any sport, sports participation was dichotomised, with 'no': not doing any sports weekly with at least moderate intensity (moderate intensity=4–6 MET for 18–55 years old; 3–5 MET for 55+ years old) versus 'yes': doing sports at least once a week with moderate or high intensity. Logistic regression analyses were done with sports participation as binary outcome (no vs. yes), i.e. respondents not doing any moderate or high intensity sports at least once a week were classified as nonparticipants.

We found a clear gradient between SEP and no sports participation, with the lowest educated (odds ratio OR=3.99; 95 % confidence interval (CI): 2.99–5.31) and lowest income group (OR=3.02; 95 % CI: 2.36–2.86) most likely to report no sports participation (Kamphuis et al. 2008b). With regard to possible explanatory factors for this gradient, participants from lower SEP groups were more likely to report that their neighbourhood was not safe and unattractive and had insufficient places for physical activity compared to higher SEP groups (Table 12.2). Also, they were more likely to experience a small social network and low social cohesion in their neighbourhood. All of these characteristics increased the risk of doing no sports. People indicating not feeling at home in their neighbourhood were also more likely to do no sports, but this was not significantly more prevalent among any of the educational groups ($p=0.093$).

Two out of three indicators of material deprivation (crowding and having financial problems) and all three indicators of social deprivation increased the likelihood of doing no sports (see Table 12.2). Also, these factors showed higher prevalence among lower socioeconomic groups. Furthermore, all individual cognitions of recommended physical activity were significantly related to sports participation, and unfavourable cognitions were more prevalent among lower socioeconomic groups. As an exception, the negative outcome expectancy "physical activity requires too much time" was more frequently reported by people from higher than lower socioeconomic groups. Of all factors examined, self-efficacy and intention showed the strongest associations with sports participation.

Table 12.1 Neighbourhood, household, and individual factors as measured in the GLOBE postal survey 2004

Factors in logistic regression models	Measurement of factors in GLOBE postal survey 2004	Answering categories in the analyses
Neighbourhood		
Neighbourhood physical factors		
Neighbourhood safety	"My neighbourhood is unsafe"	Agree, disagree
Neighbourhood attractiveness	"My neighbourhood is unattractive"	Agree, disagree
Availability of facilities	"There are insufficient places for physical activity in my neighbourhood"	Agree, disagree
Poor weather	"It is often poor weather"	Agree, disagree
Neighbourhood social factors		
Social network (the extent to which one is interconnected and embedded in a community (McNeill et al. 2006))	The first factor constructed by a factor analysis with 13 items concerning aspects of social relationships, which we referred to as 'social network'. Items that loaded on this factor were e.g. "I borrow stuff from my neighbours", "I visit my neighbours in their house", and "I ask my neighbours for advice" (five-point scale: totally agree—totally disagree)	Large, medium, small
Social capital in the neighbourhood (the extent of connectedness and solidarity among groups (McNeill et al. 2006))	Second factor constructed by a factor analysis with 13 items concerning aspects of social relationships, which we referred to as 'social capital'. Items that loaded on this factor were e.g. "People in this neighbourhood agree on norms and values", "People in this neighbourhood are willing to help each other", and "People in this neighbourhood can be trusted" (five-point scale: totally agree—totally disagree)	High, medium, low
Feeling at home in one's neighbourhood	Third factor constructed by a factor analysis with 13 items concerning aspects of social relationships, which we referred to as "feeling at home in one's neighbourhood". Items that loaded on this factor were e.g. "I feel alone in this neighbourhood", "(f) I feel at home in this neighbourhood", (g) "I want to move out of this neighbourhood" (five-point scale: totally agree—totally disagree)	High, medium, low

(continued)

Table 12.1 (continued)

Factors in logistic regression models	Measurement of factors in GLOBE postal survey 2004	Answering categories in the analyses
Social disorganisation (the inability of residents of an area to regulate everyday public behaviours and physical conditions (McCulloch 2003))	One factor constructed by a factor analysis with 11 items concerning the frequency with which adverse neighbourhood events occurred (often, sometimes, (almost) never). Items referred to e.g. litter, graffiti, vandalism, people being hassled on the streets, drunken people in the streets	High, medium, low
Length of residence	"For how long have you lived in this neighbourhood?"	0–2; 2–5; 5–15; 15 ≥ years
Household		
Indicators for material deprivation		
Indicator 1: financial problems	"Did you have financial problems last year, e.g. problems paying bills, food or rent?"	None, some, many
Indicator 2: car possession	"Is there a car available in your household?"	Yes, no
Indicator 3: crowding	Crowding was calculated from 2 items, i.e. "With how many people do you live together in your household? (including yourself)", and "How many rooms has the house you live in?" (excluding kitchen, corridor, cellar, bathroom, toilet, garage, attic)	1 < person per room, 1 ≥ persons per room,
Indicators for social deprivation		
Indicator 1: friends/family for dinner monthly	"Do you have friends/family over for dinner at least monthly?"	Yes; no, for financial reasons; no, for other reasons;
Indicator 2: going out fortnightly	"Do you go for a night out with friends/family at least fortnightly?"	Yes; no, for financial reasons; no, for other reasons;
Indicator 3: going on holiday yearly	"Do you go on holiday for at least 1 week per year?"	Yes; no, for financial reasons; no, for other reasons;
Individual		
Positive outcome expectancies of recommended PA[a]	Measured with six items on a five-point scale (very important—very unimportant)[b]: "It makes me feel less stressed", "I get in a good mood", "I enjoy being active", "I'm more confident with my body", "It is good for my fitness", "I feel energized".	(Very) important, not important/unimportant, (very) unimportant,

(continued)

Table 12.1 (continued)

Factors in logistic regression models	Measurement of factors in GLOBE postal survey 2004	Answering categories in the analyses
Negative outcome expectancies of recommended PA	Measured with six items on a five-point scale (very important—very unimportant)[b] : "It requires too much time", "It requires too much discipline", "It requires too much energy", "I'm afraid of injuries", "I feel uncomfortable when others see me exercising", "Doing sports is expensive".	(Very) important, not important/ unimportant, (very) unimportant,
Subjective norm	"Significant others think that I should be physically active for at least 30 min/day"	Agree, partly agree/ disagree, disagree,
Social support	"Significant others support me to be physically active for at least 30 min/day"	Agree, partly agree/ disagree, disagree,
Modelling	"Significant others are physically active for at least 30 min/day themselves"	Agree, partly agree/ disagree, disagree,
Self-efficacy	"How sure are you that you can be physically active for at least 30 min/day?" (measured on a five-point scale (very sure—very unsure)[b]	(Very) sure, not sure/ unsure, (very) unsure,
Intention	"Do you plan to be physically active for at least 30 min/day?" (measured on a five-point scale (surely yes—surely no)[b]	(Surely) yes, maybe, (surely) no,

Source: Kamphuis, C.B., Van Lenthe, F.J., Giskes, K., Huisman, M., Brug, J., Mackenbach, J.P. (2008b). Socioeconomic status, environmental and individual factors, and sports participation. *Medicine and Science in Sports and Exercise* 40(1):71–81; reprinted by permission of the publisher

[a]All items regarding individual factors were asked in relation to the following definition of recommended physical activity (PA): "being physically active with at least moderate intensity on at least 30 min per day"

[b]Items were measured in the questionnaire on a five-point scale, though reduced to a three-point scale for the analyses

Factors that were significantly associated with sports participation *and* with SEP, were included in further explanatory analyses (see Table 12.3). Taking these neighbourhood, household and individual factors into account reduced socioeconomic inequalities in sports participation to a large extent, i.e. the ORs of doing no sports for the lowest educational group reduced by 57 %, for the second lowest by 48 % and for the second highest by 26 %.

Although neighbourhood factors seemed to account for only a small proportion of the reduction in equalities (i.e. 7 % for the lowest educational group), this does

Table 12.2 Adjusted odds ratios (OR)[a] for doing no sports, and prevalence rates of response categories of neighbourhood, household and individual factors by educational level

Independent factors	OR[a] for doing no sports	95 % CI	p^b	Educational level 1 (low)	2	3	4 (high)	p^b
Neighbourhood								
Neighbourhood physical factors								
Neighbourhood is unsafe								
Disagree	1.00		0.005	92.9[c]	96.4	97.7	97.8	0.000
Agree	1.77	(1.18–2.65)		7.1	3.6	2.3	2.2	
Neighbourhood is unattractive								
Disagree	1.00		0.000	72.4	83.9	88.4	87.2	0.000
Agree	1.45	(1.20–1.75)		27.6	16.1	11.6	12.8	
Insufficient places for physical activity								
Disagree	1.00		0.106	68.7	80.1	84.7	89.4	0.000
Agree	1.16	(0.97–1.37)		31.1	19.9	15.3	10.6	
Often poor weather								
Disagree	1.00		0.051	72.8	82.0	84.0	82.1	0.000
Agree	1.19	(1.00–1.41)		27.2	18.0	16.0	17.9	
Neighbourhood social factors								
Social network								
Large	1.00		0.006	32.8	39.5	36.5	29.1	0.000
Medium	1.27	(1.09–1.49)		35.8	31.4	34.2	33.3	
Small	1.23	(1.05–1.45)		31.3	29.1	29.3	37.6	
Social cohesion								
High	1.00		0.000	30.9	36.1	36.1	36.9	0.028
Medium	0.85	(0.72–0.99)		30.5	32.9	33.5	35.5	
Low	1.17	(1.00–1.38)		38.7	31.0	30.4	27.6	
Feeling at home in neighbourhood								
High	1.00		0.018	30.1	37.0	36.6	35.3	0.093
Medium	1.16	(0.99–1.35)		31.2	34.2	33.5	34.2	
Low	1.26	(1.07–1.48)		38.7	28.9	29.9	30.5	
Social disorganisation								
Low	1.00		0.552	43.9	52.1	51.2	54.5	0.058
Medium	1.16	(0.89–1.50)		8.9	6.7	6.8	7.2	
High	1.02	(0.89–1.17)		47.2	41.2	42.1	38.3	
Length of residence								
0–2 Years	1.08	(0.85–1.36)	0.681	12.5	8.7	14.5	19.0	0.000
2–5 Years	0.95	(0.77–1.17)		12.1	13.6	22.0	22.9	
5–15 Years	1.05	(0.88–1.24)		28.7	32.2	34.0	35.0	
15≥ Years	1.00			46.8	45.5	29.5	23.2	
Household								
Indicators of material deprivation								
1. Financial problems								
No	1.00		0.000	53.0	61.8	63.4	79.7	0.000
Some	1.36	(1.17–1.59)		34.3	30.2	30.8	17.3	
Many	2.13	(1.59–2.87)		12.7	8.0	5.8	3.0	

(continued)

Table 12.2 (continued)

Independent factors	OR[a] for doing no sports	95 % CI	p^b	Educational level 1 (low)	2	3	4 (high)	p^b
2. Car possession								
Yes	1.00		0.105	79.9	91.9	94.4	95.0	0.000
No	1.27	(0.96–1.62)		20.1	8.1	5.6	5.0	
3. Crowding								
<1 Per room	1.00		0.001	78.4	82.0	80.1	85.8	0.000
≥1 Person per room	1.37	(1.14–1.64)		21.6	18.0	19.9	14.2	
Indicators of social deprivation								
1. Friends/family for dinner monthly								
Yes	1.00		.052	43.7	50.7	55.2	67.7	.000
No, for financial reasons	1.31	(1.02–1.69)		18.7	10.9	8.0	2.8	
No, for other reasons	1.13	(0.98–1.30)		37.7	38.4	36.8	29.5	
2. Going out fortnightly								
Yes	1.00		0.000	27.7	29.4	40.3	46.2	0.000
No, for financial reasons	1.57	(1.30–1.91)		35.4	22.8	19.0	9.3	
No, for other reasons	1.31	(1.13–1.51)		37.7	47.8	40.8	44.5	
3. Going on holiday yearly								
Yes	1.00		0.000	50.2	76.1	81.6	90.1	0.000
No, for financial reasons	1.68	(1.35–2.10)		31.6	13.4	11.7	5.0	
No, for other reasons	1.33	(1.04–1.77)		18.2	10.5	6.7	4.9	
Individual								
Positive outcome expectancies of PA								
Makes me feel less stressed								
Important	1.00		0.000	59.7	63.2	70.5	69.3	0.000
Unimportant	2.13	(1.85–2.46)		40.3	36.8	29.5	30.7	
Get in good mood								
Important	1.00		0.000	59.9	67.4	71.4	68.6	0.003
Unimportant	2.17	(1.87–2.50)		40.1	32.6	28.6	31.4	
Like being active								
Important	1.00		0.000	64.7	64.8	64.2	65.2	0.966
Unimportant	2.61	(2.27–3.00)		35.3	35.2	35.8	34.8	
More confident with body								
Important	1.00		0.000	61.9	67.9	68.3	67.4	0.257
Unimportant	1.89	(1.64–2.18)		38.1	32.4	31.7	32.6	
Good for fitness/condition								
Important	1.00		0.000	80.3	87.0	91.5	92.0	0.000
Unimportant	2.45	(1.94–3.08)		19.7	13.0	8.5	8.0	
Feel energized								
Important	1.00		0.000	71.6	80.4	85.1	84.4	0.000
Unimportant	2.23	(1.86–2.67)		28.4	19.6	14.9	15.6	
Negative outcome expectancies of PA								
Requires too much time								
Unimportant	1.00		0.000	47.4	53.1	45.3	37.7	0.000
Important	1.43	(1.25–1.64)		52.6	46.9	54.7	62.3	

(continued)

Table 12.2 (continued)

Independent factors	OR[a] for doing no sports	95 % CI	p^b	Educational level 1 (low)	2	3	4 (high)	p^b
Requires too much discipline								
Unimportant	1.00		0.000	49.1	51.4	45.6	44.8	0.005
Important	1.55	(1.36–1.77)		50.9	48.6	54.4	55.2	
Requires too much energy								
Unimportant	1.00		0.000	47.7	58.5	65.3	74.1	0.000
Important	1.85	(1.61–2.13)		52.3	41.5	34.7	25.9	
Afraid to get injured								
Unimportant	1.00		0.000	55.0	67.2	75.1	81.9	0.000
Important	1.31	(1.13–1.53)		45.0	32.8	24.9	18.1	
Feel uncomfortable when exercising								
Unimportant	1.00		0.000	65.3	78.9	84.4	90.0	0.000
Important	1.89	(1.57–2.26)		34.7	21.1	15.6	10.0	
Doing sports is expensive								
Unimportant	1.00		0.000	48.5	68.2	76.7	82.4	0.000
Important	1.81	(1.55–2.12)		51.5	31.8	23.3	17.6	
Social influences								
Subj. norm: other think I should do PA								
True	1.00		0.000	54.1	57.5	58.6	65.0	0.000
Not true/false	1.31	(1.12–1.53)		19.8	24.3	25.0	22.5	
False	1.48	(1.23–1.78)		26.1	18.2	16.4	12.5	
Soc. support: others support me in PA								
True	1.00		0.000	46.3	41.2	37.7	40.2	0.000
Not true/false	1.40	(1.20–1.62)		25.7	34.4	36.7	39.2	
False	1.87	(1.59–2.22)		28.0	24.4	25.7	20.6	
Modelling: others do PA								
True	1.00		0.000	51.3	48.6	44.4	46.9	0.175
Not true/false	1.32	(1.15–1.52)		37.9	39.2	44.6	41.6	
False	1.30	(1.05–1.61)		10.8	12.2	11.0	11.5	
Self-efficacy								
How sure to get sufficient PA?								
(Very) sure	1.00		0.000	57.5	70.6	73.6	79.0	0.000
Not sure/unsure	2.25	(1.91–2.66)		33.2	24.9	20.8	15.2	
(Very) unsure	2.81	(2.08–3.81)		9.3	4.5	5.6	5.8	
Intention: Plan to get sufficient PA?								
Yes	1.00		0.000	46.3	60.4	65.9	75.3	0.000
Maybe	2.73	(2.35–3.57)		44.0	34.6	30.7	21.4	
No	3.39	(2.36–4.87)		9.7	5.0	3.4	3.3	

Source: Kamphuis, C.B., Van Lenthe, F.J., Giskes, K., Huisman, M., Brug, J., Mackenbach, J.P. (2008b). Socioeconomic status, environmental and individual factors, and sports participation. *Medicine and Science in Sports and Exercise* 40(1):71–81; reprinted by permission of the publisher

[a]Models were adjusted for age, sex, educational level, and country of origin

[b]*n.s.* not significant; * = $p \leq 0.050$; ** = $p \leq 0.010$; *** = $p \leq 0.001$

[c]This is the percentage of respondents that agreed on the statement per socioeconomic group; for example, 92.9 % of those in the lowest group disagreed with the statement "My neighbourhood is unsafe"

Table 12.3 Effect of adjustment for neighbourhood, household, and individual level factors on clustering of sports participation in neighbourhoods (random effects), and on the association between educational level and no sports participation[a] (fixed effect)[b]

		Area (random effects)		Educational level[c] (fixed effect)						
				1—low (*N*=347)		2 (*N*=1,346)		3 (*N*=984)		4—high (*N*=1,244)
	Factors included in the model (significant)	Area level variance (SE)	MOR (95 % CrI)	OR	95 % C.I.	OR	95 % C.I.	OR	95 % C.I.	OR
Model 0 (empty)	–	0.157 (0.047)	1.46 (1.30–1.63)							
Model 1: Basic	Education + age + sex + country of origin	0.067 (0.032)	1.28 (1.15–1.43)	3.99	(2.99–5.31)	2.19	(1.86–2.59)	1.65	(1.39–1.96)	1.00
Model 2: Basic + neighbourhood	Neighbourhood attractiveness + neighbourhood safety + social network + social cohesion	0.060 (0.031)	1.26 (1.10–1.40)	3.77 *7 %*[d]	(2.83–5.02)	2.18 *1 %*	(1.84–2.59)	1.71 *0 %*	(1.45–2.02)	1.00
Model 3: Basic + household	Material deprivation (ind. 1 + 3) + social deprivation (ind. 2 + 3)	0.049 (0.024)	1.23(1.12–1.36)	3.16 *28 %*	(2.34–4.26)	1.89 *25 %*	(1.58–2.26)	1.54 *17 %*	(1.29–1.84)	1.00
Model 4: Basic + individual	PA makes me feel less stressed + I get in a good mood + PA is good for my fitness + PA costs too much energy + I feel uncomfortable during PA + PA is too expensive + social support + modelling + self-efficacy + intention	0.052 (0.036)	1.24 (1.05–1.40)	2.67 *44 %*	(1.96–3.63)	1.75 *37 %*	(1.45–2.12)	1.54 *17 %*	(1.27–1.87)	1.00

Model 5: Basic + neighbourhood + household + individual	Neighbourhood safety + social cohesion + material deprivation (ind. 3) + social deprivation (ind. 2 + 3) + PA makes me feel less stressed + I get in a good mood + PA is good for my fitness + PA costs too much energy + I feel uncomfortable during PA + PA is too expensive + social support + modelling + self-efficacy + intention	0.046 (0.024)	1.22 (1.12–1.36)	2.29 *57 %*	(1.70–3.07)	1.62 *48 %*	(1.34–1.96)	1.48 *26 %*	(1.23–1.78)	1.00

Source: Kamphuis et al. (2008b). *Medicine and Science in Sports and Exercise* 40(1):71–81; reprinted by permission of the publisher

[a]Doing sports (no vs. yes), with 'no': not doing any sports, with at least moderate intensity (i.e. 3–5 MET for 55+ years old and 4–6.5 MET for 18–55 years old)

[b]Multilevel models were estimated with the Markov Chain Monte Carlo method implemented in MlwiN (version 2.02) ; CrI, credible interval; MOR, median odds ratio; OR, odds ratio; SE, standard error

[c]Education: highest attained education, with 1 = no education or primary education; 2 = lower secondary; 3 = higher secondary; 4 = tertiary

[d]Percentages in *italic* show the percentages reduction in odds ratio's compared to the basic model, per educational group. For instance, the reduction in the OR for the lowest educational group when adding neighbourhood factors into the basic model, is [(3.99–3.77)/(3.99–1.00] × 100 = 7 %

not mean that neighbourhood factors require less attention in policy and intervention development. From a population perspective, even small odds ratios for neighbourhood characteristics may imply that changes to (perceptions of) the neighbourhood context may have a significant effect on physical activity levels. In particular, since we found that higher reports of unfavourable neighbourhood factors were more prevalent among lower socioeconomic groups, these may offer important opportunities to reduce socioeconomic inequalities in physical activity.

Socioeconomic Inequalities in Recreational Walking

Further, socioeconomic differences in another physical activity outcome were studied, namely, recreational walking, and we examined to what extent neighbourhood perceptions and individual cognitions mediated the SES-walking relationship (Kamphuis et al. 2009). For these analyses, we used the same data as the former study; however, we selected only on older adults (55 years of age or older, $N=1,994$), as they represent a rapidly increasing share of the general population and physical activity is important to preserve their health, functioning and social participation.

A moderate socioeconomic gradient in recreational walking was observed, with the lowest educated being about 1,5 times more likely not to engage in any recreational walking than their higher status counterparts (see Table 12.4). Three out of seven neighbourhood perceptions were significantly associated with no recreational walking, i.e. poor neighbourhood aesthetics, high social cohesion and a small social network. As the latter two risk factors were more prevalent among high SEP groups, these factors could not serve as possible explanatory factors for the raised odds for no recreational walking among low SEP groups. All four individual cognitions were significantly associated with no recreational walking, and risk categories (i.e. negative attitude, negative social influences, low perceived behaviour control and no intention to be regularly physically active) were most prevalent among the lowest SEP groups. Therefore, all individual cognitions and one neighbourhood perception (neighbourhood aesthetics) were taken into account in further explanatory models.

The association between SEP and recreational walking attenuated when neighbourhood aesthetics was included in the model and largely reduced when individual cognitions were added to the model (with largest effects of attitude and intention regarding). The association between poor neighbourhood aesthetics and no recreational walking attenuated to (borderline) insignificance when individual cognitions were taken into account. So, although individual cognitions towards physical activity (e.g. attitude, perceived behavioural control) contributed most to the explanation of socioeconomic differences in recreational walking, perceived neighbourhood aesthetics also had a significant contribution and mediated the association between SEP and recreational walking largely via individual cognitions.

Table 12.4 Odds ratios with 95 % confidence intervals (OR, 95 % CI) for no recreational walking by education, mediated by neighbourhood perceptions and individual cognitions

		Model 1 (base model): education + age + sex OR (95 % CI)	Model 2: base + neighbourhood OR (95 % CI)	Model 3: base + individual OR (95 % CI)	Model 4: base + neighbourhood + individual OR (95 % CI)
Education	% no walking				
1. Low (*n*=281)	38.5	1.67 (1.18–2.35)	1.60 (1.13–2.27)	1.33 (0.93–1.90)	1.30 (0.91–1.87)
2. (*n*=908)	34.7	1.49 (1.17–1.90)	1.48 (1.16–1.89)	1.35 (1.04–1.75)	1.29 (0.99–1.68)
3. (*n*=366)	22.1	0.84 (0.60–1.18)	0.84 (0.60–1.19)	0.80 (0.57–1.13)	0.75 (0.53–1.06)
4. High (*n*=439)	29.2	1.00	1.00	1.00	1.00
Neighbourhood perceptions					
My neighbourhood is unattractive					
Disagree			1.00		1.00
Agree			1.32 (1.06–1.65)		1.19 (0.95–1.50)
Individual cognitions					
Attitude towards regular physical activity					
Positive				1.00	1.00
Neutral				1.12 (0.87–1.45)	1.11 (0.86–1.43)
Negative				2.30 (1.59–3.32)	2.26 (1.57–3.26)
Social influences for regular physical activity					
Positive				1.00	1.00
Neutral				1.24 (1.01–1.52)	1.24 (1.02–1.532)
Negative				1.54 (1.11–2.14)	1.54 (1.11–2.14)
Perceived behaviour control to be regularly active					
(Very) sure				1.00	1.00
Not sure/unsure				1.21 (0.95–1.55)	1.20 (0.94–1.54)
(Very) unsure				1.57 (1.11–2.22)	1.56 (1.10–2.21)

(continued)

Table 12.2 (continued)

	Model 1 (base model): education + age + sex OR (95 % CI)	Model 2: base + neighbourhood OR (95 % CI)	Model 3: base + individual OR (95 % CI)	Model 4: base + neighbourhood + individual OR (95 % CI)
Intention to be regularly active				
(Very) likely			1.00	1.00
Maybe			1.31 (0.99–1.73)	1.30 (0.98–1.72)
(Very) unlikely			2.38 (1.59–3.57)	2.38 (1.59–3.57)
Random effects[a]				
Level-2 variance (SE)	0.000 (0.000)	0.000 (0.000)	0.000 (0.000)	0.000 (0.000)

Source: Kamphuis, C.B., van Lenthe, F.J., Giskes, K., Huisman, M., Brug, J., Mackenbach, J.P. (2009). Socioeconomic differences in lack of recreational walking among older adults: the role of neighbourhood and individual factors. Int J Behav Nutr Phys Act 6:1; reprinted by permission of the publisher

[a]Weighted multilevel models were estimated with the iterative generalized least squares procedure implemented in MlwiN version 2.02

Socioeconomic Differences in Neighbourhood Perceptions: The Role of Objective Neighbourhood Factors

In the studies described so far, we noticed that lower socioeconomic groups were more likely to perceive their neighbourhood as unattractive and unsafe than higher socioeconomic groups, which was related to more physical inactivity among low socioeconomic groups (Kamphuis et al. 2008b; 2009). Studies that have investigated neighbourhood perceptions in association with physical activity often assume—either implicitly or explicitly—that these perceptions reflect actual, objective neighbourhood circumstances. Indeed, objective neighbourhood factors have been found to be associated with physical activity (Li et al. 2005; Saelens et al. 2003) and to contribute to socioeconomic variations in physical activity (Kamphuis et al. 2008a; Van Lenthe et al. 2005). However, other studies that have investigated the level of agreement between objective and perceived environmental factors found this agreement to be moderate or low (Giles-Corti and Donovan 2002; Kirtland et al. 2003; Kweon et al. 2006). This suggests that factors other than the objective neighbourhood environment may play a role in the formation of residents' perceptions.

Therefore, in a subsequent study we examined whether objectively measured neighbourhood characteristics (i.e. design, traffic safety, social safety, aesthetics and destinations) and/or other factors (i.e. social neighbourhood environment and psychosocial factors) could explain these socioeconomic differences in neighbourhood perceptions (Kamphuis et al. 2010). For this study, we used the same GLOBE survey data from 2004, as described in the first study on sports participation, but we only selected participants residing in seven of the most deprived and seven of the most advantaged neighbourhoods of the city of Eindhoven ($N=814$).

Socioeconomic position (SEP), demographic characteristics, possible explanatory factors (psychosocial factors and social neighbourhood factors) and perceived neighbourhood attractiveness and safety were self-reported in the postal survey. Objective neighbourhood characteristics with respect to aesthetic, design, traffic safety, social safety and destination features were not self-reported, but assessed by means of a systematic audit instrument by trained observers that visited the 14 neighbourhoods during field observations. The audit instrument was developed based on other audit instruments (Caughy et al. 2001; Day et al. 2006; Pikora et al. 2002; Weich et al. 2001; Zenk et al. 2007), and its development has been described in more detail elsewhere (Kamphuis 2008) (pp. 25–43). For each neighbourhood, 10 % of the total number of streets in the neighbourhood was randomly selected, resulting in 75 streets to be audited. Specific audit items measured five domains of objective neighbourhood characteristics that are hypothesised to influence physical activity based on the framework of Pikora and colleagues (Pikora et al. 2003, 2006), i.e. aesthetics, design, traffic safety, social safety and destinations. Audit scores of all items belonging to a specific domain were summed, and the mean street-level sum scores for each of the five domains were aggregated to the neighbourhood level, resulting in a database with scores for $N=14$ neighbourhoods. Table 12.5 shows the specific items that were summed in each sum score, the reliability of the

Table 12.5 Descriptives of objective neighbourhood characteristics measured in 14 neighbourhoods in the city of Eindhoven—inter-rater reliability, mean score, range [minimum, maximum score], *p* value[a]

	Inter-rater reliability[a]	Mean score	[range]	p^d
Sum score design (functional) features		2.28	[1.60–3.38]	*
Sidewalks present (0 = no, 1 = yes)	0.97	0.95	[0.50–1.00]	**
Quality of sidewalks (0 = bad-moderate, 1 = good)	0.70[b]	0.50	[0.00–1.00]	n.s.
Cycling track present (0 = no, 1 = yes)	0.93	0.12	[0.00–0.40]	n.s.
Quality of cycling tracks (0 = bad-moderate, 1 = good)	0.93[b]	0.71	[0.00–1.00]	n.s.
Speed-limit zone (max. 30 km/h) (0 = no, 1 = yes)	0.77	0.18	[0.00–0.60]	n.s.
Traffic control devices (0 = no; 1 = yes)	0.87	0.46	[0.00–1.00]	**
Sum score social unsafety		0.98	[0.50–1.80]	n.s.
Houses for sale (0 = no, 1 = yes)	0.80[b]	0.26	[0.00–0.57]	n.s.
Empty houses (0 = no, 1 = yes)	0.70[b]	0.18	[0.00–0.60]	*
Height of fences (0 = lager dan ooghoogte; 1 = hoger dan ooghoogte)	0.73	0.13	[0.00–0.40]	n.s.
Visibility of the street from surrounding houses (0 = ≥½ of the street is visible, 1 = <1/2 of the street is visible)	0.73[b]	0.17	[0.00–0.60]	n.s.
Vandalism (0 = none, 1 = some, 2 = many)[c]	0.97[b]	[c]–	–	–
Street lighting (0 = on both sides, 1 = on one side)	0.83	0.15	[0.00–0.40]	n.s.
Youth hanging around in the streets (0 = no, 1 = yes)[c]	0.90	[c]–	–	–
Signs of alcohol/drugs use (0 = no; 1 = yes)	0.83	0.12	[0.00–0.40]	n.s.
Sum score traffic unsafety		1.07	[0.00–2.60]	*
Traffic (0 = bestemmingsverkeer only, 1 = through traffic)	0.80	0.27	[0.00–1.00]	*
Crossovers present (0 = no, 1 = yes)	0.93	0.08	[0.00–0.20]	n.s.
Traffic signs painted on the road (0 = no, 1 = yes)	0.67[b]	0.20	[0.00–0.50]	n.s.
Traffic control devices (0 = yes, 1 = no)	0.87	0.52	[0.00–1.00]	**
Sum score aesthetics		3.90	[1.20–7.25]	***
Graffiti (0 = yes, 1 = no)	0.70[b]	0.55	[0.20–1.00]	n.s.
Vandalism (0 = none, 1 = some, 2 = many)[c]	0.97[b]	[c]–	–	–
Litter on the streets (0 = yes, some or a lot, 1 = no, nothing much)	0.67[b]	0.55	[0.00–1.00]	**
Maintenance of best buildings (0 = bad-moderate, 1=excellent)	0.67[b]	0.78	[0.40–1.00]	*
Maintenance of worst buildings (0 = bad-moderate, 1 = excellent)	0.67[b]	0.48	[0.00–1.00]	***
Gardens (0 = not with all houses, 1 = with all houses)	0.87[b]	0.59	[0.00–1.00]	***
Maintenance of best-maintained gardens (0 = bad-moderate, 1 = excellent)	0.80[b]	0.61	[0.20–1.00]	*
Green diversity (0 = ≤1 kind of green, 1 = ≥2 kinds of green, e.g. trees, field, bushes)	0.83[b]	0.44	[0.00–0.60]	n.s.
Maintenance of public green areas (0 = bad-moderate, 1 = excellent)	0.80	0.18	[0.00–0.75]	***
Sum score destinations		0.46	[0.00–1.20]	**
Destinations (0 = none, 1 = one or more)	0.77[b]	0.31	[0.00–1.00]	n.s.
Public transport (0 = no; 1 = yes)	0.73	0.13	[0.00–0.40]	***

(continued)

Table 12.5 (continued)

Source: Kamphuis, C.B.M., Mackenbach, J.P., Giskes, K., Huisman, M., Brug, J., Van Lenthe, F.J. (2010) Why do poor people perceive poor neighbourhoods? Socioeconomic differences in perceptions of neighbourhood safety and attractiveness: the role of objective neighbourhood features and residents' psychosocial characteristics. Health Place 16:744–754; reprinted by permission of the publisher)

[a]Inter-rater reliability is represented by the percentage agreement between two observers (consensus score). Percent agreement for each specific item was calculated by adding up the number of cases that received the same rating by both judges and dividing that number by the total number of cases rated by the two judges

[b]Originally, there were more than two response categories for this audit item. However, categories were dichotomized in order to calculate meaningful sum scores. Inter-rater reliability scores were calculated for the original items, and therefore, are actually higher for the dichotomised items

[c]Item has not been included in the sum score as the prevalence was very low, i.e. in all neighbourhoods the prevalence of signs of vandalism and youth in the streets was close to zero

[d]*p* value indicates whether mean score for the item or sum score differed significantly between the 14 neighbourhoods, with ***= $p \leq 0.001$, **= $p \leq 0.010$, *= $p \leq 0.050$, n.s.=not significant (analysed by ANOVA in SPSS 15.0)

items and whether the mean sum scores for each domain differed significantly between the 14 neighbourhoods. Sum scores were dichotomised for analytic purposes. Dichotomised sum scores for each neighbourhood were merged with the resident-level (postal survey) data.

Being male, unmarried, having a lower household income and having a lower education were associated with an increased likelihood of perceiving the neighbourhood as unattractive. In multivariate models, only household income and sex remained significantly associated with neighbourhood unattractiveness (therefore, all subsequent models were sex adjusted, and household income was chosen as SEP indicator). The lowest income group had an odds of 1.75 (95 % CI: 0.85–3.58) to perceive their neighbourhood as unattractive, compared to the highest income group (although differences between income groups fell short of significance). Women, elderly, unemployed and those with lower incomes and lower levels of education were significantly less likely to perceive their neighbourhood as safe in bivariate analyses (results not shown). Only household income, age and sex remained significant in the multivariate model (therefore, age and sex were taken into account in subsequent models, and household income was chosen as SEP indicator). Low-income residents were more likely to perceive their neighbourhoods as unsafe (OR = 2.97; 95 % CI: 1.55–5.67).

The elevated ORs for neighbourhood unattractiveness observed among the lowest income group decreased by 33 % when objective neighbourhood factors were added (Kamphuis et al. 2010). Adding self-reported social neighbourhood and psychosocial factors reduced the ORs for perceived neighbourhood unattractiveness among the lowest income group by 81 % to 1.14 (95 % CI: 0.57–2.25). In the full model, two objective neighbourhood factors (aesthetics and destinations), and social cohesion and depressed mood remained statistically significant. The odds for perceived neighbourhood unsafety among the lowest compared to the highest income group was attenuated by 11 % when objective neighbourhood aesthetics was included in the model and with 66 % when self-reported social neighbourhood and psychosocial factors were added. In this full model, one objective neighbourhood factor (aesthetics), and social cohesion and depressed mood remained statistically significant.

Additionally, we found in multilevel analyses that residents' perceptions of neighbourhood unattractiveness and safety clustered within neighbourhoods (Kamphuis et al. 2010). This clustering reduced to a great extent when objective neighbourhood characteristics were taken into account and only limitedly by differences in neighbourhood composition (age, sex, income level).

Challenges for Future Research

Several challenges for the next decades of research in this field derived from the limitations of the studies as described in this chapter need to be addressed.

Measurement of Neighbourhood Characteristics

There is a debate in the literature about what matters most for physical activity: perceptions of neighbourhood characteristics as reported by residents or objective neighbourhood features (van Lenthe and Kamphuis 2011). For bringing this debate a step further, it is important in the first place to measure both factors in an adequate way.

Neighbourhood perceptions should be measured as specific as possible and—where necessary—with regard to the specific (physical activity) behaviour studied. It is, for example, insufficient to ask whether a respondent feels safe in his/her neighbourhood, but rather this should be inquired with regard to traffic safety and safety from crime. Perceptions of footpaths should, for instance, be asked for as possible determinant of walking behaviour and perceptions of cycling paths for cycling behaviour. Also, it is not the mere presence of facilities like paths and green spaces should be investigated, but their quality should be assessed as well.

Furthermore, one can discuss what the appropriate measurement unit is in order to measure area effects and how this scale should vary by health behaviour. The attractiveness of the area within a 5-min walk from home may affect recreational walking; however, for recreational cycling, likely, a much larger area will matter. Also, characteristics of destinations that people walk or cycle to may be at least as important as characteristics of one's area of residence. These issues show that the objective measurement of neighbourhood characteristics is a very young field of research with many opportunities for improvement.

Measurement of Physical Activity

In the current literature on neighbourhood and physical activity, physical activity is nearly always measured by self-report questionnaires, in which respondents are asked to recall their physical activity over some period of time (e.g. the previous week) and fill in their own estimations in the questionnaire (Beenackers et al. under review). Physical activity, however, is a complex, multidimensional behaviour and it is therefore difficult to recall retrospectively. Self-reported physical activity questionnaires are therefore prone to recall biases, which can lead to the misclassification of physical activity levels (Prince et al. 2008). Therefore, it would be better if future studies could also make use of objective physical activity measurements, such as accelerometers or a combination of heart rate and movement sensors, which are seen as best practices for accurate physical activity measurement. Currently, due to practical and monetary reasons, it is hardly ever possible to measure physical activity with these types of devices in large-scale epidemiological studies and intervention studies. Hopefully in the future, small, accurate and inexpensive physical activity sensors will be developed that can be easily worn by research participants and which automatically transfer their summary data to databases for easy data handling.

Mechanisms Underlying the Association of Neighbourhood Factors with Physical Activity

Knowing of an association between neighbourhood characteristics and physical activity is a first step; however, in order to understand the relationship, we should have more insight in the *causal* mechanisms underlying this association. Far and foremost, this research field is in need of studies with a longitudinal design, with multiple measurements of neighbourhood determinants, physical activity behaviour and possible confounders, preferably before and after an environmental change. One approach for this is for researchers to take advantage of "natural experiments" that provide exogenous sources of contextual variation.

Regarding possible mechanisms, it is, for instance, possible that an attractive, green neighbourhood with many destinations leads to a more positive attitude towards walking for transport among residents, which results in more walking behaviour. This possible mediation of attitude in the neighbourhood-activity association is based on the long tradition to consider health behaviours as the result of planned, deliberate cognitive processes. However, from the new perspective of dual-process model, environmental exposures may also directly influence health behaviours, i.e. through an automatic, non-reflective mechanism (Kremers et al. 2006). For instance, it is suggested that when viewing an elevator one may automatically use the elevator, without any conscious consideration of whether or not taking the stairs instead.

It is suggested in the literature that the unconscious, automatic response is more likely to dominate over cognitive decision making when a person is under stress, tired or preoccupied or is overloaded with information. In these situations, one's resources for deliberative choices that require self-regulation can get depleted (Baumeister 2003). Since low socioeconomic groups generally have fewer resources for information processing (i.e. less education) and may be exposed to more stressful social, cultural, physical and economic environments, this may result in more automatic, "default" choices. In our current obesogenic environment (i.e. supportive of eating as well as physical inactivity), active self-control or self-regulation is needed not to automatically fall back into our evolutionary-determined default options: eating items high in sugar and fat and being inactive (Peters et al. 2002). This raises the intriguing question as to whether differential exposures to environmental factors between high and low socioeconomic groups result in different health behaviours via planned or to more automatic mechanisms.

Conclusion

We found moderate to large socioeconomic inequalities in sports participation and recreational walking in the Netherlands, with those from most disadvantaged backgrounds being least active. Unfavourable perceptions of the neighbourhood, particularly with respect to attractiveness, safety and social cohesion, were related to these physical inactivity outcomes and were more prevalent among lower SEP groups. Largely in line with these findings, the current literature shows that the objective and perceived availability and accessibility of facilities, as well as the objective and perceived general design of neighbourhoods (e.g. the presences of sidewalks) and perceived aesthetics are positively associated with various types and levels of physical activity (McCormack et al. 2004). In conclusion, findings suggest that the neighbourhood environment has a moderate but significant contribution to the explanation of socioeconomic differences in several types of physical inactivity. Although most of the neighbourhood factors we studied were perceptions (i.e. self-reported by residents), the results suggested that these are at least partly a reflection of actual (objective) characteristics of neighbourhoods.

References

Ajzen, I. (1991). The theory of planned behaviour. *Organizational Behavior and Human Decision Processes, 50*, 179–211.

Andersen, L. B., Schnohr, P., Schroll, M., & Hein, H. O. (2000). All-cause mortality associated with physical activity during leisure time, work, sports, and cycling to work. *Archives of Internal Medicine, 160*(11), 1621–1628.

Antonovsky, A. (1967). Social class, life expectancy and overall mortality. *The Milbank Memorial Fund Quarterly, 45*, 31–73.

Armitage, C. J., & Conner, M. (2001). Efficacy of the theory of planned behaviour: a meta-analytic review. *British Journal of Social Psychology, 40*(Pt 4), 471–499.

Ball, K., Timperio, A., Salmon, J., Giles-Corti, B., Roberts, R., & Crawford, D. (2007). Personal, social and environmental determinants of educational inequalities in walking: a multilevel study. *Journal of Epidemiology and Community Health, 61*(2), 108–114.

Baranowski, T., Cullen, K. W., Nicklas, T., Thompson, D., & Baranowski, J. (2003). Are current health behavioral change models helpful in guiding prevention of weight gain efforts? *Obesity Research, 11*(Suppl), 23–43.

Batty, G. D. (2002). Physical activity and coronary heart disease in older adults. A systematic review of epidemiological studies. *European Journal of Public Health, 12*, 171–176.

Baumeister, R. F. (2003). Ego depletion and self-regulation failure: a resource model of self-control. *Alcoholism, Clinical and Experimental Research, 27*(2), 281–284.

Beenackers, M. A., Kamphuis, C. B., Giskes, K, Brug, J, Kunst, A. E., Burdorf, A, & van Lenthe, F. J. (2012) Socioeconomic inequalities in occupational, leisure-time, and transport related physical activity among European adults: a systematic review. Int J Behav Nutr Phys Act. 2012 Sep 19(9)116.

Bosma, H., Van de Mheen, H. D., Borsboom, G. J., & Mackenbach, J. P. (2001). Neighborhood socioeconomic status and all-cause mortality. *American Journal of Epidemiology, 153*, 363–371.

Caughy, M. O., O'Campo, P. J., & Patterson, J. (2001). A brief observational measure for urban neighborhoods. *Health & Place, 7*(3), 225–236.

Crespo, C. J., Ainsworth, B. E., Keteyian, S. J., Heath, G. W., & Smit, E. (1999). Prevalence of physical inactivity and its relation to social class in U.S. adults: results from the Third National Health and Nutrition Examination Survey, 1988–1994. *Medicine and Science in Sports and Exercise, 31*(12), 1821–1827.

Day, K., Boarnet, M., Alfonzo, M., & Forsyth, A. (2006). The Irvine-Minnesota inventory to measure built environments: development. *American Journal of Preventive Medicine, 30*(2), 144–152.

Diez-Roux, A. V., Link, B. G., & Northridge, M. E. (2000). A multilevel analysis of income inequality and cardiovascular disease risk factors. *Social Science & Medicine, 50*(5), 673–687.

Dowler, E. (2001). Inequalities in diet and physical activity in Europe. *Public Health Nutrition, 4*(2B), 701–709.

Droomers, M., Schrijvers, C. T., & Mackenbach, J. P. (2001). Educational level and decreases in leisure time physical activity: predictors from the longitudinal GLOBE study. *Journal of Epidemiology and Community Health, 55*(8), 562–568.

Droomers, M., Schrijvers, C. T., van de Mheen, H., & Mackenbach, J. P. (1998). Educational differences in leisure-time physical inactivity: a descriptive and explanatory study. *Social Science & Medicine, 47*(11), 1665–1676.

Ecob, R., & Macintyre, S. (2000). Small area variations in health related behaviours; do these depend on the behaviour itself, its measurement, or on personal characteristics? *Health & Place, 6*(4), 261–274.

Franco, O. H., de Laet, C., Peeters, A., Jonker, J., Mackenbach, J., & Nusselder, W. (2005). Effects of physical activity on life expectancy with cardiovascular disease. *Archives of Internal Medicine, 165*(20), 2355–2360.

Giles-Corti, B., & Donovan, R. J. (2002). Socioeconomic status differences in recreational physical activity levels and real and perceived access to a supportive physical environment. *Preventive Medicine, 35*(6), 601–611.

Kamphuis, C. B. M. (2008). *Explaining socioeconomic inequalities in health behaviours—the role of environmental factors*. Rotterdam: Erasmus University Medical Centre.

Kamphuis, C. B., Giskes, K., Kavanagh, A. M., Thornton, L. E., Thomas, L. R., van Lenthe, F. J., et al. (2008a). Area variation in recreational cycling in Melbourne: a compositional or contextual effect? *Journal of Epidemiology and Community Health, 62*(10), 890–898.

Kamphuis, C. B. M., Mackenbach, J. P., Giskes, K., Huisman, M., Brug, J., & Van Lenthe, F. J. (2010). Why do poor people perceive poor neighbourhoods? Socioeconomic differences in perceptions of neighbourhood safety and attractiveness: the role of objective neighbourhood features and residents' psychosocial characteristics. *Health & Place, 16*, 744–754.

Kamphuis, C. B., Van Lenthe, F. J., Giskes, K., Huisman, M., Brug, J., & Mackenbach, J. P. (2008b). Socioeconomic status, environmental and individual factors, and sports participation. *Medicine and Science in Sports and Exercise, 40*(1), 71–81.

Kamphuis, C. B., van Lenthe, F. J., Giskes, K., Huisman, M., Brug, J., & Mackenbach, J. P. (2009). Socioeconomic differences in lack of recreational walking among older adults: the role of neighbourhood and individual factors. *International Journal of Behavioral Nutrition and Physical Activity, 6*, 1.

Kirtland, K. A., Porter, D. E., Addy, C. L., Neet, M. J., Williams, J. E., Sharpe, P. A., et al. (2003). Environmental measures of physical activity supports: perception versus reality. *American Journal of Preventive Medicine, 24*(4), 323–331.

Kremers, S. P., de Bruijn, G. J., Visscher, T. L., van Mechelen, W., de Vries, N. K., & Brug, J. (2006). Environmental influences on energy balance-related behaviors: a dual-process view. *International Journal of Behavioral Nutrition and Physical Activity, 3*, 9.

Kweon, B. S., Ellis, C. D., Lee, S. W., & Rogers, G. O. (2006). Large-scale environmental knowledge: investigating the relationship between self-reported and objectively measured physical environments. *Environment and Behavior, 38*(1), 72–91.

Li, F., Fisher, K. J., Brownson, R. C., & Bosworth, M. (2005). Multilevel modelling of built environment characteristics related to neighbourhood walking activity in older adults. *Journal of Epidemiology and Community Health, 59*(7), 558–564.

Lindstrom, M., Hanson, B. S., & Ostergren, P. O. (2001). Socioeconomic differences in leisure-time physical activity: the role of social participation and social capital in shaping health related behaviour. *Social Science & Medicine, 52*(3), 441–451.

Lynch, J. W., Kaplan, G. A., & Salonen, J. T. (1997). Why do poor people behave poorly? Variation in adult health behaviours and psychosocial characteristics by stages of the socioeconomic lifecourse. *Social Science & Medicine, 44*(6), 809–819.

Macintyre, S., Ellaway, A., & Cummins, S. (2002). Place effects on health: how can we conceptualise, operationalise and measure them? *Social Science & Medicine, 55*(1), 125–139.

Mackenbach, J. P., Bos, V., Andersen, O., Cardano, M., Costa, G., Harding, S., et al. (2003). Widening socioeconomic inequalities in mortality in six Western European countries. *International Journal of Epidemiology, 32*(5), 830–837.

Mackenbach, J. P., Stirbu, I., Roskam, A. J., Schaap, M. M., Menvielle, G., Leinsalu, M., et al. (2008). Socioeconomic inequalities in health in 22 European countries. *The New England Journal of Medicine, 358*(23), 2468–2481.

Marshall, S. J., Jones, D. A., Ainsworth, B. E., Reis, J. P., Levy, S. S., & Macera, C. A. (2007). Race/ethnicity, social class, and leisure-time physical inactivity. *Medicine and Science in Sports and Exercise, 39*(1), 44–51.

McCormack, G., Giles-Corti, B., Lange, A., Smith, T., Martin, K., & Pikora, T. J. (2004). An update of recent evidence of the relationship between objective and self-report measures of the physical environment and physical activity behaviours. *Journal of Science and Medicine in Sport, 7*(1 Suppl), 81–92.

McCulloch, A. (2003). An examination of social capital and social disorganisation in neighbourhoods in the British household panel study. *Social Science & Medicine, 56*(7), 1425–1438.

McNeill, L. H., Kreuter, M. W., & Subramanian, S. V. (2006). Social environment and physical activity: a review of concepts and evidence. *Social Science & Medicine, 63*(4), 1011–1022.

Peters, J. C., Wyatt, H. R., Donahoo, W. T., & Hill, J. O. (2002). From instinct to intellect: the challenge of maintaining healthy weight in the modern world. *Obesity Reviews, 3*(2), 69–74.

Pickett, K. E., & Pearl, M. (2001). Multilevel analyses of neighbourhood socioeconomic context and health outcomes: a critical review. *Journal of Epidemiology and Community Health, 55*(2), 111–122.

Pikora, T. J., Bull, F. C., Jamrozik, K., Knuiman, M., Giles-Corti, B., & Donovan, R. J. (2002). Developing a reliable audit instrument to measure the physical environment for physical activity. *American Journal of Preventive Medicine, 23*(3), 187–194.

Pikora, T., Giles-Corti, B., Bull, F., Jamrozik, K., & Donovan, R. (2003). Developing a framework for assessment of the environmental determinants of walking and cycling. *Social Science & Medicine, 56*(8), 1693–1703.

Pikora, T. J., Giles-Corti, B., Knuiman, M. W., Bull, F. C., Jamrozik, K., & Donovan, R. J. (2006). Neighborhood environmental factors correlated with walking near home: Using SPACES. *Medicine and Science in Sports and Exercise, 38*(4), 708–714.

Prince, S. A., Adamo, K. B., Hamel, M. E., Hardt, J., Gorber, S. C., & Tremblay, M. (2008). A comparison of direct versus self-report measures for assessing physical activity in adults: a systematic review. *International Journal of Behavioral Nutrition and Physical Activity, 5*, 56.

Rothenbacher, D., Koenig, W., & Brenner, H. (2006). Lifetime physical activity patterns and risk of coronary heart disease. *Heart, 92*, 1319–1320.

Saelens, B. E., Sallis, J. F., & Frank, L. D. (2003). Environmental correlates of walking and cycling: findings from the transportation, urban design, and planning literatures. *Annals of Behavioral Medicine, 25*(2), 80–91.

Sallis, J. F., Cervero, R. B., Ascher, W., Henderson, K. A., Kraft, M. K., & Kerr, J. (2006). An ecological approach to creating active living communities. *Annual Review of Public Health, 27*, 297–322.

Sallis, J. F., & Owen, N. (2002). Ecological models of health behaviour. In K. Glanz, F. M. Lewis, & B. K. Rimer (Eds.), *Health behaviour and health education. Theory, research and practice* (pp. 462–484). San Francisco: Jossey-Bass.

Schnohr, P., Lange, P., Scharling, H., & Jensen, J. S. (2006). Long-term physical activity in leisure time and mortality from coronary heart disease, stroke, respiratory diseases, and cancer. The Copenhagen City Heart Study. *European Journal of Cardiovascular Prevention and Rehabilitation, 13*(2), 173–179.

Schnohr, P., Scharling, H., & Jensen, J. S. (2003). Changes in leisure-time physical activity and risk of death: an observational study of 7,000 men and women. *American Journal of Epidemiology, 158*, 639–644.

Stringhini, S., Sabia, S., Shipley, M., Brunner, E., Nabi, H., Kivimaki, M., et al. (2010). Association of socioeconomic position with health behaviors and mortality. *Journal of the American Medical Association, 303*(12), 1159–1166.

Sundquist, J., Malmstrom, M., & Johansson, S. E. (1999). Cardiovascular risk factors and the neighbourhood environment: a multilevel analysis. *International Journal of Epidemiology, 28*(5), 841–845.

Swain, D. P., & Franklin, B. A. (2006). Comparison of cardioprotective benefits of vigorous versus moderate intensity aerobic exercise. *The American Journal of Cardiology, 97*, 141–147.

Swinburn, B., Egger, G., & Raza, F. (1999). Dissecting obesogenic environments: the development and application of a framework for identifying and prioritizing environmental interventions for obesity. *Preventive Medicine, 29*(6 Pt 1), 563–570.

Trost, S. G., Owen, N., Bauman, A. E., Sallis, J. F., & Brown, W. (2002). Correlates of adults' participation in physical activity: review and update. *Medicine and Science in Sports and Exercise, 34*(12), 1996–2001.

van der Lucht, F., & Polder, J. J. (2010). *Kernrapport van de Volksgezondheid Toekomst Verkenning 2010 Van gezond naar beter*. Bilthoven: Rijksinstituut voor Volksgezondheid en Milieu.

Van Lenthe, F. J., Brug, J., & Mackenbach, J. P. (2005). Neighbourhood inequalities in physical inactivity: the role of neighbourhood attractiveness, proximity to local facilities and safety in the Netherlands. *Social Science & Medicine, 60*(4), 763–775.

van Lenthe, F. J., & Kamphuis, C. B. (2011). Mismatched perceptions of neighbourhood walkability: need for interventions? *Health & Place, 17*(6), 1294–1295.

Wannamethee, S. G., & Shaper, A. G. (2001). Physical activity in the prevention of cardiovascular disease: an epidemiological perspective. *Sports Medicine, 31*(2), 101–114.

Wannamethee, S. G., Shaper, A. G., & Walker, M. (1998). Changes in physical activity, mortality and incidence of coronary heart disease in older men. *The Lancet, 351*, 1603–1608.

Wardle, J., & Steptoe, A. (2003). Socioeconomic differences in attitudes and beliefs about healthy lifestyles. *Journal of Epidemiology and Community Health, 57*, 440–443.

Weich, S., Burton, E., Blanchard, M., Prince, M., Sproston, K., & Erens, B. (2001). Measuring the built environment: validity of a site survey instrument for use in urban settings. *Health & Place, 7*(4), 283–292.

Weinstein, N. D. (1993). Testing four competing theories of health-protective behavior. *Health Psychology, 12*(4), 324–333.

Wendel-Vos, W., Droomers, M., Kremers, S., Brug, J., & van Lenthe, F. (2007). Potential environmental determinants of physical activity in adults: a systematic review. *Obesity Reviews, 8*(5), 425–440.

Wendel-Vos, G. C., Schuit, A. J., Saris, W. H., & Kromhout, D. (2003). Reproducibility and relative validity of the short questionnaire to assess health-enhancing physical activity. *Journal of Clinical Epidemiology, 56*(12), 1163–1169.

Zenk, S. N., Schulz, A. J., Mentz, G., House, J. S., Gravlee, C. C., Miranda, P. Y., et al. (2007). Inter-rater and test-retest reliability: methods and results for the neighborhood observational checklist. *Health & Place, 13*(2), 452–465.

Chapter 13
Building in Prevention: Nudging Towards Physical Activity and Public Health

Jens Troelsen

Introduction

It is obvious that our physical surroundings—given by the air we breathe, the food we eat and the environment we move around in—have a direct influence on our health. This knowledge has been available since ancient times (Aristotle 1996). It was, however, only in the nineteenth century that there appeared a willingness on the part of central governments to make more systematic efforts to tackle poor-quality physical surroundings, e.g. basic sanitation and water supplies. In an initiative to promote hygiene, physical surroundings were to be clean and secure to be in, so that coming generations would get a better and a longer life (Porter 1997). Since then, attempts to prevention have, therefore, aimed at changing conditions of life for the better, so that cities, the environment, traffic, etc. should not have a negative effect on the development of illness, accidents and mortality. While major advances were made in preventive work in the middle of the nineteenth century through physical structural prevention by means of sewerage systems, slum clearance and access to running water, light and fresh air, the focus in the twenty-first century has been placed more on the regulation of inappropriate individual health behaviours through restrictive legislation. Prohibition and taxation policy have been typical mechanisms for regulation for keeping our late-modern lifestyle illnesses under control with the focus on regulating the use of tobacco, alcohol and unhealthy foods (Shibuya et al. 2003; Room et al. 2005). Either by banning unhealthy lifestyle habits or by making them costly, structural prevention initiatives have contributed to ensuring that the risk to public health has been reduced. As a result we can expect to live longer than previous generations, and we can look forward to a life that is less burdened by life-threatening illnesses.

J. Troelsen (✉)
Institute of Sports Science and Clinical Biomechanics, University of Southern Denmark, Campusvej 55, 5230 Odense M, Denmark
e-mail: jtroelsen@health.sdu.dk

C. Stock and A. Ellaway (eds.), *Neighbourhood Structure and Health Promotion*,
DOI 10.1007/978-1-4614-6672-7_13,

The question is, however, whether to simply continue to subject individual choice to bans, taxes or prejudice is a suitable course of action to follow in future preventive work. A society based on prohibitive legislation that limits people's freedom may not be the sort of society we wish to pass down to future generations. At the same time, it is questionable whether active policies of limitation and containment will have an effect when seen in relation to the new public health challenges we are facing. Legislation and taxation policy combined with fear arousing campaigns have proved to be a success as regards limiting smoking. With regard to physical inactivity however, which is the fourth biggest risk factor for mortality across the world (WHO 2010a, b), the same approach would be grotesque. Legislation that dictated the maximum levels of physical inactivity in public spaces or placed a tax on sedentary work would require as its ultimate consequence the sanction of actual physical compunction. Generally speaking, there would seem to be compelling reasons for thinking new thoughts with regard to preventive strategies in the twenty-first century, when health risks are associated more with deselection of healthy lifestyles than the selection of unhealthy ones.

Taking these public health challenges as my starting point, I shall discuss in this chapter why and how physical structural prevention can be a well-chosen strategy seen in relation to the challenges of the future. Physical structural prevention is defined as interventions in the natural and built environments that support and value healthy choices. This will be discussed in relation to the unintended consequences that current health discourse brings with it. The chapter consists of three sections, of which the first will be a discussion of the choice between an active and a passive prevention strategy. This will be followed by an argumentation for the strength of passive prevention through physical structuring in combating health epidemics seen from a historical perspective. In the concluding section, the nudging of physical activity is discussed in relation to countering the development of the growing epidemic of obesity in the western world.

The Scale of Health Challenges

The occurrence of noncommunicable diseases is increasing on the global scale. As WHO asserts:

> [...] tackling it constitutes one of the major challenges for development in the twenty-first century. Noncommunicable diseases, principally cardiovascular diseases, diabetes, cancers, and chronic respiratory diseases, caused an estimated 35 million deaths in 2005. This figure represents 60 % of all deaths globally [...] Total deaths from noncommunicable diseases are projected to increase by a further 17 % over the next 10 years. (WHO 2008, p. 5)

To address this development in disease patterning, WHO presents proposals for a global strategy, which on the one hand charts the causes of this development and on the other strengthens the health-care system. Basically what is needed is prevention in relation to the risk factors that bring about noncommunicable diseases.

The strategy is explained in the report "Prevention and control of noncommunicable diseases: implementation of the global strategy":

> Reducing the level of exposure of individuals and populations to the common modifiable risk factors for noncommunicable diseases—namely, tobacco use, unhealthy diet and physical inactivity, and the harmful use of alcohol—and their determinants, while at the same time strengthening the capacity of individuals and populations to make healthier choices and follow lifestyle patterns that foster good health. (WHO 2008, p. 3)

In other words what is being suggested is a strategic approach both for prevention and for health promotion that at the same time reduces risk factors and educates people how to make those choices most advantageous to health. Physical structural prevention is not explicitly mentioned in the global strategy, but since there is evidence that physical environments can both promote and prevent health (Jackson 2003), it would be an appropriate long-term strategy to focus to a greater extent on ways in which we design the physical environment that surrounds us in our everyday lives.

Prevention and Health Promotion in Public Spaces: Two Sides of the Same Coin

One aspect often absent from overall considerations about health strategy is the fact that, quite apart from their tendency to promote disease as a result of pollution, pesticides, noise and so on, our physical surroundings also have a direct effect on public health as a consequence of the health behaviour they appeal to. If an individual nurses the intention to live healthy, the environment can be experienced as presenting a restrictive factor in the realisation of a healthy lifestyle. A decrepit, vapid built environment may fail to arouse the desire or the need to live healthy in the first place.

USA is often used as frightening example in this context. For example, can certain areas be characterised as food deserts as a way of saying that access to shops with good raw materials is negligible compared to the mountain of chain stores that thrust junk food over the counter (Walker et al. 2010). There it will be more difficult, more expensive and more time-consuming to serve, for example, a good and nourishing meal for your children. In the same way, both the geography and the infrastructure of those unending American suburbs make walking and cycling impossible. If someone has the desire to be physically active in their leisure time, then this has to be done in one of the expensive commercial fitness centres or in the park that has to be within reasonable driving distance. Physical surroundings demand, then, two or more cars if the daily business of an American family is to be accomplished within the 24 h that are available. This has had severe consequences. A diet with an excess of calories combined with an everyday life with reduced physical activity has led to American in particular being hit by what is seen as an obesity epidemic. The same development of excessive weight applies to the whole of the western world (Philip et al. 2010). An underlying culture of indolent comfort underpinned by a favourable economic climate and technological development that has minimised physical work in production can be seen as part of the explanation.

Physical surroundings – and these include urban development, infrastructure and land use – must, however, also be factored into obesity calculations. Generally, physical planning in the western world over the past 50 years has been steered by commercial interest in being able to sell attractive plots to be used for housing or business. This has resulted in urban sprawl with zones divided into separate sectors. This form of urban development is simultaneously supported by an infrastructure that is constantly extended to link to ever-greater distances without loss of time, and this leads to the construction of road systems that are extremely demanding in terms of space (Frumkin et al. 2004).

Criticisms of inappropriate urban development have been raised from various quarters. Since the beginning of the 1980s, the movement known as New Urbanism, which consists of professionals such as architects, planners, sociologists and psychologists, has argued stridently for urban densification and for mixed land use with a broadly ramified infrastructure to promote activity (Haas 2008). Arguments in favour of this approach have been based in particular on the opportunities for urban space to improve quality of life, identification with the local environment and sense of belonging to physical and social frameworks. Since that time, arguments in favour of public health have been added, supported by evidence from many studies showing improved health in loc.l areas that enable and appeal to physical activity (Kawachi and Berkman 2003).

An opposite tendency is, however, also in the process of spreading among larger American and Australian cities, whereby large-scale campaigns and building projects are being established to revitalise the urban space. Europe is no exception. Here virtually all large coastal cities are in the process of refashioning antiquated harbours and old industrial factory areas. Market towns alter market places and squares into places for physical and cultural activity. There is a general move towards establishing harbour swimming pools, cycling lanes, green city oasis, car-free zones and so on in order to create a more appealing urban space. It is questionable, however, whether such examples of passive prevention are sufficient to counteract the epidemic of obesity the contemporary western world.

Personal Freedom or Tyranny of Health?

One bone of contention in preventive work is the question of how invasive any actions to tackle poor health behaviours should be. This is the question of where the limits to personal freedom should be drawn. Should individuals have the freedom to smoke, drink and grow fat as much as they like, or should there be strict rules and actual bans on inappropriate health behaviours? The chair of the Danish Prevention Commission, Mette Wier, makes herself a spokesperson for the need for active prevention:

> In many areas it is good as a starting point to allow as much as possible to be left to the individual's free choice. The question is, however, whether situations of choice are that simple in the area of health. Children, for example, do not themselves decide how often unhealthy food should be served, whether they drink too much or whether people smoke in

> the home. Before anti-smoking legislation came in, people did not decide for themselves whether they were passive smokers in a café or not. And the great majority [of smokers] already start smoking when they are teenagers—the question is whether they understand the consequences of their choice. I would go so far as to say that it does not always make sense to talk about 'freedom' of choice, and that not taking active prevention even involved elements of neglect. In my view it is getting to be high time for us to take the lead and create new frameworks that promote citizens' health choices. (Wier 2008)

Active prevention would to a greater or lesser extent involve an invasion of personal freedom. One example is the Danish anti-smoking legislation introduced as of 15 August 2007, which prohibits smoking in workplaces; in school and institutions; in bars and restaurants; in trains, buses and taxis; and in places with public access. The ban creates freedom from passive smoking for the majority of the Danish population but must be experienced as a clear limitation of freedom of activity for the 12 % of the population of Denmark who smoke every day. A popular Danish rock star, Kim Larsen, was one among other popular icons who made no secret of their dislike and in a protest against the anti-smoking laws spoke of "a battle for freedom and democracy". Backed by his own private funds, the rock star then took the initiative to set up an expensive campaign with the slogan "Gesundheit macht frei", as an allegory for Nazi processes of purification in their aim to achieve a pure race (TV2News 2008). Central government involvement in the private sphere is seen in these terms as health fascism (Hybel 2008).

Interventions Limiting Freedom and Their Limitations

Health fascism or not, it is in the national interest to create living conditions that can generally help human behaviour to move in a healthier direction. Where formerly the motive was driven by the desire for a large and powerful military force, for a state in society, today it would be the desire to create a large, self-regulating and productive workforce (Hobsbawm 1994). More important, in the transition to a knowledge society, the desire will be to create a creative class with a high degree of well-being and quality of life (Florida 2004). A welfare system with a tightly woven safety net combined with the absence of negative stress can create the conditions for growth for the innovative thinking that can ensure that a society is in the vanguard of developments in the global knowledge market. And there are signs that the Danish social model has succeeded in this part of the project. A number of studies award Danes the honour of being the world's happiest people, with room for creative thinking. And, as a side effect, one of the studies records that this happiness has a positive effect on the population's general blood pressure (Blanchflower and Oswald 2008).

Seen in through the eyes of a social cynic, however, citizens who are a burden on the health service and die young but happy are not useful citizens. If a health problem is judged to be burdensome for the interest of the whole community, then restrictions must be placed on individual happiness. Seen in this light, then, it can come as no surprise that the state becomes a "nanny state". In a democratic society, it is the majority that decides at the expense of the minority.

Active prevention is, therefore, a form of action that presents restrictions to quality of life for some people while being experienced as an improvement for the remaining majority. Banning smoking is one example, and having speed limits for traffic is another one. Active prevention through the use of restrictive intervention can be seen as necessary when considered in the light of a common set of values and, if taken to the extreme, involve the removal of people's freedom and imprisonment when an individual is assessed to represent a danger for the community. In Europe there is legislation that prohibits firearms on account of the risk of accidental shooting or of murder due to "crime passionnel", but a republican Texan would see it as invasion of his right to defend himself and thereby of his freedom. A secondary consequence of active prevention would, therefore, be that behaviour in one situation would be normalised, while in another it would be criminalised when the legal requirements are transgressed.

Whether it constitutes neglect not to employ active preventive measures, as chairperson Mette Wier expressed it, must be democratic decision. There is much to suggest that people are willing to go a long way down the road that leads to tighter prevention policies. According to a Danish study "Prevention in the future—according to Danes", 78 % of Danes are of the opinion that sweets and soda vending machines should be banned from schools and sports centres (Mandagmorgen 2008). Almost three quarters believe that it should be compulsory for children to be outdoors during school breaks, and 63 % think that students should not be allowed to leave school during all breaks. Active prevention using prohibition and coercion has, therefore, considerable support. The study also shows, however, that almost half of all Danes would rather enjoy life than live healthily. It says something about the positive attitude to active prevention that the study is based on responses from over 2,000 Danes in the age range 18–74 who in the examples named here are expressing opinions about other target groups than their own. By comparison, restrictions on making car journeys over short distances and a total smoking ban are only supported by 27 % and 15 % of adults Danes, respectively (Mandagmorgen 2008). Based on this study, active prevention seems to be a good solution as long it does not involve oneself.

Clear restrictions are demanded when risk behaviour has to be restricted. It would be naïve to imagine that appeals could be made for considerate driving in order to minimise the number of traffic accidents. In the same way, restrictions are needed to restrict the development of lifestyle-related diseases brought on by smoking, alcohol or other health-damaging substances. At the same time, it has to be recognised that restrictions are not always the answer to regulating behaviour. This can lead to vigilantism and common defiance and may have the opposite effects to that intended.

In relation to physical activity, it would be difficult to lay down restrictions for how physically inactive people were allowed to be. The smoking of tobacco is traditionally reckoned to be the most important threat to public health in the western world, but the rankings have been under dispute since 2000. Physical inactivity ranks between the second and sixth most important risk factor in contributing to the population burden of disease in westernised countries (Bauman and Craig 2005). This is due to the fact that the number of regular smokers has fallen over just a few years, while physical inactivity is increasing due to the changing nature of work and leisure activities. Physical inactivity has the potential to develop into our greatest challenge to health (Oldridge 2008; Roger et al. 2011).

The result of active prevention in smoking cannot be denied, but the same strategy would be difficult to maintain in relation to prevent the lack of exercise in people's everyday lives. Parents can lay down rules for their children's use of TV and computers, and the school's board of governors can decide that pupils should be outside during breaks, but for the remainder of the population, making physical inactivity illegal would mean far-reaching intervention using prohibition and coercion.

Targeted prevention must, therefore, make use of a variety of initiatives tailored to the risk behaviour that we wish to alter. An alternative to active prevention characterised by legislation, overprotection and admonishment would be a more passive prevention supporting desirable behaviours rather than prohibiting undesirable ones. And if such suggested prevention is translated onto a physical structural plane, then good physical planning will ensure that the healthy choice becomes the natural choice—a choice that does not arouse a sense of guilt at one's own poor health but which takes place at a nonconscious level as being the instinctive correct choice in the moment.

Historically, physical structural prevention has had huge significance for the public health. At the same time, improvements in the physical framework of people's lives can be a practical way to address social differences in health, whereby a minority of the population monopolises the great majority of the total resources devoted to health care. In Denmark, for example, it has been shown that 70 % of the population does not make use of hospital services, while the 10 % of the population that use the most services used 85 % of public resources allotted to hospitals (Interior and Health Ministry 2007). This means, then, that there is a definable group of citizens making heavy demands on the health system, and this is an imbalance that information campaigns, individually oriented intervention or active prevention has not managed to even out.

Prevention is a requirement, but seen in the light of future demands, physical, structural intervention should be given higher priority. In what follows I shall, therefore, clarify the significance of physical planning and, using a theoretical perspective, illustrate how physical, structural prevention makes an impact on health behaviour.

Physical Structural Prevention of Epidemics

In December 2006 the British Medical Journal gave their readers the opportunity to vote on which out of 15 decisive milestones should be designated the greatest medical advance since 1840, the year in which the British Medical Journal was first published. The 11,331 highly qualified and competent readers gave their verdict: sanitation. Sewerage systems and the piping of fresh water were singled out as having been responsible for the greatest medical advance since 1840 (Ferriman 2007). What is noteworthy is that in the ranking order, this first place was contested by other medical advances such as antibiotics, anaesthesia, the introduction of vaccines and the discovery of the structure of DNA. On the face of it, we may be surprised that readers assessed access to water and sewage as the greatest medical advances at the expense of these other areas that were more prestigious and heavier on research. However, seen in the light of extremely high mortality in the nineteenth century caused by cholera and epidemic disease (and not least in view of the current prospects in developing countries), the choice seems natural.

Doctor John Snow, who showed that cholera bacteria were transmitted through water, and the social reformer Sir Edwin Chadwick, who was among those campaigning for running water and sewage systems in the most deprived urban areas, can be regarded as pioneers in this area. With their research and their dedication, they paved the way for this sanitary revolution of the mid-nineteenth century. It was a physical structural change that has had huge implications for subsequent public health (Mackenbach 2007). For example, in 1853, almost 5,000 citizens of Copenhagen died during a cholera epidemic, which corresponded to almost 5 % of the city's population. Action was, then, essential at a time when drinking water was fetched from the market well and excrement driven away by the nightman.

In developed countries sanitation is taken for granted, a comfort in our everyday lives that only comes to our attention when the drain is blocked or the water polluted. In comparison with more high-tech treatment methods, we will often underestimate the significance of sanitation. This makes the result in the British Medical Journal particularly pleasing to Johan Mackenbach, professor of public health:

> I'm delighted that sanitation is recognised by so many people as such an important milestone. The general lesson which still holds is that passive protection against health hazards is often the best way to improve population health. (Ferriman 2007, p. 111)

We in the west are no longer fighting cholera epidemics in the twenty-first century. The structural improvements made since the 1850s that have ensured that drinking water and waste water, for example, are separated have removed that health risk. With the majority of hygiene problems having been solved in western countries, however, we have to accept that, as a result of a high-tech affluent society, a new epidemic brought about by obesity has been generated.

The term obesity epidemic is used to describe the way the rapid spread of obesity is taking place, particularly among North American and European population groups. This development is regarded by many health experts as constituting a significant threat to public health in the western world (Seidell 1995; James 2004; Kosti and Panagiotakos 2006; Ogden et al. 2006; Prentice 2006). It is estimated that almost 70 % of the adult American population are overweight, having a body mass index of over 25 ($BMI = kg/m^2$), with a third of them being classified as obese with a BMI of over 30 (WHO 2000). This is a level of obesity in the USA that has more than doubled in the course of just 30 years (Flegal et al. 2010).

In Europe we are well on the way to matching conditions in America. According to country estimates for 2008, over 50 % of both men and women in the WHO European Region were overweight, and approximately 23 % of women and 20 % of men were obese (WHO 2010a, b). If we look at the next generation, children and adolescents are also becoming fatter. Estimates of the number of overweight infants and children in the WHO European Region rose steadily from 1990 to 2008. Over 60 % of children who are overweight before puberty will be overweight in early adulthood (WHO 2010a, b).

The causes of obesity can be stated very simply. Over a prolonged period, the intake of energy is greater than consumption of energy. In other words, there is a permanent imbalance between a calorie-rich diet and the degree of physical activity (Stubbs and Lee 2004). This imbalance causes large deposits of fat, which constitute a risk of coronary and arterial disease, of type 2 diabetes, of excessive strain on the skeletal and motor apparatus and of a whole range of other lifestyle diseases (Kissebah et al. 1989; Nguyen et al. 2010).

Preventive Measures Against Physical Inactivity

In the twenty-first century then, there is particular need for measures that can reduce or, at best, eradicate the general imbalance between energy intake and energy consumption and thereby prevent the development of an ongoing epidemic of obesity. As was true in the decisive role played by sanitation since the mid-nineteenth century, today there is the need to set in motion physical structural preventive measures that can have a positive influence on western lifestyle diseases. One area to be focused on in particular is the lack of energy consumption, brought about by physical inactivity. If people use their bodies more actively in their daily lives, they may also eat more healthily, smoke fewer cigarettes and consume less alcohol in their overall desire to achieve a better functioning body (Sallis and Owen 1999). This pattern, in which some life choices bring others in their wake, is called cluster behaviour by epidemiologists (Schuit et al. 2002; Chiolero et al. 2006; Poortinga 2007). In that sense increased physical activity can be regarded as being the provoking factor in the attempt to improve public health. This is supported by epidemiological studies and trials showing that it is better to be fat and fit than slim and slack (Pedersen 2003; Berentzen et al. 2006; Pedersen 2006). In other words it has been shown that, as regards overweight, inactivity has marked significance for the relative risk of mortality of any cause (Farrell et al. 2002; Katzmarzyk et al. 2005).

As shown in a number of other chapters in this book, there are many investigations and intervention studies showing that the environment has an influence on physical activity. Physical structural prevention can, therefore, make a difference. The question is simply how the environment shapes our behaviour, and a theoretically constructed perspective in the second half of the chapter aims to provide an overview of the way in which physical structural preventive measures have both a direct and an indirect influence on our behaviour. This knowledge can be used to create environments that encourage greater degrees of physical activity and, by extension, promote the establishment of a form of prevention that, instead of directing attention at individual physical shortcomings, creates a framework in which individuals can master their own lives.

Nudging Physical Activity: The Direct and Indirect Influence of the Environment

Physical structural prevention can be characterised by the construction of environments that support and value healthy choices. The motto for appropriate physical structural preventive measures is they make the healthy choice into an easy and natural choice, whether we are aware of it or not. Running water in our taps and flushing toilets do away with the village pump and the nightman—and with them the risk of developing cholera and other epidemic diseases. In the same way, society in the twenty-first century can be organised in such a way that physical activity becomes the easy choice. Urban planners, engineers and health professionals can, within reason, become the "choice architects" of our day to nudge physical activity. Professors R.H. Thaler and C.R. Sunstein define "nudging" in this context as:

> A nudge, as we will use the term, is any aspect of choice architecture that alters people's behavior in a predictable way without forbidding any options or significantly changing their economic incentives. To count as a mere nudge, the intervention must be easy and cheap to avoid. Nudges are not mandates. Putting the fruit at eye level counts as a nudge. Banning junk food does not. (Thaler and Sunstein 2009, p. 6)

With this as a starting point, road and footpath systems, the sitting of housing, schools, workplaces, parks, playgrounds, sports facilities and so on can be organised in such a way as to reduce distance and increase accessibility, making it likely that motorised, passive transport, for example, will be made redundant in everyday life. The decision as to whether the car remains in the carport, however, is weighted against our purpose with the planned trip, our attitude to pollution such as CO_2 emissions, our wish to send a symbolic signal, our experience of weather conditions, our need to take the children and so on. The nature of our environment can lead us both directly and unconsciously towards particular behaviours, just as our environment can indirectly influence our intention about a particular form of behaviour. This complex relation can be illustrated in a model of the direct and indirect influence of the environment on physical activity (PA) (Fig. 13.1).

In general the model in Fig. 13.1 shows that physical activity in relation to the surrounding environment is influenced in part directly, illustrated by the lower direct route, and influenced in part indirectly, illustrated in the upper route, where cognitive processes mediate behaviour. This twofold influence can be described as a dual process, in that behaviour caused by a particular environment comes about both through intentional actions and through an "automatic pilot", who at an unreflective level steers it in certain directions. The behaviour is moderated in this dual process by individual conditions, which can have either a positive or a negative influence in respect of the likelihood of being physically active.

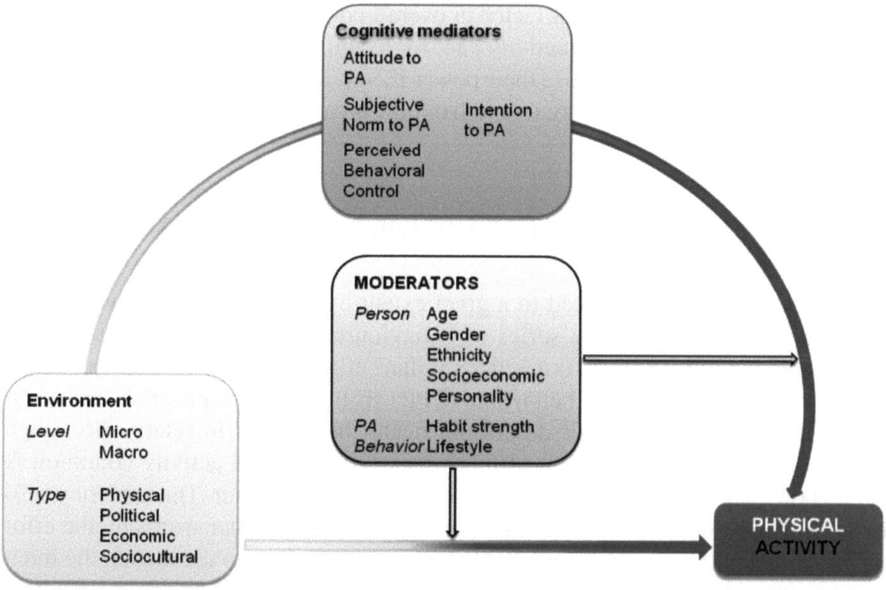

Fig. 13.1 Nudging physical activity—the direct and indirect influence of the environment. (Source: adapted from Kremers, S.P., de Bruijn, G.J., Visscher, T.L., van Mechelen, W., de Vries, N.K., Brug, J. (2006) Environmental influences on energy balance-related behaviors: a dual-process view. *International Journal of Behavioral Nutrition and Physical Activity 3*, 9; reprinted by permission of the publisher)

Physical structural preventive measures are directed at interventions in the physical environment. In addition to being influenced by the physical environment, physical activity is also subject to the influence of a social, political and cultural domain (Sallis et al. 2006). Physical planning must, therefore, be seen in and must take account of a whole picture in which other domains have a role to play (Troelsen et al. 2008). The Dutch and the Danes, for example, boast of having a cycling culture in which most people are experienced and confident cyclists. This culture is on the one hand upheld by a political environment that prioritises the maintenance and extension of a cycling infrastructure and on the other is under the influence of social currents campaigning for the importance of cycling. In countries like the USA and the United Kingdom, the cycling culture disappeared during the 1950s, as the political and social climate favoured the car culture, so in that particular political and cultural context, physical planning that favours cycling, for example, will have far less support than in other places where the culture of cycling is still intact. This means that, in our efforts to examine which interventions are physically possible, how they can be realised and who they are aiming at, environment must be seen in a broader context (Salli et al. 2008).

In our approach to the environment, we must at the same time distinguish between a micro and a macro level, depending on whether the intervention is local and residential in character or on a more generalised regional or national level. A physical structural measure will have limited effect if its focus is limited to the local environment and does not factor in overall considerations. Walking as a form of transport or as recreational activity can, for example, be increased using targeted local interventions, but they lose their power if, say, a particular decision relating to traffic policy makes commuting to and from the area difficult.

The Environment's Mediated Influence on Physical Activity

Human behaviour is influenced to a great extent by our awareness of what we do and what we want. A whole series of behavioural theories are about surveying factors that have an effect on our actions (Glanz et al. 2008). In this context we can highlight theory of planned behaviour (TPB) in that, like others, this theory has been found to be suitable for describing health behaviours in relation to weight control, including the balancing of food intake and physical activity (Baranowski et al. 2003). The aim of TPB is to explain and predict behaviour. The tendency is for behaviour to be determined by the intention to behave, in other words by the effort an individual will make to act out that behaviour. According to the model, the intention to behave is regulated to take account of the attitude to the behaviour, of subjective norms and of the sense of control that is experienced over behaviour. An attitude to behaviour here is the result of deliberations in which positive and negative perceptions of a given form of behaviour are weighed up. Subjective norms are an expression of the experience of social pressure that a given form of behaviour is expected to generate. The perceived control experienced over behaviour is the individual's perception of how difficult or easy it will be to evince a given form of behaviour, a perceived control that can also have direct influence on the actual behaviour (Ajzen 2005).

The environment can stimulate the arousal or reduce the intention to be physically active. Seeing Nordic pole walkers, runners, children playing, the presence of footpaths or even just an attractive park can direct attention to the fact that physical activity in a particular environment is a potential form of activity. Depending on their composition, the individual's attitude, norms and perceived behavioural control can either reinforce or reduce the intention to be physically active. The environment will also affect cognitive mediators, so that the conscious behavioural filter will in time change its nature. An individual's attitude, norms and perceived control will, then, also reflect the environment and the behaviour that takes place in it.

The Environment's Influence on Unconscious Behaviour

There are upper limits on what we can grasp consciously. To take a stance on every one of our actions would be to disable all activity (Thaler and Sunstein 2009). For that reason a large proportion of our behaviour is relegated to daily routines that do not demand controlled awareness in relation to what we do. Similarly, spontaneous actions happen without conscious deliberation, as we move in new directions that only make sense the moment the action is rationalised after the event. The pivotal area of research into behavioural automatism is what promotes unintended actions (Moskowitz et al. 1999). This research field has focused, for example, on our unconscious tendency to imitate our social surroundings, which is a central part of children's learning and socialisation. The unconscious searching to satisfy physical needs is something that has particularly occupied criminologists, in the same way as the decoding of signals and consumer behaviour have particular interest for marketing research (Kardes et al. 2011). Automatism in behaviour is marked by undercurrent feedback loops between the body and the environment that make themselves felt through a sudden, routine or spontaneous action. In that sense the environment can play a role when the shaping of settings creates recognisability, trust and curiosity, and it will come to play a role when the setting upsets or requires a controlled, conscious awareness (Kaplan et al. 1998).

As far as making physical activity into an automatic action, then, it is a matter of creating settings in which the opportunity to be active is hard to ignore. A stairway, a pathway, a ball, the skateboard, the vantage point and so on can be the triggering factor by inviting to physical activity without conscious will.

Moderators Regarding Physical Activity

Physical activity is influenced by the environment both directly and indirectly, but this dual process is moderated by individual preconditions determining whether an individual is physically active or not. The intention to indulge in physical activity may be aroused by the environment, but the type, extent and intensity of the activity is moderated by individual features, in which demographic background, character make-up, habits and lifestyle all play their part.

The influence of the environment will be dependent on age, gender, ethnicity and socio-economic status. The individual's demographic profile will influence the way in which the environment is perceived. When, for example, older people estimate how far it is to the nearest park, they assess an objectively measured distance as being longer than a young age group will do. Seen subjectively, this can be seen as being the result of the difference in their perception of the time needed to traverse the distance to the park at speed. In the same way, well-planned and well-lit paths play a larger role in women's sense of security and thereby in their desire to cycle than is the case for men. A high level of education and income also has a positive influence on physical activity as a result of greater resources, dedication and knowledge as regards health benefits. The appeal of the environment will vary according to demographic profile. Children and pensioners, therefore, have hugely different expectations as to the environment in which physical activity can be realised.

Individual traits of character can also moderate dedication in the interplay between environment and physical activity. Studies have shown that extrovert people have greater motivation for physical activity than more introvert people, who do not wish to dedicate and expose themselves to the same extent (Rhodes and Smith 2006). Correspondingly, people with a conscientious nature show greater endurance in meeting expectations in regard to health. Furthermore, studies have also shown that traits of character such as emotional stability, indolence and readiness for experience have an effect as regards choosing or declining opportunities for physical activity (Huang et al. 2007).

Lifestyle and habit may bring about reluctance in people's readiness to change. Many years of practising and experiencing particular patterns of behaviour can make alteration difficult. Habits can be seen as actions that are subconscious, so that despite any awareness of the surrounding milieu, habits have to be reviewed before they can be altered. In the same way, lifestyle changes require a review that takes issue not only with an individual's actions but also with the identity the person wishes to be inscribed by. Physical activity in that context can be trendy, but it can also be associated with negative bodily experiences by the individual.

Hidden Prevention

From a theoretical perspective, the model indicates how physical activity is affected by the environment both on a direct, unconscious level and on an indirect, conscious one. From a restricted preventive perspective, the way the environment affects physical activity is secondary as long as an altered use of space plays a part in increasing the level of activity. In a more extended preventive perspective, however, a longer-term option would be to invest in structures that underpin the direct, unconscious route to physical activity. If physical activity occurs in a way that is unsolicited or unforced, it is more likely that the activity level will be maintained when reminded about it. What is more central, however, is that physical activity should take place without the notion of becoming healthy being set up as a target. When physical activity is overlaid by a utilitarian ethos denoting the value of health, it could compromise the desire to take active part. Setting up a framework whereby physical activity becomes the natural thing to do at a particular moment in time and in particular circumstances allows the health aspect to fade into the background. Prevention is driven by a prophylactic rationalism, e.g. stimulating physical activity, but, in contrast to active, admonitory prevention, physical structural preventions are passive and optimally visible to those they are targeting in an immediate way. In the same way as sanitary installations are preventive for epidemic diseases, urban planning and architecture can be preventive for physical inactivity without it crossing our minds in our everyday lives.

Just as motorways, escalators, suburbs and technology have made the population inactive without their being immediately aware of it, marketplaces, streets and stairways can generate activity. Such hidden prevention creates connotations about a Big Brother society with concealed interest groupings and a population of puppets. It can, however, also be seen as an alternative way to mastering preventive initiatives and thereby minimising the unintended consequences of traditional prevention.

Mastering Prevention

Globally, the development of noncommunicable disease has brought with it an increase in focus on the need for prevention. Sedentary lifestyles present a significant risk factor here, especially in high-income countries. Such countries had more than double the prevalence of inactivity compared with low-income countries for both men and women, with 41 % of men and 48 % of women insufficiently physically active (Ala Alwan et al. 2011).

Those advocating preventive initiatives typically make use of philanthropic arguments about creating quality of life and improved living conditions for individuals, but the bottom line of the social equation is also the question of preserving the basis for the survival of a welfare state. It is a matter of creating a strong, healthy workforce placing a minimum of strain on the health services. Prevention becomes, therefore, an unavoidable project, which will always have a democratic majority behind it in attempts to achieve what is best for the common good. The entire preventive project can in continuation of this be described as a common project to create a social order, in which the prophylactic rationalism determines what good and correct actions commonly are. This gives rise to a preventive discourse that establishes the premises for legitimate health behaviour.

Adults, for example, are recommended to walk a minimum of 10,000 paces a day or to be moderately physically active for at least 150 min per week (WHO 2010a, b, p.26). Several studies show, however, that only 10–15 % of the adult population in different countries follow this recommendation (Orsini et al. 2008; Chastin et al. 2009; Tucker et al. 2011). There is, then, a rest of 85–90 % of the population that can be characterised as having inappropriate health behaviour—a group that can be given the blame for their lack of ability in following such a recommendation. At the individual level, preventive discourse of this kind contributes to increased self-recrimination driven by pangs of conscience at one's own lack of effort in maintaining health. At the group level, the discourse contributes to increased social control and stigmatisation, since deviant health behaviours can be measured and registered by the lack of activity and bodily appearance. At the social level, it can lead to "blaming the victim" and to the marginalisation of vulnerable groups, who are unable to follow instructions for health living. At the same time, prophylactic rationalism is linked to a form of inertia that means that preventive work is an ever-expanding and never-ending project. To follow the prophylactic rationalism requires ever more invasive prevention, and in the final analysis, a medical police force would have to be established to ensure and enforce good order in the domain of health.

Prophylactic rationalism of this kind based on campaigns, health recommendations and active intervention has, therefore, a number of limitations and undesirable consequences which have to be taken into account if we are to hope to reach even those with limited resources. A discursive countermove would be to shift the health focus away from the individual and focus instead on the physical environment surrounding the individual. In this chapter it has been argued that physical surroundings can act as a restrictor or as a spur to activity, regardless of whether we are aware of it or not. And this means that it is possible to design the physical environment in accordance with the health imperative that dictates that physical activity is a goal in itself and not simply a means to achieve health. Making it easy, attractive and natural to be physically active at an unconscious, automatic level will allow the phrase "to take ten" to move away from its meaning of "putting one's feet up for 10 min" towards getting one's feet pumping by moving 10 min.

References

Ajzen, I. (2005). *Attitudes, personality, and behavior*. Maidenhead, Berkshire, England, New York: Open University Press.

Ala Alwan, T.A., Cowan, M., Riley, L. (2011). Noncommunicable diseases. *Country profiles 2011*. WHO, pp. 1–209.

Aristoteles. (1996). *The politics, and the institution of Athens*. Cambridge: Cambridge University Press.

Baranowski, T., Cullen, K. W., Nicklas, T., Thompson, D., & Baranowski, J. (2003). Are current health behavioral change models helpful in guiding prevention of weight gain efforts? *Obesity Research, 11*, 23s–43s.

Bauman, A., & Craig, C. L. (2005). The place of physical activity in the WHO global strategy on diet and physical activity. *The International Journal of Behavioral Nutrition and Physical Activity, 1186*(1479–5868), 2–10.

Berentzen, T., Sørensen, M. S., Sørensen, T. I., & Astrup, A. V. (2006). The importance of physical activity and fitness in avoiding the complications of obesity. *Ugeskrift for Laeger, 168*(2), 144–149.

Blanchflower, D. G., & Oswald, A. J. (2008). Hypertension and happiness across nations. *Journal of Health Economics, 27*(2), 18–233.

Chastin, S., Dall, P., Tigbe, W., Grant, M., Ryan, C., Rafferty, D., & Granat, M. (2009). Compliance with physical activity guidelines in a group of UK-based postal workers using an objective monitoring technique. *European Journal of Applied Physiology, 106*(6), 893–899.

Chiolero, A., Wietlisbach, V., Ruffieux, C., Paccaud, F., & Cornuz, J. (2006). Clustering of risk behaviors with cigarette consumption: A population-based survey. *Preventive Medicine, 42*(5), 348–353.

Farrell, S., Braun, L., Barlow, C. E., Cheng, Y. J., & Blair, S. N. (2002). The relation of body mass index, cardiorespiratory fitness, and all-cause mortality in women. *Obesity Research, 10*(6), 417–423.

Ferriman, A. (2007). BMJ readers choose the "sanitary revolution" as greatest medical advance since 1840. *BMJ, 334*(7585), 111.

Flegal, K. M., Carroll, M. D., Ogden, C. L., & Curtin, L. R. (2010). Prevalence and trends in obesity among US adults, 1999–2008. *JAMA, 303*(3), 235–241.

Florida, R. (2004). *The rise of the creative class: and how it's transforming work, leisure, community and everyday life*. New York: Basic Books.

Frumkin, H., Frank, L., & Jackson, R. (2004). *Urban sprawl and public health. Designing, planning, and building for healthy communities*. Washington: Island Press.

Glanz, K., Rimer, B. K., & Viswanath, K. (2008). *Health behavior and health education: theory, research, and practice*. San Francisco, CA: Jossey-Bass.

Haas, T. (2008). *New urbanism and beyond: designing cities for the future*. New York: Rizzoli.

Hobsbawm, E. J. (1994). *The age of extremes: a history of the world, 1914–1991*. London: Pantheon Books.

Huang, C. H., Lee, L. Y., & Chang, M. (2007). The influences of personality and motivation on exercise participation and quality of life. *Social Behavior and Personality, 35*(9), 1189–1209.

Hybel, K. (2008). *Det er en parallel til Nazityskland [It's analogous to Nazi-Germany]*. Copenhagen: Politiken.
Interior and Health Ministry. (2007). *The Danish Health Sector in Figures*. Copenhagen: Interior and Health Ministry.
Jackson, R. J. (2003). The impact of the built environment on health: an emerging field. *American Journal of Public Health, 93*(9), 1382–1384.
James, P. T. (2004). Obesity: the worldwide epidemic. *Clinics in Dermatology, 22*(4), 276–280.
Kaplan, R., Kaplan, S., & Ryan, R. L. (1998). *With people in mind: design and management of everyday nature*. Washington, D.C.: Island Press.
Kardes, F.R., Cronley, M.L., Cline, T.W. (2011). *Consumer Behavior: Science and Practice*. South-Western, Cengage Learning, p. 480
Katzmarzyk, P. T., Ross, R., Church, T. S., Blair, S. N., & Janssen, I. (2005). Metabolic syndrome, obesity, and mortality—Impact of cardiorespiratory fitness. *Diabetes Care, 28*(2), 391–397.
Kawachi, I., & Berkman, L. F. (2003). *Neighborhoods and health*. New York: Oxford University Press.
Kissebah, A. H., Freedman, D. S., & Peiris, A. N. (1989). Health risks of obesity. *The Medical Clinics of North America, 73*(1), 111–138.
Kosti, R. I., & Panagiotako, D. B. (2006). The epidemic of obesity in children and adolescents in the world. *Central European Journal of Public Health, 14*(4), 151–159.
Kremers, S. P., de Bruijn, G. J., Visscher, T. L., van Mechelen, W., de Vries, N. K., & Brug, J. (2006). Environmental influences on energy balance-related behaviors: a dual-process view. *International Journal of Behavioral Nutrition and Physical Activity, 3*, 9.
Mackenbach, J. P. (2007). Sanitation: pragmatism works. *BMJ, 334*(suppl 1), s17.
Mandagmorgen (2008). Fremtidens Forebyggelse—ifølge danskerne. Copenhagen
Moskowitz, G. B., Skurnik, I., & Galinsky, A. (1999). The history of dual process notions. The future of preconscious control. In S. Chaiken & Y. Trope (Eds.), *Dual process models in social psychology* (pp. 12–36). New York: Guilford.
Nguyen, N. T., Nguyen, X. M. T., Wooridge, J. B., Slone, J. A., & Lane, J. S. (2010). Association of obesity with risk of coronary heart disease: Findings from the National Health and Nutrition Examination Survey, 1999–2006. *Surgery for Obesity and Related Diseases, 6*(5), 465–469.
Ogden, C. L., Carroll, M. D., Curtin, L. R., McDowell, M. A., Tabak, C. J., & Flegal, K. M. (2006). Prevalence of overweight and obesity in the United States, 1999–2004. *Journal of the American Medical Association, 295*(13), 1549–1555.
Oldridge, N. B. (2008). Economic burden of physical inactivity: healthcare costs associated with cardiovascular disease. *European Journal of Cardiovascular Prevention and Rehabilitation, 15*(2), 130–139.
Orsini, N., Bellocco, R., Bottai, M., Hagstromer, M., Sjostro, M., & Pagano, M. (2008). Profile of physical activity behaviors among Swedish women aged 56–75 years. *Scandinavian Journal of Medicine & Science in Sports, 18*(1), 95–101.
Pedersen, B. K. (2003). Rather fat and fit than thin and boring. *Ugeskrift for Laeger, 165*(51), 4947–4950.
Pedersen, B. K. (2006). Fitness, physical activity and death from all causes. *Ugeskrift for Laeger, 168*(2), 137–144.
Philip, W. J., Jackson-Leach, R., & Rigby, N. (2010). An international perspective on obesity and obesogenic environments. In T. G. T. Amelia, A. Lake, & S. Alvanides (Eds.), *Obesogenic environments: complexities perceptions and objective measures* (pp. 1–9). Oxford: Wiley.
Poortinga, W. (2007). The prevalence and clustering of four major lifestyle risk factors in an English adult population. *Preventive Medicine, 44*(2), 124–128.
Porter, R. (1997). *The greatest benefit to mankind: A medical history of humanity from Antiquity to the present*. London: Fontana.
Prentice, A. M. (2006). The emerging epidemic of obesity in developing countries. *International Journal of Epidemiology, 35*(1), 93–99.
Rhodes, R. E., & Smith, N. E. I. (2006). Personality correlates of physical activity: a review and meta-analysis. *British Journal of Sports Medicine, 40*(12), 958–965.

Roger, V. L., Go, A. S., Lloyd-Jones, D. M., Adams, R. J., Berry, J. D., & Brown, T. M. (2011). Heart disease and stroke statistics-2011 update a report from the American Heart Association. *Circulation, 123*(4), E18–E209.
Room, R., Babor, T., & Rehm, J. (2005). Alcohol and public health. *The Lancet, 365*(9458), 519–30.
Salli, J. F., Owen, N., & Fisher, E. B. (2008). Ecological models of health behavior. In K. Glanz, B. K. Rimer, & K. Viswanath (Eds.), *Health behavior and health education: Theory, research, and practice*. San Francisco, CA: Jossey-Bass. xxxiii, 552.
Sallis, J. F., Cervero, R. B., Ascher, W., Henderson, K. A., Kraft, M. K., & Kerr, J. (2006). An ecological approach to creating active living communities. *Annual Review of Public Health, 27*, 297–322.
Sallis, J. F., & Owen, N. (1999). *Physical activity and behavioral medicine*. Thousand Oaks, CA: Sage.
Schuit, A. J., van Loon, A. J., Tijhuis, M., & Ocke, M. C. (2002). Clustering of lifestyle risk factors in a general adult population. *Preventive Medicine, 35*(3), 219–224.
Seidell, J. C. (1995). Obesity in Europe: scaling an epidemic. *International Journal of Obesity and Related Metabolic Disorders, 3*(19), 1–4.
Shibuya, K., Ciecierski, C., Guindon, E., Bettcher, D. W., Evans, D. B., & Murray, C. J. (2003). WHO framework convention on tobacco control: development of an evidence based global public health treaty. *BMJ, 327*(7407), 154–157.
Stubbs, C. O., & Lee, A. J. (2004). The obesity epidemic: both energy intake and physical activity contribute. *The Medical Journal of Australia, 181*(9), 489–491.
Thaler, R. H., & Sunstein, C. R. (2009). *Nudge: improving decisions about health, wealth, and happiness*. New York: Penguin.
Troelsen, J., Roessler, K., Nielsen, G., & Toftager, M. (2008). *De bolignære områders betydning for sundhed: hvordan indvirker bolignære områder på sundheden—og hvordan kan udformningen gøres bedre. Institut for Idræt og Biomekanik*. Odense: [Odense], Syddansk Universitet.
Tucker, J. M., Welk, G. J., & Beyler, N. K. (2011). Physical activity in US adults: compliance with the physical activity guidelines for Americans. *American Journal of Preventive Medicine, 40*(4), 454–461.
TV2News (2008). Gesundheit macht frei—Battle against smoking cessation act. Retrieved 22 December, 2011, from http://nyhederne-dyn.tv2.dk/article.php/id-14473435:kim-larsen-til-kamp-mod-rygeloven.html?infomedia.
Walker, R. E., Keane, C. R., & Burke, J. G. (2010). Disparities and access to healthy food in the United States: A review of food deserts literature. *Health & Place, 16*(5), 876–884.
WHO. (2000). Obesity: preventing and managing the global epidemic. Report of a WHO consultation. *World Health Organization Technical Report Series, 894*, 1–253.
WHO (2008). Prevention and control of noncommunicable diseases: implementation of the global strategy. *Sixty first World Health Assembly*
WHO (2010). Global recommendations on physical activity for health. *WHO Library Cataloguing-in-Publication Data*
WHO (2010). *Global status report on noncommunicable diseases 2010*:1–8
Wier, M. (2008). *Liberty to choose?* Altinget

Chapter 14
Rethinking Exposure in Area Studies on Social Inequities in Smoking in Youth and Young Adults

Martine Shareck and Katherine L. Frohlich

Introduction

Smoking prevalence has decreased considerably since the 1980s in many developed countries including a number of European ones such as England (NHS Information Centre 2011), Germany, Italy, Spain and Scandinavia (Giskes et al. 2005). In England, for example, in 2009, 21 % of people aged 16 years or more smoked compared to 39 % in 1980 (NHS Information Centre 2011). This is encouraging news from a public health standpoint since tobacco smoking is the principal risk factor for cancer, cardiovascular diseases and tuberculosis which together are responsible for 70 % of all deaths that occur in adults over 30 years old worldwide (Jha 2009). From a health promotion and equity-focused perspective, however, this overall population decline in smoking comes accompanied by a darker reality: the decline in smoking has not been equitably distributed across socio-demographic groups and geographic areas within countries and cities (Giskes et al. 2005; Smith et al. 2009; Hiscock et al. 2011; Hotchkiss et al. 2011; NHS Information Centre 2011).

In fact, in countries with a long-standing smoking epidemic, youth and young adults (defined as people less than 18 years old and those between 18 and 25 years old, respectively) consistently register the highest smoking prevalence of all age groups (Backinger et al. 2003; NHS Information Centre 2011). For example, in 2009, 28 % of young adults in England smoked compared to 21 % of the overall population (NHS Information Centre 2011). Smoking is also increasingly associated with lower socio-economic status, whether measured as educational attainment, occupation or income (Barbeau et al. 2004; Federico et al. 2007; Gilman et al. 2008; Smith et al. 2009; Norwegian Institute of Public Health 2010; Hiscock et al. 2011;

M. Shareck (✉) • K.L. Frohlich
Département de médecine sociale et préventive, Université de Montréal (IRSPUM), C.P. 6128, succ. Centre-ville, Montréal, QC H3C 3J7, Canada
e-mail: martine.shareck@umontreal.ca; katherine.frohlich@umontreal.ca

C. Stock and A. Ellaway (eds.), *Neighbourhood Structure and Health Promotion*,
DOI 10.1007/978-1-4614-6672-7_14,

NHS Information Centre 2011). As well, there exist geographic differences in smoking prevalence whereby smoking tends to be concentrated in more socially and materially deprived areas (Giskes et al. 2006; Hiscock et al. 2011; NHS Information Centre 2011; The Scottish Government 2011). These differences in smoking prevalence across age and socio-economic groups, as well as geographic areas, can be referred to as social inequities in smoking: systematic differences in smoking between groups that occupy unequal positions in the social hierarchy based on their wealth, power and/or prestige (Braveman 2006). Since these inequities are socially produced, they are deemed to be modifiable and should be reduced (Graham 2004; Braveman 2006).

Reducing social inequities in smoking is crucial for at least two reasons. First, being socially produced and remediable, social inequities in smoking are simply unfair and should be addressed as a matter of social justice (Organisation mondiale de la santé 2008). Second, social inequities in smoking have important public health implications. The concentration of smoking among youth and young adults is particularly critical since early smoking initiation is associated with less success in quitting and thus a longer smoking duration (Breslau and Peterson 1996; Pierce and Gilpin 1996). Inequities in smoking across socio-economic groups also contribute significantly to the burden of smoking-related health problems. Individuals from lower socio-economic groups or more disadvantaged areas tend to start smoking at a younger age compared to their less deprived counterparts; they smoke more cigarettes per day, inhale more nicotine, smoke for more years and have more difficulty quitting the habit (Schaap and Kunst 2009; Hiscock et al. 2011). Socially deprived smokers thus suffer from significantly more smoking-related diseases and subsequent mortality than their less deprived counterparts (Choiniere et al. 2000; Barbeau et al. 2004). In fact, smoking is responsible for roughly 20–50 % of the difference in mortality between lower and higher social classes (Marmot 2006).

Importantly, these social determinants of smoking (age, socio-economic status and geographic area) often interact. Some individuals might therefore suffer from the double or triple burden of being young, of a low socio-economic status and living in a disadvantaged area. For example, social gradients across educational level, income, occupation and employment status have been observed in studies limited to young adults (Harman et al. 2006; Lawrence et al. 2007; Solberg et al. 2007). Similarly, being young and living in a poor area have been associated with a higher likelihood of smoking than being a young resident of a less deprived area (Matheson et al. 2011). In fact, it has been stated in a 2010 World Health Organization report that "there are two stages of life where inequities in vulnerability and exposure to tobacco use are most evident: during adolescence, with those from lower socioeconomic backgrounds most at risk of taking up tobacco; and during adulthood, especially young adulthood, where tobacco use cessation is more difficult for those from disadvantaged backgrounds" (Blas et al. 2010, p. 200). This entails that socially deprived youth and young adults are at particularly high risk of smoking and of suffering from its adverse consequences. The issue of social inequities in smoking among youth and young adults should therefore be addressed sooner rather than later.

Fortunately, youth and young adulthood are windows of opportunity during which health promotion efforts to prevent smoking initiation and continuation, as well as to promote cessation, could be particularly fruitful (Backinger et al. 2003). Indeed, although smoking initiation usually occurs during youth, young adulthood is also a key period during which non-smokers may be initiating smoking. In fact, although a considerable proportion of adult smokers will have started smoking in adolescence, estimates suggest that up to 38 % of smokers aged 18–25 years old will have started smoking after the age of 18, once they entered college, university or the workforce (Lantz 2003; Freedman et al. 2012). As well, during young adulthood, experimental smokers may transition to become established smokers or to quit smoking, and non-dependent smokers may go on to develop a strong nicotine addiction (Adlaf et al. 2003; Backinger et al. 2003). Socio-economic inequities have been documented for all these different transition phases (Blas et al. 2010). Youth and young adulthood therefore encompass a range of smoking milestones to which health promotion efforts could be targeted to reduce social inequities in smoking. To better tailor our health promotion interventions to youth and young adults, however, we must first deepen our understanding of what influences social inequities in smoking in these age groups and how to reduce them. Part of the answer could lie in characteristics of areas or "neighbourhoods".[1]

Research on area effects on inequities in health and health behaviours such as smoking has traditionally focused on the influence of one's neighbourhood of residence (Leal and Chaix 2011). However, during adolescence and young adulthood, social and physical bonds to one's residential area have been said to decrease because of increased mobility, independence and the development of relationships outside the residential neighbourhood (Rainham et al. 2010). In fact, during older youth and young adulthood, a transition occurs in which individuals are entering new places of study (e.g. going from college to university) or workplaces, as well as places of leisure and social activities (Lantz 2003). Youth and young adults thus experience various non-residential life environments which might also influence their smoking, such as their school or work areas. Before designing area-level interventions to reduce social inequities in smoking in youth and young adults, we must therefore identify which areas to study and intervene upon. This may require that we move beyond the residential neighbourhood and include other areas encompassing relevant life environments. A review of the literature can help us identify relevant areas and area-level characteristics to study.

In this chapter, we review the literature on area effects and social inequities in smoking in youth and young adults. We highlight two main limitations of contemporary research and interventions: (1) the narrow focus on single, mainly residential areas, rather than multiple life environments and (2) the lack of research

[1] A detailed discussion of the many ways "neighbourhoods" have been defined throughout history and in different fields of research is beyond the scope of this chapter. Here, we use the terms neighbourhood and area interchangeably to refer to a local, spatially defined area in which health-relevant attributes are measured. The size and shape of this area can vary between studies and so do the life environments (residential, school, etc.) encompassed by the area. Neighbourhood or area-level features and resources are those measured within a given area.

on the differential effect of area-level interventions on smoking across social groups. We conclude by introducing a health promotion perspective which could contribute to furthering the study of area-level influences on social inequities in smoking in youth and young adults. This perspective involves two key principles integrated in an ongoing research project which will be presented for illustrative purposes. As a subcomponent of the Interdisciplinary Study on Inequalities in Smoking (ISIS), the ISIS-Activity Space project explores the influence of area-level exposures measured within multiple life environments, which together form the “activity space”, on social inequities in smoking in a sample of young adults residing in areas of varied deprivation levels in Montreal, Canada.

Why Study Area Characteristics and Social Inequities in Smoking in Youth and Young Adults?

In 1986, the Ottawa Charter for health promotion included “the creation of healthy and supportive environments” as one of its action means (Organisation mondiale de la santé 1986). The focus on environments was spawned by a desire to move beyond an individual-based approach to health and to influence health and health behaviours through action on the places where people live, work and play and on the people found within these settings (Poland et al. 2009). Area, or neighbourhood, and health studies partly stem from this setting’s approach to health promotion. The study of area effects represents a hopeful avenue for research and action that could contribute to reducing social inequities in smoking in youth and young adults. Indeed, smoking is “a social activity rooted in place” (Poland et al. 2006) and is influenced not only by micro-level factors (individual, family and peer) but also by meso-level (school, workplace, neighbourhood) and macro-level factors (policy, media) (Poland et al. 2006), which are all potential research and intervention targets. A person’s decision to smoke is thus made within this broader social and environmental context (Pokorny et al. 2003). As well, many area-level structural features and resources that have been found to influence social inequities in smoking in youth and young adults, such as the density of tobacco retailers or of cigarette advertisement (which often directly targets youth and young adults (Backinger et al. 2003), especially those of lower socio-economic status (Blas et al. 2010; Hiscock et al. 2011), could be modified to reflect healthier conditions and ultimately contribute to reducing social inequities in smoking (Feighery et al. 2008; Cohen and Anglin 2009). Intervening to modify the environment, rather than the individual, is also thought to lead to more sustainable behaviour changes and health improvements than trying to change individuals directly through standard preventive measures such as health education (Brownson et al. 2006). Finally, in response to some individual-level interventions having failed to reduce smoking in low socio-economic groups (Niederdeppe et al. 2008), area-level interventions have been suggested as potentially more useful in reaching these social groups and thus contributing to reducing social inequities in smoking (Stafford et al. 2008).

Area Effects on Social Inequities in Youth and Young Adults: Current Evidence

The literature concerning area effects on social inequities in smoking is rich in studies on smoking initiation and continuation in youth younger than 18 years of age and on smoking prevalence and cessation in adults (Backinger et al. 2003). Evidence regarding young adults between 18 and 25 years old is more scarce since they tend to be studied in combination with older adults rather than being considered of interest *per se*. In fact, young adults' smoking behaviours are often assumed to be similar to that of older adults, although it has been suggested that young adults might in fact resemble youth in their attitudes towards cessation and their responses to common behavioural interventions (Lantz 2003). Because of similarities between youth and young adults, studies of area effects on social inequities in youth smoking can help us shed light on some aspects of smoking among young adults.

A wide array of area-level exposures have been investigated for their correlation with social inequities in smoking in youth which could also be relevant to young adults. These include compositional characteristics based on the aggregate socio-demographic characteristics of residents of an area (Ennett et al. 1997; Allison et al. 1999; Ecob and Macintyre 2000; Frohlich et al. 2002; Reardon et al. 2002; Pokorny et al. 2003; Wardle et al. 2003; Milton et al. 2004; Chuang et al. 2005; Nowlin and Colder 2007; Kaestle and Wiles 2010; Matheson et al. 2011), sociocultural attributes such as smoking-related norms and measures of safety (Dowdell 2002; Gibbons et al. 2004; Lambert et al. 2004; Fagan et al. 2007; Musick et al. 2008) and more structural features including resource availability and aspects of the physical environment such as tobacco advertising (Frohlich et al. 2002; Pokorny et al. 2003; Dent and Biglan 2004; Novak et al. 2006; Leatherdale and Strath 2007; Lovato et al. 2007, 2010; Henriksen et al. 2008; McCarthy et al. 2009). Of these, area deprivation, which is commonly operationalised as an aggregate measure of residents' income, educational level, employment status or other socio-demographic characteristics, has been the most extensively studied in relation to smoking in less than 18-year-olds (Ennett et al. 1997; Allison et al. 1999; Ecob and Macintyre 2000; Frohlich et al. 2002; Reardon et al. 2002; Pokorny et al. 2003; Wardle et al. 2003; Milton et al. 2004; Chuang et al. 2005; Nowlin and Colder 2007; Kaestle and Wiles 2010; Matheson et al. 2011). Evidence however remains equivocal, with some studies having found that youth living in more deprived neighbourhoods were more likely to have ever tried smoking (Wardle et al. 2003) or to be smokers (Milton et al. 2004; Matheson et al. 2011) and other studies having not found a significant association between neighbourhood deprivation and smoking initiation (Reardon et al. 2002; Pokorny et al. 2003; Nowlin and Colder 2007) or smoking status (Ennett et al. 1997; Allison et al. 1999; Ecob and Macintyre 2000; Frohlich et al. 2002; Pokorny et al. 2003; Nowlin and Colder 2007). For example, Matheson et al. (2011) found that youth aged 12 to 18 years old who lived in deprived neighbourhoods were 22 % more likely to smoke than youth living in less deprived areas, while in their study, Ecob and Macintyre (2000) did not find an association between residential area deprivation and current smoking in a cohort of 15-year-old individuals. Contrary to what would be expected, a study by Chuang et al. (2005) found that low residential neighbourhood socio-economic status was associated with lower youth smoking.

In most of these studies, deprivation was measured within the residential area which was usually defined as the administrative unit (census tract, block group, ward or post code area) in which participants' home was located (Ennett et al. 1997; Allison et al. 1999; Ecob and Macintyre 2000; Frohlich et al. 2002; Reardon et al. 2002; Wardle et al. 2003; Milton et al. 2004; Chuang et al. 2005; Nowlin and Colder 2007; Matheson et al. 2011). In three of them, the residential neighbourhood was said to approximately match the school area; thus, these two life environments were considered as being the same (Ennett et al. 1997; Frohlich et al. 2002; Pokorny et al. 2003). Only one study has looked at deprivation within the school area which did not necessarily correspond to youth's residential area (Kaestle and Wiles 2010). In this study, Kaestle and Wiles (2010) found that smoking rates were higher among youth attending schools located in areas of lower socio-economic level measured using a composite index of poverty, unemployment and educational level compared to high socio-economic level areas.

More structural area-level characteristics have also been studied in relation to social inequities in youth smoking. These could be relevant to young adults as well and include the availability of tobacco products as well as their price and the advertisement for them. Smoking initiation or prevalence has been found to be highest in youth who resided (Pokorny et al. 2003; Novak et al. 2006) or attended school (Leatherdale and Strath 2007; Henriksen et al. 2008; McCarthy et al. 2009) in areas with the highest density of tobacco retailers. A high density of retail advertising (Henriksen et al. 2008; Lovato et al. 2007, 2010), lower cigarette prices (Lovato et al. 2010) and a higher availability of tobacco retailers willing to sell to minors (Pokorny et al. 2003; Dent and Biglan 2004) in the residential neighbourhood have also been found to be associated with higher youth smoking prevalence. It should be noted that area-level sales to minors is not as relevant for smoking among young adults who are of legal age to purchase cigarettes. Finally, in a study by Frohlich et al. (2002), youth smoking was lower in areas where a high proportion of commercial establishments discouraged smoking on their premises. In cases where this was specified, tobacco retailer density, advertising, sales to minors and low cigarette prices were more prevalent in socio-economically deprived neighbourhoods (Novak et al. 2006; Feighery et al. 2008; Henriksen et al. 2008), which could explain part of the association between area deprivation and smoking.

The research reported so far has focused on social inequities in youth smoking. Results can guide us towards the types of areas (residential and/or school) as well as the area-level exposures to study which could also influence smoking in young adults. However, studying young adults for their own sake is still warranted given the heterogeneity in their smoking behaviours as well as in the places where they might be found. For example, several youth studies have focused on the school area, but this life environment might not be relevant for older youth and young adults engaged in the workforce or those who are no longer attending school. We found only two studies which, although focusing on youth, also included young adults in their samples (Lee and Cubbin 2002; Novak et al. 2006). However, only one of these specifically reported results for young adults (Novak et al. 2006). In their study, Lee and Cubbin (2002) did not find that socio-economic status and social disorganisation were associated with a higher likelihood of smoking among 12- to 21-year-old individuals. Conversely, Novak et al. (2006) found that young people between 19 and 23 years old (who could legally buy cigarettes) who resided in neighbourhoods with a high density of tobacco retailers were approximately 20 % more likely to have smoked in the past month than those residing in neighbourhoods with a lower density of tobacco-selling outlets. Both these studies examined the residential neighbourhood exclusively, without considering the potential relevance of taking exposure to other life environments into account, as had been done in some studies on youth.

Area-Level Interventions to Address Social Inequities in Smoking in Youth and Young Adults: Current Evidence

Traditionally tobacco control interventions aiming to reduce smoking among youth and young adults have consistently involved educational programmes directly targeting individuals (Biglan and Hinds 2009; Carson et al. 2011). These interventions which aim to raise awareness on the risks of smoking have mostly been implemented in schools, viewed as containers: closely bounded settings within which a captive population of students could be found and acted upon (Carson et al. 2011). School-based interventions typically treat the school as being isolated from the wider area or community of which it is part. Other interventions commonly relied upon have taken the form of educational messages disseminated through the media in community settings. These again directly target individuals, encouraging them to change their smoking behaviours for healthier ones (Carson et al. 2011). However, a review of the effects of educational and media campaigns on social inequities in smoking has suggested that these, even when dispensed within bounded settings such as a school or a geographically defined area such as a community, were not as effective in reaching and triggering behaviour changes in lower socio-economic status groups compared to their more favoured counterparts (Niederdeppe et al. 2008). In some cases, such interventions even risked exacerbating social inequities in smoking rather than reducing them (Niederdeppe et al. 2008). This has been suggested to be due, partly, to deprived groups having fewer capacities for assimilating educational messages and subsequently taking action to change their behaviours, compared to less deprived groups (Frohlich and Potvin 2008). An individual's decision to smoke or not is actually made within a larger social context involving personal as well as structural (social, physical and political) factors which interact. Individuals are not independent from these structural resources which may promote or hamper their smoking (Poland et al. 2006). Social inequities in smoking thus arise from the joint inequities in individual capacity and in exposure to structural resources (Abel and Frohlich 2012). Interventions that aim to change not only the individuals but also the structure of areas they are found in, thereby making the healthiest choice (i.e. of not smoking) the easiest choice, may therefore be quite promising (Carson et al. 2011; Poland et al. 2006).

Despite this, interventions to change the neighbourhood structure remain rare. Most interventions have taken the form of community-based interventions targeting all age groups rather than youth and young adults specifically. In a recent Cochrane review, 25 controlled trial studies of multiple-component community interventions to reduce youth smoking were analysed, some of which could be classified as area-level interventions. Of these trials, only one concerned local smoking bans in public places and six aimed to reduce commercial tobacco sales to minors within the community, highlighting the scarcity of area interventions focused on youth. The other studies reviewed, although implemented in community settings, all primarily involved educational interventions and media campaigns which directly targeted individuals (Carson et al. 2011).

Other review articles have synthesised results from interventional and observational studies investigating the effect of smoking bans, reducing sales to minors or increasing cigarette prices on smoking in youth (Greaves et al. 2006; Forster et al. 2007; Bader et al. 2011), in young adults (Bader et al. 2011) or in low-income adults (Greaves et al. 2006; Main et al. 2008; Thomas et al. 2008; Bader et al. 2011). These are examples of policies and interventions applied to populations or areas and which aim to make the social, physical or legislative environment less conducive to smoking (Main et al. 2008). Thus, even when they are not explicitly targeted at specific areas, their implementation and effects can be felt on the ground, in geographically defined areas, which may correspond to people's residential neighbourhood or not. Review studies suggested that implementing measures to reduce sales to minors was associated with reduced youth smoking (Greaves et al. 2006; Forster et al. 2007), while increasing cigarette prices reduced smoking in youth and young adults (Forster et al. 2007; Greaves et al. 2006; Bader et al. 2011). In two reviews, banning smoking in the community was also found to be associated with less smoking initiation, less transitioning from experimental to regular smoking and more quitting among youth (Forster et al. 2007) and young adults (Greaves et al. 2006). The unintended consequences of location bans, such as the social stigma suffered by smokers and increased visibility of smoking outdoors, have however been highlighted and should not be overlooked in future intervention development (Greaves et al. 2006). Of particular interest are three of these reviews which have explicitly applied an "equity lens" to tobacco control interventions (Greaves et al. 2006; Main et al. 2008; Thomas et al. 2008) in an attempt to unveil the differential effect of tobacco control interventions across social groups. Unfortunately, the evidence base was generally deemed too limited to draw conclusions relative to a differential effect of smoking bans in public places, increasing tobacco prices and restricting youth access to tobacco products on smoking among young people or adults of various socio-economic groups (Main et al. 2008; Thomas et al. 2008). The limited data available for comparing intervention effects across different social groups and geographic areas compounds the fact that very few area-level interventions were found that had specifically aimed to address smoking among young people, especially young adults. As well, in cases where interventions had been duly evaluated, it was not specified whether effects had been observed among residents of the areas receiving the intervention or among the general population at large.

An alternative type of intervention implemented at the area level and used to address social inequities in smoking, directly or not, is neighbourhood renewal programmes such as the New Deal for Communities (Stafford et al. 2008) or Health Action Zones in the United Kingdom (Adams et al. 2000). Renewal programmes have explicitly tried to "narrow the gap between the most deprived neighbourhoods and the rest of the country" by targeting efforts to improve the conditions in highly deprived areas (Stafford et al. 2008). Examples of interventions implemented in the context of renewal programmes include the provision of employment and educational opportunities and environmental and road safety improvements or the implementation of smoking cessation services (Woods et al. 2003; Stafford et al. 2008; Blackman et al. 2001). The overarching aim of renewal programmes is to improve the social conditions at the root of social inequities in health and health behaviours. In theory, renewal programmes thus hold great promise in reducing social inequities in smoking. However, practical evidence would suggest otherwise. For example, an evaluation study of the New Deal for Communities Programme has found that 2 years after the programme had been implemented, there was an increase in inequities in smoking within the targeted areas. This was suggested to be due to the fact that the more educated people living in target areas benefited more from smoking cessation services and were thus more likely to have stopped smoking than the less educated residents (Stafford et al. 2008).

The Health Action Zones programme attempted to prevent this from happening by locating smoking cessation services in public buildings already used by other community-based organisations in order to reach highly deprived smokers more effectively. Nonetheless, it has been suggested that smoking cessation services implemented as part of Health Action Zones failed to meet the needs of disadvantaged groups and ultimately to reduce social inequities in smoking (Woods et al. 2003). In fact, although they targeted geographic areas characterised by high deprivation levels, Health Action Zones, similarly to what had been done in the New Deal for Communities Programme, attempted to reduce social inequities in smoking through the implementation of smoking cessation services. Unfortunately, these services, in lieu of making the neighbourhood structure more health promoting itself, still influenced smoking through the intermediary of the individuals who would access them. This could partly explain the limited impact these large neighbourhood renewal programmes had in decreasing social inequities in smoking. Indeed, they might have ignored social contextual factors of smoking such as structural barriers for lower socio-economic groups to access and benefit from smoking cessation services (Woods et al. 2003).

Alternatively, other programmes such as the Neighbourhood Renewal Area Programme have involved the improvement of aspects of the physical environment such as housing, roads and sidewalks in a deprived neighbourhood (Blackman et al. 2001). Results from its evaluation suggested that 5 years after the programme was implemented, smoking prevalence among residents had fallen by more than half to reach 28 %. Smokers also reported smoking fewer cigarettes per day. It was hypothesised that the programme had had this effect through a reduction in the stress experienced by residents. Unfortunately, the evaluation study could not reveal if smoking had decreased equally among all socio-economic groups within the targeted area nor if the observed success in reducing smoking prevalence was attributable to the intervention itself since there was no comparison neighbourhood (i.e. a comparable area which had not received the intervention) (Blackman et al. 2001).

Limitations of Current Etiologic Research and Interventions

The Residential and Single Environment Traps

A first limitation of current research and interventions on social inequities in smoking in youth and young adults concerns the focus on single, mainly residential areas. In the field of area and health research, this has been termed the "residential trap" (Chaix et al. 2009). Most etiologic studies of youth smoking have indeed focused on the residential neighbourhood (Ennett et al. 1997; Allison et al. 1999; Ecob and Macintyre 2000; Frohlich et al. 2002; Reardon et al. 2002; Pokorny et al. 2003; Wardle et al. 2003; Dent and Biglan 2004; Milton et al. 2004; Chuang et al. 2005; Novak et al. 2006; Henriksen et al. 2008; Lovato et al. 2010; Matheson et al. 2011), which in a few cases also corresponded to the school area (Ennett et al. 1997; Frohlich et al. 2002; Pokorny et al. 2003). The two studies which did include young adults in their samples investigated structural features of the residential neighbourhood exclusively (Lee and Cubbin 2002; Novak et al. 2006). Area-level interventions such as neighbourhood renewal programmes have also attempted to reduce social inequities in smoking by providing services to residents of deprived areas (Adams et al. 2000; Stafford et al. 2008). Interventions were implicitly aimed at residents of the targeted areas, although these areas may have corresponded to the residential neighbourhood for some people and to the education or work area for others. Similarly, community-based interventions have typically defined a "community" as the area in which the target population resided (Woods et al. 2003; Stafford et al. 2008; Blackman et al. 2001; Carson et al. 2011). Although community-based interventions could theoretically entail acting upon an area encompassing several of residents' life environments (residential, school, workplace, etc.), this has not been explicitly explored.

Underlying this focus on the residential area is the assumption, albeit implicit, that youth and young adults are most exposed to, and influenced by, their residential area. This life environment is thus considered as being the most salient for understanding and acting upon areas to influence social inequities in smoking in these age groups, regardless of how much time they spend in their residential neighbourhood. However, this residential focus overlooks the fact that individuals are mobile and move between various life environments, which might not be included in their residential area or “community”. During youth and young adulthood, a transition occurs in which individuals are entering new places of study (e.g. going from college to university) or workplaces, as well as places of leisure and social activities (Lantz 2003). Youth and young adults may therefore be found in a diverse range of non-residential areas which may be located large distances from their residential neighbourhood (Matthews 2011). Mobility across space and distance travelled daily have in fact been shown to peak between 20 and 35 years old (Morency et al. 2011). This mobility entails that young people, and young adults in particular, may not be highly nor solely exposed to their residential neighbourhood (Morency et al. 2011; Schönfelder and Axhausen 2003). Mobility and daily distance travelled also vary with income and employment status. For example, low-income and part-time employed individuals (all age groups combined) have been shown to travel shorter distances, on a daily basis, than their less deprived or fully employed counterparts (Morency et al. 2011). Young people of varied socio-economic groups may thus be differentially exposed to their residential area. Importantly, according to work in time geography, the strongest determinants of area-level exposure are the places where individuals undertake their daily activities as well as how much time they spend there (Kwan 2009). Logically, if individuals spend time at school or work, exposure to smoking-relevant characteristics of their residential area is reduced. Therefore, the residential area may in these cases influence smoking less than other life environments would. Similarly, interventions implemented in people’s residential neighbourhood may have less of an effect on those who are not exclusively or extensively exposed to this area.

Some researchers have attempted to address this limited focus on the residential neighbourhood, although implicitly, by studying youth smoking in relation to area deprivation measured within the school district (Kaestle and Wiles 2010) or the density of tobacco retailers in a circular area of a given radius surrounding a school (Leatherdale and Strath 2007; Henriksen et al. 2008; McCarthy et al. 2009). This is interesting since it recognises that the school context is, for those youth who attend school, their primary social context outside of the home (Kim and McCarthy 2006). However, the focus still remained on a single environment even though during youth and young adulthood, the areas young people are exposed to in their daily activities become diversified: some individuals may be attending establishments of higher education and/or become engaged in paid work, while others may be out of school or unemployed, albeit momentarily (Backinger et al. 2003). This entails that young people may not be exposed to resources or interventions in what would be their school area (Lantz 2003). This lack of evidence regarding social inequities in smoking among youth and young adults not attending school or university has previously been highlighted as a major limitation of contemporary research on social inequities in smoking (Lantz 2003). Indeed, youth and young adults who are attending school may differ considerably in terms of their socio-economic characteristics and smoking behaviours from those who are enrolled in paid work or not employed at all (Backinger et al. 2003; Hiscock et al. 2011). For example, youth who leave school early are more likely to be (1) smokers and (2) heavy smokers compared to those enrolled in college (Lantz 2003). Focusing on the school area exclusively as a way to better understand area-level influences on social inequities in smoking among this age group may therefore fall short because it excludes subgroups of individuals not enrolled in education.

Measuring exposure to smoking-relevant characteristics within the residential neighbourhood or school area exclusively may therefore lead to misclassification errors and an underestimation of area effects on social inequities in smoking. Unfortunately, few if any studies and interventions have explicitly acknowledged that different life environments such as the residential, school and work environments may together influence social inequities in smoking (Cook 2003). We also did not find any study that had investigated exposure to area-level features measured within non-residential areas of potential relevance to smoking among those youth and young adults not attending school. Focusing narrowly on the residential or school areas may thus overlook socio-economic groups not found within these settings. In addition to being a heterogeneous group in terms of the smoking milestones they have reached, youth and young adults of varied socio-economic levels may differ in terms of the areas they might be exposed to. Expanding our conceptualisation of "areas" in the study of area effects and smoking so that it includes the influence of life environments other than the residential or school areas may therefore be useful to further our understanding of social inequities in smoking in youth and young adults. To do so, viewing areas as systems composed of multiple and interconnected life environments rather than static entities limited to where people live warrants further study. This would help design etiologic studies and interventions which could be more effective in reaching a diversity of people found in various environments.

Handling Social Equity Inadequately

A second limitation of current research and interventions on areas and social inequities in smoking concerns the scarcity of evidence regarding the differential effect of area-level interventions across social groups and areas of varied deprivation levels. Our review has shown that the field of area-level interventions to prevent smoking and promote cessation among youth and young adults is still in its infancy. Most importantly, interventions have not always been designed, implemented and evaluated in a way that is attentive to equity across age and social groups. For example, interventions such as neighbourhood renewal programmes have typically targeted highly deprived neighbourhoods (Woods et al. 2003; Stafford et al. 2008; Blackman et al. 2001). This is of limited utility if the aim is to uncover the effect of an intervention on differences in smoking across social groups found in more and less deprived areas, since the only data available concern deprived areas. As well, although the inclusion of comparable areas of various deprivation levels with which to compare intervention effects would allow to attribute the observed effects, if there are any, to the intervention itself rather than to other, unspecified circumstances, this has rarely been done (Blackman et al. 2001). Even in cases where population-level policies such as smoking bans in the home, school, workplace and public places or restrictions in tobacco retail licencing have been implemented, implicitly covering a wide range of both individual- and area-level deprivation levels, few studies had provided data that would permit the assessment of their differential effect by social and age group. This has therefore limited the conclusions which could be drawn relative to their influence on social inequities in smoking (Ogilvie and Petticrew 2004; Greaves et al. 2006; Main et al. 2008; Thomas et al. 2008; Blas et al. 2010). Thoroughly thinking through the design, implementation and evaluation of area-level interventions so that they would further our understanding of area effects on social inequities in smoking among youth and young adults is therefore warranted.

A special note should also be made of the unintended consequences which area-level interventions can potentially have on social inequities in smoking. Banning smoking in the home, school or workplace (Greaves and Jategaonkar 2006) or increasing cigarette prices in retailers across a neighbourhood might reduce smoking in some individuals and groups. However, it has been suggested that these interventions might also leave out other smokers who might subsequently suffer adverse consequences (Greaves et al. 2006). For example, cases have been reported where smokers suffered from social stigmatisation following bans on the grounds of educational institutions (Greaves et al. 2006) or where they had to turn to alternative sources, such as social sources or contraband, to purchase their tobacco products, following access restrictions (Dent and Biglan 2004). The risk of such drawbacks occurring should thus be acknowledged and prevented when possible.

The Way Forward: Area Effects and Interventions and Social Inequities in Smoking Under a Health Promotion Lens

We have argued so far that current research on area effects on social inequities in smoking in youth and young adults is plagued by two limitations: (1) the somewhat narrow focus on the residential or school area solely, at the expense of other life environments and (2) the lack of data to uncover how area-level interventions differentially influence smoking across age and social groups. These limitations must be dealt with if social inequities in smoking are to be well understood and addressed in a way that respects basic health promotion tenets. Below, we present a health promotion perspective which can stimulate reflection and innovation in the field of area effects and social inequities in smoking, specifically, and in health more generally. This perspective also provides a means to address the limitations previously discussed. It involves two principles which we describe below.

First Principle: Health Is Produced in Everyday Life Environments

According to the 1986 Ottawa Charter for Health Promotion, "health is produced in everyday life, where people live, work and play" (Organisation mondiale de la santé 1986). This means that the neighbourhood people live in as well as the places where they undertake various daily activities may provide exposures to structural features influencing their health and health behaviours. This principle calls for a broader conceptualisation of “areas” than the one currently used in research on area effects on social inequities in smoking in youth and young adults.

This basic tenet of health promotion is supported by work in behavioural and space-time geography which has shown that most people are mobile and experience their residential neighbourhood as well as other non-residential environments, such as places of work, education or leisure (Schönfelder and Axhausen 2004). Although people may confer a strong sense of attachment to their place of residence, these other life environments may also provide exposures to smoking-influencing factors (Schönfelder and Axhausen 2003; Kwan 2009). One way to operationalise this combination of residential and non-residential areas relevant for social inequities in smoking is through the concept of “activity space”. A person’s activity space can be defined as “the subset of all locations with which an individual has direct contact as a result of his day-to-day activities” (Kamruzzaman et al. 2011, p. 2). It might thus include a person’s residential neighbourhood as well as her places of study, work, physical activity or leisure, among others. Studying individuals’ exposure to area-level features measured within the activity space has the advantage of taking into account the spatial configuration of exposure experienced by an individual. Activity spaces may also inform us as to the extent to which individuals are confined to their residential area and on their exposure to resources found in the non-residential life environments they experience. The publication of studies on the influence of structural exposures measured within the activity space on various health outcome and behaviours has recently increased (Inagami et al. 2007; Kestens et al. 2010; Vallee et al. 2010; Zenk et al. 2011), but we found no study that had examined social inequities in smoking specifically.

An ongoing research project, the ISIS-Activity Space project, is therefore applying this concept to the study of social inequities in smoking in young adults. The concept of activity space is particularly relevant to the study of this issue since, as it has been argued previously, smoking is a “practice rooted in place” (Poland et al. 2006) and young adults are a highly mobile group. As such, their exposure to smoking-relevant features, when measured within their residential neighbourhood, may not accurately represent their actual exposure. For example, a young adult residing in a deprived area characterised by a high density of tobacco retailers might attend school in an area with a lower density of this resource. This individual’s actual (average) exposure to tobacco retailers would thus be lower than his exposure measured within the residential area uniquely. Similarly, two young adults residing in the same neighbourhood may be exposed to different levels of smoking-related resources in the course of their daily routines. Given this evidence, measuring area-level characteristics within the activity space rather than within the residential area alone may provide more valid measures of exposures and limit exposure misclassification (Miller 2007). It is in this context that the ISIS-Activity Space project is attempting to answer several questions such as the following: how do smoking-related area-level exposures compare between the residential neighbourhood and other areas included in a person’s activity space? How do these resources relate to social inequities in smoking when measured within the residential as compared to the activity space areas? This kind of research is required in order to better understand if taking young adults' mobility through various life environments into account improves our understanding of what the relevant area(s) is/are for better understanding social inequities in smoking. This research can also shed light onto which life environments should be the targets of future interventions to reduce social inequities in smoking in youth and young adults.

Second Principle: An Explicit Focus on Equity

The second basic principle of the health promotion perspective put forth here concerns the requirement for an explicit focus on equity. In this chapter, inequities were understood as differences in smoking (in this case) across groups occupying unequal positions in the social hierarchy. Thus, in research and intervention work, if the aim is to uncover area-level influences on social inequities in smoking, studies must involve a sample of groups and areas of diverse socio-economic positions. They should ideally cover the full range between the very deprived and the very well off. The ISIS-Activity Space project has been developed to take this into account. Indeed, participants to the study have been sampled based on the social and material deprivation level (low, medium or high) of their residential area. This area has been operationalised as the dissemination area, the smallest administrative unit in Canada which encompasses between 400 and 700 individuals (Statistics Canada 2009). Without this socio-economic variability in areas, the social conditions and neighbourhood features patterned by deprivation level which are relevant to social inequities in smoking would be equally shared by all participants. This would hamper our ability to reveal their influence on smoking behaviours since, as basic epidemiology teaches us, there must be variation in an exposure if effects of this exposure are to be detected (Rothman and Greenland 1998). This explicit focus on equity as concerning a wide range of deprivation levels is also required to address the shortcomings on neighbourhood interventions which have been exclusively implemented in deprived areas of neighbourhoods or for which the effects have not been evaluated across social groups. Future evaluation of interventions should thus ensure that they produce the data required to estimate socially differentiated effects, either to show that an intervention has had the desired effect of reducing social inequities in smoking or to uncover unintended consequences such as an increase in inequities in smoking.

Conclusion

Reducing smoking prevalence in all age and social groups will require that our attention and efforts be invested in studying young people, especially young adults, and intervening upon them. We suggest that etiologic research and interventions at the area-level offer great promise in addressing inequities in smoking across socio-economic and age groups, as well as geographic areas. However, in order to do so more effectively and in an innovative way, researchers will need to adopt a lens explicitly informed by basic health promotion principles which entails expanding the conceptualisation of "areas" as more than single, mainly residential areas to include other life environments and explicitly focusing on uncovering the differential effect of interventions across socio-economic groups and geographic areas of varied deprivation levels.

References

Abel, T., & Frohlich, K. L. (2012). Capitals and capabilities: Linking structure and agency to reduce health inequalities. *Social Science & Medicine, 74*(2), 236–244. doi:10.1016/j.socscimed.2011.10.028.

Adams, C., Bauld, L., & Judge, K. (2000). *Smoking cessation services: Early experiences from health action zones*. Canterbury: PSSRU, University of Kent.

Adlaf, E. M., Gliksman, L., Demers, A., & Newton-Taylor, B. (2003). Cigarette use among Canadian undergraduates. *Canadian Journal of Public Health, 94*(1), 22–24.

Allison, K. W., Crawford, I., Leone, P. E., Trickett, E., Perez-Febles, A., Burton, L. M., et al. (1999). Adolescent substance use: Preliminary examinations of school and neighborhood context. *American Journal of Community Psychology, 27*(2), 111–141.

Backinger, C. L., Fagan, P., Matthews, E., & Grana, R. (2003). Adolescent and young adult tobacco prevention and cessation: Current status and future directions. *Tobacco Control, 12*(Suppl 4), iv46–iv53.

Bader, P., Boisclair, D., & Ferrence, R. (2011). Effects of tobacco taxation and pricing on smoking behavior in high risk populations: A knowledge synthesis. *International Journal of Environmental Research and Public Health, 11*, 4118–4139.

Barbeau, E. M., Krieger, N., & Soobader, M. J. (2004). Working class matters: Socioeconomic disadvantage, race/ethnicity, gender, and smoking in NHIS 2000. *American Journal of Public Health, 94*(2), 269–278.

Biglan, A., & Hinds, E. (2009). Evolving prosocial and sustainable neighborhoods and communities. *Annual Review of Clinical Psychology, 5*, 169–196.

Blackman, T., Harvey, J., Lawrence, M., & Simon, A. (2001). Neighbourhood renewal and health: Evidence from a local case study. *Health & Place, 7*(2), 93–103.

Blas, E., Kurup, A. S., & World Health Organization. (2010). *Equity, social determinants and public health programmes*. Geneva: World Health Organization.

Braveman, P. (2006). Health disparities and health equity: Concepts and measurement. *Annual Review of Public Health, 27*, 167–194.

Breslau, N., & Peterson, E. L. (1996). Smoking cessation in young adults: Age at initiation of cigarette smoking and other suspected influences. *American Journal of Public Health, 86*(2), 214–220.

Brownson, R. C., Haire-Joshu, D., & Luke, D. A. (2006). Shaping the context of health: A review of environmental and policy approaches in the prevention of chronic diseases. *Annual Review of Public Health, 27*, 341–370.

Carson, K. V., Brinn, M. P., Labiszewski, N. A., Esterman, A. J., Chang, A. B., & Smith, B. J. (2011). Community interventions for preventing smoking in young people. *Cochrane Database System Review*, (7), CD001291. doi:10.1002/14651858.CD001291.pub2.

Chaix, B., Merlo, J., Evans, D., Leal, C., & Havard, S. (2009). Neighbourhoods in eco-epidemiologic research: Delimiting personal exposure areas. A response to Riva, Gauvin, Apparicio and Brodeur. *Social Science & Medicine, 69*(9), 1306–1310.

Choiniere, R., Lafontaine, P., & Edwards, A. C. (2000). Distribution of cardiovascular disease risk factors by socioeconomic status among Canadian adults. *Canadian Medical Association Journal, 162*(9 Suppl), S13–S24.

Chuang, Y.-C., Ennett, S. T., Bauman, K. E., & Foshee, V. A. (2005). Neighborhood influences on adolescent cigarette and alcohol use: Mediating effects through parent and peer behaviors. *Journal of Health and Social Behavior, 46*(2), 187–204.

Cohen, J. E., & Anglin, L. (2009). Outlet density: A new frontier for tobacco control. *Addiction, 104*(1), 2–3.

Cook, T. D. (2003). The case for studying multiple contexts simultaneously. *Addiction, 98*, 151–155.

Dent, C., & Biglan, A. (2004). Relation between access to tobacco and adolescent smoking. *Tobacco Control, 13*(4), 334–338.

Dowdell, E. B. (2002). Urban seventh graders and smoking: A health risk behavior assessment. *Issues in Comprehensive Pediatric Nursing, 25*(4), 217–229.

Ecob, R., & Macintyre, S. (2000). Small area variations in health related behaviours: Do these depend on the behaviour itself, its measurement, or on personal characteristics? *Health & Place, 6*(4), 261–274.

Ennett, S. T., Flewelling, R. L., Lindrooth, R. C., & Norton, E. C. (1997). School and neighborhood characteristics associated with school rates of alcohol, cigarette, and marijuana use. *Journal of Health and Social Behavior, 38*(1), 55–71.

Fagan, A. A., Van Horn, M. L., Hawkins, J. D., & Arthur, M. (2007). Using community and family risk and protective factors for community-based prevention planning. *Journal of Community Psychology, 35*(4), 535–555.

Federico, B., Costa, G., & Kunst, A. E. (2007). Educational inequalities in initiation, cessation, and prevalence of smoking among 3 Italian birth cohorts. *American Journal of Public Health, 97*(5), 838–845.

Feighery, E. C., Schleicher, N. C., Cruz, T. B., & Unger, J. B. (2008). An examination of trends in amount and type of cigarette advertising and sales promotions in California stores, 2002–2005. *Tobacco Control, 17*(2), 93–98.

Forster, J. L., Widome, R., & Bernat, D. H. (2007). Policy interventions and surveillance as strategies to prevent tobacco use in adolescents and young adults. *American Journal of Preventive Medicine, 33*(6 Suppl), 335–339.

Freedman, K. S., Nelson, N. M., & Feldman, L. L. (2012). Smoking initiation among young adults in the United States and Canada, 1998–2010: A systematic review. *Preventing Chronic Disease, 9*, 110037. doi:10.5888/pcd9.110037.

Frohlich, K. L., & Potvin, L. (2008). Transcending the known in public health practice: The inequality paradox: The population approach and vulnerable populations. *American Journal of Public Health, 98*(2), 216–221.

Frohlich, K. L., Potvin, L., Gauvin, L., & Chabot, P. (2002). Youth smoking initiation: Disentangling context from composition. *Health & Place, 8*(3), 155–166.

Gibbons, F. X., Gerrard, M., Lune, L. S. V., Wills, T. A., Brody, G., & Conger, R. D. (2004). Context and cognitions: Environmental risk, social influence, and adolescent substance use. *Personality and Social Psychology Bulletin, 30*(8), 1048–1061.

Gilman, S. E., Martin, L. T., Abrams, D. B., Kawachi, I., Kubzansky, L., Loucks, E. B., et al. (2008). Educational attainment and cigarette smoking: A causal association? *International Journal of Epidemiology, 37*(3), 615–624.

Giskes, K., Kunst, A. E., Benach, J., Borrell, C., Costa, G., Dahl, E., et al. (2005). Trends in smoking behaviour between 1985 and 2000 in nine European countries by education. *Journal of Epidemiology and Community Health, 59*(5), 395–401.

Giskes, K., van Lenthe, F. J., Turrell, G., Brug, J., & Mackenbach, J. P. (2006). Smokers living in deprived areas are less likely to quit: A longitudinal follow-up. *Tobacco Control, 15*(6), 485–488.

Graham, H. (2004). Tackling inequalities in health in England: Remedying health disadvantages, narrowing health gaps or reducing health gradients? *Journal of Social Policy, 33*(1), 115–131.

Greaves, L., & Jategaonkar, N. (2006). Tobacco policies and vulnerable girls and women: Toward a framework for gender sensitive policy development. *Journal of Epidemiology and Community Health, 60*(Suppl 2), 57–65.

Greaves, L., Johnson, J., Bottorff, J., Kirkland, S., et al. (2006). What are the effects of tobacco policies on vulnerable populations? A better practices review. *Canadian Journal of Public Health, 97*(4), 310–315.

Harman, J., Graham, H., Francis, B., & Inskip, H. M. (2006). Socioeconomic gradients in smoking among young women: A British survey. *Social Science & Medicine, 63*(11), 2791–2800.

Henriksen, L., Feighery, E. C., Schleicher, N. C., Cowling, D. W., Kline, R. S., & Fortmann, S. P. (2008). Is adolescent smoking related to the density and proximity of tobacco outlets and retail cigarette advertising near schools? *Preventive Medicine, 47*(2), 210–214.

Hiscock, R., Bauld, L., Amos, A., Fidler, J. A., & Munafo, M. (2011). Socioeconomic status and smoking: A review. *Annals of the New York Academy of Sciences*. doi:10.1111/j.1749-6632.2011.06202.x.

Hotchkiss, J. W., Davies, C., Gray, L., Bromley, C., Capewell, S., & Leyland, A. H. (2011). Trends in adult cardiovascular disease risk factors and their socio-economic patterning in the Scottish population 1995 to 2008: Cross-sectional surveys. *BMJ Open, 1*(1). doi:10.1136/bmjopen-2011-000176.

Inagami, S., Cohen, D. A., & Finch, B. K. (2007). Non-residential neighborhood exposures suppress neighborhood effects on self-rated health. *Social Science & Medicine, 65*(8), 1779–1791.

Jha, P. (2009). Avoidable global cancer deaths and total deaths from smoking. *Nature Reviews. Cancer, 9*(9), 655–664.

Kaestle, C. E., & Wiles, B. B. (2010). Targeting high-risk neighborhoods for tobacco prevention education in schools. *American Journal of Public Health, 100*(9), 1708–1713.

Kamruzzaman, M., Hine, J., Gunay, B., & Blair, N. (2011). Using GIS to visualise and evaluate student travel behaviour. *Journal of Transport Geography, 19*(1), 13–32.

Kestens, Y., Lebel, A., Daniel, M., Thériault, M., & Pampalon, R. (2010). Using experienced activity spaces to measure foodscape exposure. *Health & Place, 16*(6), 1094–1103.

Kim, J., & McCarthy, W. J. (2006). School-level contextual influences on smoking and drinking among Asian and Pacific Islander adolescents. *Drug and Alcohol Dependence, 84*(1), 56–68.

Kwan, M. P. (2009). From place-based to people-based exposure measures. *Social Science & Medicine, 69*(9), 1311–1313.

Lambert, S. F., Brown, T. L., Phillips, C. M., & Ialongo, N. S. (2004). The relationship between perceptions of neighborhood characteristics and substance use among urban African American adolescents. *American Journal of Community Psychology, 34*(3–4), 205–218.

Lantz, P. M. (2003). Smoking on the rise among young adults: Implications for research and policy. *Tobacco Control, 12*(Suppl 1), i60–i70.

Lawrence, D., Fagan, P., Backinger, C. L., Gibson, J. T., & Hartman, A. (2007). Cigarette smoking patterns among young adults aged 18–24 years in the United States. *Nicotine & Tobacco Research, 9*(6), 687–697.

Leal, C., & Chaix, B. (2011). The influence of geographic life environments on cardiometabolic risk factors: A systematic review, a methodological assessment and a research agenda. *Obesity Reviews, 12*(3), 217–230.

Leatherdale, S., & Strath, J. (2007). Tobacco retailer density surrounding schools and cigarette access behaviors among underage smoking students. *Annals of Behavioral Medicine, 33*(1), 105–111.

Lee, R. E., & Cubbin, C. (2002). Neighborhood context and youth cardiovascular health behaviors. *American Journal of Public Health, 92*(3), 428–436.

Lovato, C. Y., Hsu, H. C., Sabiston, C. M., Hadd, V., & Nykiforuk, C. I. (2007). Tobacco point-of-purchase marketing in school neighbourhoods and school smoking prevalence: A descriptive study. *Canadian Journal of Public Health, 98*(4), 265–270.

Lovato, C. Y., Zeisser, C., Campbell, H. S., Watts, A. W., Halpin, P., Thompson, M., et al. (2010). Adolescent smoking: Effect of school and community characteristics. *American Journal of Preventive Medicine, 39*(6), 507–514.

Main, C., Thomas, S., Ogilvie, D., Stirk, L., Petticrew, M., Whitehead, M., et al. (2008). Population tobacco control interventions and their effects on social inequalities in smoking: Placing an

equity lens on existing systematic reviews. *BMC Public Health, 8*(1), 178. doi:10.1186/1471-2458-8-178.
Marmot, M. (2006). Smoking and inequalities. *Lancet, 368*(9533), 341–342.
Matheson, F. I., LaFreniere, M. C., White, H. L., Moineddin, R., Dunn, J. R., & Glazier, R. H. (2011). Influence of neighborhood deprivation, gender and ethno-racial origin on smoking behavior of Canadian youth. *Preventive Medicine, 52*(5), 376–380.
Matthews, S. A. (2011). Spatial polygamy and the heterogeneity of place: Studying people and place via egocentric methods: Communities, neighborhoods, and health. In L. M. M. Burton, S. A. P. Matthews, M. Leung, S. P. A. Kemp, & D. T. T. Takeuchi (Eds.), *Social disparities in health and health care* (Vol. 1, pp. 35–55). New York: Springer.
McCarthy, W. J., Mistry, R., Lu, Y., Patel, M., Zheng, H., & Dietsch, B. (2009). Density of tobacco retailers near schools: Effects on tobacco use among students. *American Journal of Public Health, 99*(11), 2006–2013.
Miller, H. (2007). Place-based versus people-based geographic information science. *Geographic Compass, 1*(3), 503–535.
Milton, B., Cook, P. A., Dugdill, L., Porcellato, L., Springett, J., & Woods, S. E. (2004). Why do primary school children smoke? A longitudinal analysis of predictors of smoking uptake during pre-adolescence. *Public Health, 118*(4), 247–255.
Morency, C., Paez, A., Roorda, M. J., Mercado, R., & Farber, S. (2011). Distance travelled in three Canadian cities: Spatial analysis from the perspective of vulnerable population segments. *Journal of Transport Geography, 19*(1), 39–50.
Musick, K., Seltzer, J. A., & Schwartz, C. R. (2008). Neighborhood norms and substance use among Teens. *Social Science Research, 37*(1), 138–155.
NHS Information Centre (2011). *Lifestyles statistics*. England: Statistics on Smoking.
Niederdeppe, J., Kuang, X., Crock, B., & Skelton, A. (2008). Media campaigns to promote smoking cessation among socioeconomically disadvantaged populations: What do we know, what do we need to learn, and what should we do now? *Social Science & Medicine, 67*(9), 1343–1355.
Norwegian Institute of Public Health (2010). Smoking in Norway – fact sheet. http://www.fhi.no/eway/default.aspx?pid=238&trg=Area_5954&MainArea_5811=5895:0:15,4993:1:0:0:::0:0&MainLeft_5895=5954:0:15,4993:1:0:0:::0:0&Area_5954=5825:84434::1:5955:1:::0:0. Accessed 2 Dec 2011.
Novak, S. P., Reardon, S. F., Raudenbush, S. W., & Buka, S. L. (2006). Retail tobacco outlet density and youth cigarette smoking: A propensity-modeling approach. *American Journal of Public Health, 96*(4), 670–676.
Nowlin, P. R., & Colder, C. R. (2007). The role of ethnicity and neighborhood poverty on the relationship between parenting and adolescent cigarette use. *Nicotine & Tobacco Research, 9*(5), 545–556.
Ogilvie, D., & Petticrew, M. (2004). Reducing social inequalities in smoking: Can evidence inform policy? A pilot study. *Tobacco Control, 13*(13), 129–131.
Organisation mondiale de la santé (1986). Charte d'Ottawa pour la promotion de la santé. http://www.euro.who.int/AboutWHO/Policy/20010827_2?language=french.
Organisation mondiale de la santé (2008). Commission des déterminants sociaux de la santé. Combler le fossé dans une génération. Instaurer l'équité en santé en agissant sur les déterminants sociaux de la santé.
Pierce, J. P., & Gilpin, E. (1996). How long will today's new adolescent smoker be addicted to cigarettes? *American Journal of Public Health, 86*(2), 253–256.
Pokorny, S. B., Jason, L. A., & Schoeny, M. E. (2003). The relation of retail tobacco availability to initiation and continued smoking. *Journal of Clinical Child and Adolescent Psychology, 32*(2), 193–204.
Poland, B., Frohlich, K., Haines, R. J., Mykhalovskiy, E., Rock, M., & Sparks, R. (2006). The social context of smoking: The next frontier in tobacco control? *Tobacco Control, 15*(1), 59–63.
Poland, B., Krupa, G., & McCall, D. (2009). Settings for health promotion: An analytic framework to guide intervention design and implementation. *Health Promotion Practice, 10*(4), 505–516.

Rainham, D., McDowell, I., Krewski, D., & Sawade, M. (2010). Conceptualizing the healthscape: Contributions of time geography, location technologies and spatial ecology to place and health research. *Social Science & Medicine, 70*(5), 668–676. doi:10.1016/j.socscimed.2009.10.035.
Reardon, S. F., Brennan, R. T., & Buka, S. L. (2002). Estimating multi-level discrete-time hazard models using cross-sectional data: Neighborhood effects on the onset of adolescent cigarette use. *Multivariate Behavioral Research, 37*(3), 297–330.
Rothman, K. J., & Greenland, S. (1998). *Modern epidemiology* (2nd ed.). Philadelphia: Lippincott-Raven.
Schaap, M. M., & Kunst, A. E. (2009). Monitoring of socio-economic inequalities in smoking: Learning from the experiences of recent scientific studies. *Public Health, 123*(2), 103–109.
Schönfelder, S., & Axhausen, K. W. (2003). Activity spaces: Measures of social exclusion? *Transport Policy, 10*, 273–286.
Schönfelder, S., & Axhausen, K. W. (2004). *Structure and innovation of human activity spaces, Arbeitsbericht Verkehrs- und Raumplanung* (Vol. 258). Zürich: IVT, ETH.
Smith, P., Frank, J., & Mustard, C. (2009). Trends in educational inequalities in smoking and physical activity in Canada: 1974–2005. *Journal of Epidemiology and Community Health, 63*(4), 317–323.
Solberg, L. I., Asche, S. E., Boyle, R., McCarty, M. C., & Thoele, M. J. (2007). Smoking and cessation behaviors among young adults of various educational backgrounds. *American Journal of Public Health, 97*(8), 1421–1426.
Stafford, M., Nazroo, J., Popay, J. M., & Whitehead, M. (2008). Tackling inequalities in health: Evaluating the new deal for communities initiative. *Journal of Epidemiology and Community Health, 62*(4), 298–304.
Statistics Canada (2009). Dissemination area (DA). http://www12.statcan.ca/census-recensement/2006/ref/dict/geo021-eng.cfm. Accessed 19 Dec 2011.
The Scottish Government (2011). *Health of Scotland's population – Smoking*. http://www.scotland.gov.uk/Topics/Statistics/Browse/Health/TrendSmoking. Accessed 19 Dec 2011.
Thomas, S., Fayter, D., Misso, K., Ogilvie, D., Petticrew, M., Sowden, A., et al. (2008). Population tobacco control interventions and their effects on social inequalities in smoking: Systematic review. *Tobacco Control, 17*(4), 230–237.
Vallee, J., Cadot, E., Grillo, F., Parizot, I., & Chauvin, P. (2010). The combined effects of activity space and neighbourhood of residence on participation in preventive health-care activities: The case of cervical screening in the Paris metropolitan area (France). *Health & Place, 16*(5), 838–852.
Wardle, J., Jarvis, M. J., Steggles, N., Sutton, S., Williamson, S., Farrimond, H., et al. (2003). Socioeconomic disparities in cancer-risk behaviors in adolescence: Baseline results from the health and behaviour in teenagers study (HABITS). *Preventive Medicine, 36*(6), 721–730.
Woods, S. E., Lake, J. R., & Springett, J. (2003). Tackling health inequalities and the HAZ smoking cessation programme: The perfect match? *Critical Public Health, 13*(1), 61–76.
Zenk, S. N., Schulz, A. J., Matthews, S. A., Odoms-Young, A., Wilbur, J., Wegrzyn, L., et al. (2011). Activity space environment and dietary and physical activity behaviors: A pilot study. *Health & Place, 17*(5), 1150–1161.

Chapter 15
Neighbourhood Structure and Alcohol and Other Drug Use: Implications for Prevention

Kim Bloomfield and Christiane Stock

Introduction

Adolescence and young adulthood is a period when many young people start to experiment with and consume alcohol. It is also the typical age for experimentation with or taking up use of certain drugs, most commonly tobacco and cannabis, and less commonly for illicit drugs such as ecstasy, amphetamines, LSD and other hallucinogens, inhalants, crack, cocaine and heroin (Hibell et al. 2009). Initiation into the use of legal substances such as alcohol and tobacco can be seen as normal for this time in life. However, it is also a vulnerable age to begin use as research has demonstrated, especially for tobacco and alcohol, that the earlier the initiation, the more likely it is that use will become problematic and/or addictive later in life (Mathers et al. 2006). Furthermore, there are concerns that use of alcohol and tobacco in youth can function as "gateway" drugs to illegal substances especially cannabis. Cannabis, in turn, is also seen as a gateway drug to experimentation and use of harder substances such as cocaine, heroin and amphetamines (Degenhart et al. 2009; Kokkevi et al. 2007b). Given these concerns over early initiation to substance use as well as over misuse in general, a major focus of alcohol and drug research has been on young people to develop ways to prevent or delay alcohol and other drug use and/or misuse.

The majority of alcohol and other drug (AOD) research addresses trends in use, effects of AOD use and misuse as well as on identifying risk factors that lie within

K. Bloomfield (✉)
Center for Alcohol and Drug Research, School of Business and Social Science, Aarhus University, Artillerivej 90, 2300 Copenhagen S, Denmark
e-mail: kb@crf.au.dk

C. Stock
Unit for Health Promotion Research, Institute of Public Health, University of Southern Denmark, Niels Bohrs Vej 9-10, 6700 Esbjerg, Denmark
e-mail: cstock@health.sdu.dk

C. Stock and A. Ellaway (eds.), *Neighbourhood Structure and Health Promotion*,
DOI 10.1007/978-1-4614-6672-7_15,

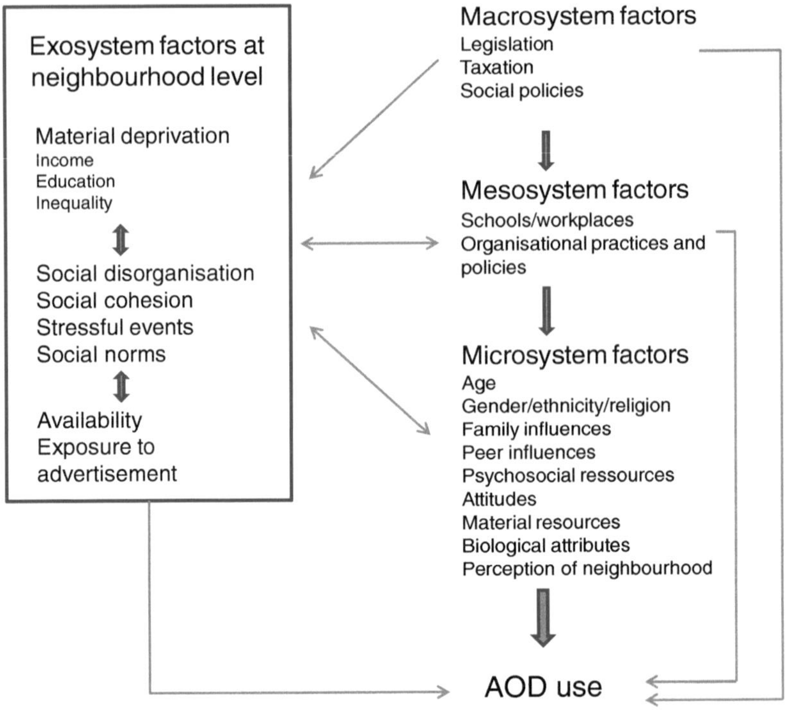

Fig. 15.1 Conceptual model on factors influencing AOD use in youth

individuals and their interpersonal environments. AOD use has been recognised as shaped by social processes and contexts. Bronfenbrenner's Social Ecological Model provides a conceptual framework for studying such social contexts in a developmental perspective by defining person-environment interrelations in terms of micro-, meso-, exo- and macrosystems. While the microsystem comprises individual or interpersonal features, the mesosystem comprises the organisational or institutional factors shaping the environment within which the individual and interpersonal relations occur. Mesosystems in term operate in the larger sphere of exosystems. Exosystems refer to the community level influences and thus comprise neighbourhood influences. Macrosystems are the cultural contexts that structure the environment in which the other system levels operate. Figure 15.1 illustrates the interaction of the different system levels.

While AOD research has been broadly concentrated on studying risk factors at the micro- and meso-level such as predictors of adolescents' alcohol use within families, the school classroom and peer groups (Hawkins et al. 1986, 1992; Kandel 1986; Newcomb et al. 1986), research on the influences of the more remote social environments, the exosystem, such as neighbourhoods still is less common (Ennett et al. 2008). In this chapter, we will therefore summarise research on neighbourhood influences on AOD use while leaving out neighbourhood influences on smoking (for this, see Chap. 14 in this book). Furthermore, we will also explore if and how micro/mesosystem processes interact with exosystem contexts. Since neighbourhood-level theories suggest that adolescents and young people are particularly vulnerable to the effects of living in disadvantaged areas (Leventhal and Brooks-Gunn 2000, 2003), this chapter focuses primarily on AOD use among youth.

Microlevel Social, Behavioural and Mental Health Correlates of Alcohol and Other Drug Use

The correlates of alcohol and drug use are to some extent similar, but they also differ in important ways partially due to the differing marketing, availability, accessibility, social acceptance and legislation of the substance in question (Babor et al. 2010).

Gender

For both alcohol and other drugs, there is overwhelming research which shows that males engage in alcohol use (e.g. Wicki et al. 2010) and other drug use (Babor et al. 2010) more often and in greater amounts than females. Among adolescents, however, the gender gap appears to be rather small. The European School Survey Project on Alcohol and other Drugs (ESPAD) has surveyed school students aged 15–16 years in 1995, 1999, 2003 and 2007 (Hibell et al. 2009). For prevalence of alcohol use in the last 12 months and last 30 days, there are virtually no differences according to ESPAD data, and regarding prevalence of heavy episodic drinking, there has been a marked closing of the gender gap over the study period (i.e. 1995–2007) (Hibell et al. 2009). Gender differences are clearer regarding prevalence of illicit drug use based on ESPAD data, but they are smaller among younger people (Babor et al. 2010).

Ethnicity and Religious Affiliation

Few studies examine ethnicity and alcohol use in Europe. Among studies of university students, those who drink the most and most frequently are Europeans. Those from lower to middle income countries, e.g. Turkey (Stock et al. 2009) and/or Asian countries, tend to drink the least. Those students affiliating with religions that discourage alcohol consumption also drink less or not at all (Wicki et al. 2010). Regarding other drug use, surveys of adolescents in the USA report higher prevalence of use among persons of European descent than those with African, Mexican or Asian backgrounds (Bachman et al. 1991). Neither ESPAD nor the Health Behaviour in School-aged Children (HBSC) data have been analysed with regard to ethnic background within a country.

Family Structure and Social Networks

Research has shown consistently that adolescents living in non-intact family arrangements are more likely to engage in heavy drinking than those who live with both biological parents (Bjarnason et al. 2003a; Bergmark and Andersson 1999; Miller 1997). Using ESPAD data from 11 European countries, Bjarnason et al. (2003b) found that with regard to smoking, adolescents living with both biological parents are also less likely to smoke as much as adolescents living with single mothers, single fathers or mothers-stepfathers or with neither biological parent. Also using data from ESPAD, Kokkevi et al. (2007b) found a similar effect of non-intact parental living situations on the lifetime use of cannabis and other drugs among adolescents. Furthermore, adolescent dissatisfaction with either mother or father was positively associated with frequent use of alcohol and cigarettes as well as lifetime use of other drugs.

It is also widely recognised that the nature of substance use in adolescents' social networks and peer groups is highly correlated with both one's initiation into and current use of substances (e.g. Ali and Dwyer 2009, 2010; Clark and Loheac 2007; Lundborg 2006; Reifman et al. 1998). However, a problem with previous research on current substance use has been to distinguish causal pathways. That is, do social networks encourage young people to drink more or do heavy drinking young people seek out friendship circles with heavy drinking friends? Recent developments in network analysis with longitudinal data have aided in demonstrating that social network membership is not only based on self-selection but also that the networks influence one's own smoking and drinking behaviours (Rosenquist et al. 2010; Christakis and Fowler 2008). Furthermore, social networks can influence substance use behaviour in both directions: initiation/current use and also cessation (Christakis and Fowler 2008).

Personality Characteristics

The psychiatric epidemiological literature has consistently documented an association of mood, anxiety and personality disorders with substance use disorders (e.g. Merikangas et al. 1998). Research among young people has further shown that the main psychological/personality correlates of substance use, particularly illicit drug use, include indicators of antisocial behaviour and conduct problems (Kokkevi et al. 2007a, b; Agrawal et al. 2011) and to some extent anomie and depression (Kokkevi et al. 2007b). However, with regard to alcohol drinking alone, in a review of alcohol use studies involving European university students, Wicki et al. (2010) found negative relationships or no relationship between depression and alcohol consumption. Mixed results were also found regarding other personality traits. Here, the literature reveals differing relationships between personality traits and substance use, depending on the type of substance (licit vs. illicit) and the severity of the use (social use vs. misuse/disorders/dependence).

Socio-economic Status

There is a growing literature on socio-economic status (SES) and alcohol and drug use among adolescents and young adults. In such studies, socio-economic status is usually measured by asking respondents about a parent's income, education or occupation (usually the father). Some studies use an index of family resources as a proxy for parental socio-economic status, as there is a problem of validity and reliability of children's reports of the various components parents' SES (e.g. a high number of missing values or inaccurate responses) (Currie et al. 2008).

Regardless of measure of SES used, a consistent outcome is found with regard to smoking. In general, young people living in low SES households are more likely to engage in cigarette smoking (Hanson and Chen 2007). However, with regard to alcohol consumption (particularly drunkenness and heavy episodic drinking) and cannabis use, parental SES has limited influence (Andersen et al. 2006; Richter et al. 2006).

The explanation for these diverse findings is that smoking is more directly linked to parents' own health habits (i.e. their own smoking) and they serve as a role model for their teenagers (Kalesan et al. 2006). Moreover, smoking is more prevalent among low SES adults (e.g. Lynch et al. 1997). Further, psychological factors such as stress and depression may be more prevalent among low SES adolescents, thereby mediating the relationship to smoking prevalence (Hanson and Chen 2007). Drinking and cannabis use, on the other hand, appear to be influenced less by familial and parental habits and more by peer social influence (Richter et al. 2006; Hanson and Chen 2007). These 'competing' or complementary influences on adolescent use of AOD have implications for research into neighbourhood influences. A multilevel analysis could distinguish more sharply the contribution of those influences related to parents from those of school and peer groups.

Trends in Alcohol and Drug Use in Europe

Two major ongoing studies of youth health behaviour have comprehensively monitored international (mainly European) trends in school students' use of alcohol and drugs since the mid-/late 1990s. The European School Survey Project on Alcohol and other Drugs (ESPAD) has surveyed school students aged 15–16 years in 1995,

1999, 2003 and 2007 (Hibell et al. 2009). In 1995, the study included 26 European countries; by 2007, the number had increased to 35. The WHO collaborative study, Health Behaviour in School-aged Children (HBSC), was initiated by researchers from three European countries in 1982 when the first data collection took place. There have been eight data collection waves since then with the number of countries/regions increasing to 43 in 2009/2010. The latest available data are from 2005/2006. Most study countries are European (Simons-Morton et al. 2009).

Latest findings on consumption trends in the ESPAD study were published in 2009 (Hibell et al. 2009). With regard to alcohol use, the average prevalence of consumption in the last 12 months over all study countries remained relatively stable from 1995 to 2007. However, in the last observation period (2003–2007), ten countries showed decreases; these decreases were also evident among boys where the average prevalence dropped from 84 % to 80 %. For consumption in the last 30 days, the average prevalence increased through 2003 and began to decline slightly in 2007, which was also evident in 13 countries. The prevalence of heavy episodic drinking (five or more drinks on an occasion) in the last 30 days, however, showed increases, especially among girls, from 35 % to 42 % between 2003 and 2007. Increases were evident in more than half of all study countries.

There was a general decrease in both lifetime and last 30 day prevalence of cigarette smoking between 1995 and 2007. The prevalence of smoking had remained relatively stable through 2003 at around 67 % but then dropped to 59 % in 2007 (Hibell et al. 2009). This trend held for both boys and girls, but the decrease was more noticeable in Northern European countries.

The trend in the average prevalence of lifetime use of any illicit drug increased between 1995 and 2003 and decreased slightly in 2007. When looking at individual countries, most increases between 2003 and 2007 were in Eastern Europe, whereas decreases occurred mainly in Western, Northern and Central Europe. Use of cannabis (lifetime and last 30 day use) showed a similar pattern. These trends were similar for boys and girls.

With regard to alcohol use, results from European countries in the HBSC study reflect similar trends from 1998 to 2006 to those found in ESPAD. Average monthly alcohol use and average prevalence of drunkenness decreased slightly over the study period (Simons-Morton et al. 2009). Boys had a higher prevalence of both behaviours at both time points, but the gap between the genders narrowed by 2006, with boys' prevalence declining and girls' increasing. On the individual country level, there were mixed tendencies regarding monthly alcohol use. Many European countries experienced no trend or a decline, but a number of Eastern European countries as well as a few Western European countries showed increases. However, for drunkenness, trends were much clearer with increases in the prevalence exclusively being seen among Eastern European countries. For the remainder of Europe, there was either no trend or a decrease.

Exolevel Influences on Alcohol and Other Drug Use

Neighbourhood Deprivation

It is hypothesised that materially deprived neighbourhoods may be a risk factor for AOD use of their residents, independently of individual SES. There are several reasons why neighbourhood deprivation may be associated with AOD use. Firstly, in neighbourhoods with low mean income and education levels, the prevalence of distress among residents may be higher, and AOD use may occur as a relief from stress (Rhodes and Jason 1990). Research indicates that stressful life events occur more often in neighbourhoods with low levels of income and education (Fang et al. 1998) and AOD use has been suggested as a means to cope with such events (Boardman et al. 2001). Other reasons for a link between neighbourhood material deprivation and AOD use include decreased individual and social resources to cope with stress, social norms, availability of substances and targeted advertising.

Some research supports the hypothesis of neighbourhood deprivation as a risk for AOD use. A study from the USA showed that neighbourhood poverty was an important predictor of heavy episodic drinking in a cohort study of young adults (Cerdá et al. 2010). Area effects may depend on drinking level (Poortinga 2006), and most studies used problem drinking behaviour as the outcome of interest. One of the few studies on neighbourhood SES and health behaviour conducted in Asia showed an inverse relationship between neighbourhood educational level and any alcohol consumption in Taiwanese adults of all ages (Chuang et al. 2007), indicating that low neighbourhood SES may also stimulate moderate alcohol use and not only problem drinking.

However, other research indicates that the association between neighbourhood deprivation and alcohol drinking is not straightforward. Some studies found that alcohol drinking is higher in high SES neighbourhoods. A study in Finland found a positive association between well educated regions and alcohol use among teenage girls, but not among boys (Karvonen and Rimpelä 1996). Other European studies found no association between neighbourhood SES and alcohol use among Danish adolescents (Stock et al. 2011), among a Dutch sample aged 15–75 years (Monden et al. 2006) or among older people Switzerland (Cornaz et al. 2009). The reason for the inconsistencies in findings regarding neighbourhood deprivation and AOD use may lie in the different factors mediating between neighbourhood material deprivation (as measured by aggregated income or education data) and AOD use as some research suggests: Chuang et al. (2005) explored the pathways through which socio-economic characteristics of neighbourhoods may influence adolescent alcohol use. They found that low neighbourhood SES was associated with increased peer drinking, which in turn was associated with increased individual adolescent alcohol use. However, at the same time, better parental monitoring was connected with decreased drinking in low SES neighbourhoods, indicating a buffering effect of parental management practices. Moreover, high SES neighbourhoods were associated with increased parental drinking, which was further associated with increased adolescent alcohol use. We can conclude from this research that neighbourhood material deprivation has the potential to influence AOD use, but the amount and direction of the effect depends very much on the mediating factors and is likely to be complex.

Neighbourhood Disorganisation and Disorder

Neighbourhood material deprivation can lead to social disorganisation. Social disorganisation has been defined by Sampson and Groves (1989) as the 'inability of a community structure to realise the common values of its residents and maintain effective social control' (p. 777). The theory posits that disadvantaged neighbourhoods with few economic and social resources lack community control. This would lead to deviant behaviour and crime with subsequent further social and economic breakdown (Sampson and Groves 1989). Social disorganisation theory is closely linked to the family of incivility or disorder theories. These 'broken windows' theories hypothesise that physical disorder in urban neighbourhoods, such as broken windows left unattended, signal disregard for the neighbourhood surroundings and promote further damage and willingness to violate social norms among residents (Wilson and Kelling 1982; Mair and Mair 2003). Measures of social disorganisation and neighbourhood disorder are not uniform, and they include different sets of indicators such as safety, crime, racism, litter, vandalism, abandoned buildings, publicly visible AOD use, church attendance (Crum et al. 1996) or homelessness, burglary, prostitution, crime and teenage loitering (Latkin and Curry 2003). Ennett et al. (1997) measured social disorganisation by household characteristics such as the percentage of divorced males. Furr-Holden et al. (2010) suggest the Neighbourhood Inventory for Environmental Typology (NIfETy) as a valid and reliable environmental assessment tool based on disorder theories.

Neighbourhood disorganisation has indeed been found to be associated with AOD use (Winstanley et al. 2008), cannabis use (Furr-Holden et al. 2011) and exposure to cocaine (Crum et al. 1996) in US adolescents. A larger number of perceived neighbourhood problems also increased the odds for illicit drug use in low-income, young women in the USA (Sunder et al. 2007). Whereas neighbourhood disorganisation seems to increase drug use, its association with alcohol use appears to be more complex. A Taiwanese study showed a positive association of neighbourhood disorganisation with alcohol use in low SES individuals, but not in high SES individuals (Chuang et al. 2007). The authors discuss this interaction effect in the light of the double jeopardy theory, suggesting that living in neighbourhoods with high social disorganisation will intensify the effects of individual low SES. Some studies found either no association of neighbourhood disadvantage with adolescent drinking (Ennett et al. 2008; Brenner et al. 2011) or even reported a higher lifetime alcohol use in schools located in areas with higher neighbourhood attachment and safety (Ennett et al. 1997). In conclusion, neighbourhood disorganisation showed some positive association with other drug use, while its association with alcohol use is less clear.

The concept of social disorganisation is mostly used in research conducted in the United States. This may be because the major characteristics of social disorganisation such as abandoned buildings are less prominent in European urban neighbourhoods due to higher public expenditures and public housing policies preventing extreme deterioration of neighbourhoods and signs of poverty.

Neighbourhood Social Inequality

It has also been suggested that apart from neighbourhood deprivation, social inequalities at the neighbourhood level would influence population health and health behaviour. International comparisons indicate that countries with more egalitarian distribution of income have lower mortality rates (Rodgers 1979) leading to the hypothesis that inequity erodes social trust and diminishes social cohesion which in turn would have negative effects on individual well-being and health (Kawachi et al. 1997). Galea et al. (2007a, b) used coefficients measuring inequality in education and income to describe neighbourhood inequality in New York City. They found higher odds for alcohol drinking and for cannabis smoking in neighbourhoods with higher education inequality, even after controlling for both neighbourhood education and income inequality (Galea et al. 2007a). The effect was greatest in neighbourhoods with low mean education levels. However, among current drinkers, neighbourhood education inequality was associated with consuming less alcohol. Galea et al. (2007b) describe similar effects of income maldistribution on alcohol and cannabis use. The authors conclude that a complex relation exists between inequality and substance use and potential roles for social norms and availability as mediating factors.

Social Influences of Neighbourhoods

Social learning theory posits that the presence or absence of role models in neighbourhoods would be important for shaping social and health behaviour. Some research indicates that neighbourhood social context, such as neighbours' alcohol misuse, may be an important factor explaining adolescents' alcohol misuse; however, the same study did not show an effect of neighbourhood disadvantage (Ennett et al. 2008). This indicated that social norms and modelling may be important factors in how the neighbourhood context influences AOD use via social influences. Another factor examined is social cohesion. The social cohesion approach emphasises 'shared beliefs in a neighbourhood's capability for action to achieve an intended effect, and assumes an active sense of engagement among neighbourhood members' (Duncan et al. 2002, p. 126). Tobler et al. (2009) characterised social cohesion as having a strong community identity, having high levels of community resources, participation in activities and influence of residents in decisions. Such neighbourhood strengths were negatively associated with alcohol use primarily among low SES American youth (Tobler et al. 2009). In the same study, neighbourhood deprivation did not show any significant effects on youth alcohol use, indicating that social influences might be more powerful than material deprivation alone. The association between neighbourhood social cohesion and AOD use seems to be influenced by mediating factors. Structural modelling suggests that among others family management practices act as mediators. Parents may act as 'buffering' the effects of risky neighbourhoods by decreasing alcohol access at home and increasing protection (Chuang et al. 2005; Tobler et al. 2009).

Availability and Exposure to Advertising

Availability has consistently been shown to be strong predictor of youth alcohol use (Gruenewald et al. 1993; Weitzman et al. 2003). Research indicates that besides home access to alcohol, the availability in the neighbourhood promotes consumption and early initiation of drinking. It is assumed that the number of alcohol outlets indicates availability of alcohol in an environment. The density of alcohol outlets has been shown to be associated with alcohol use in the general population (Scribner et al. 2000; Gruenewald et al. 2002), in college students (Presley et al. 2002; Weitzman et al. 2003) and in adolescents (Chen et al. 2010). Although the majority of studies has been conducted in the USA, some studies from Europe support the findings of a positive association between outlet density and alcohol use (Kuntsche et al. 2008).

Another neighbourhood factor potentially influencing alcohol use might be exposure to alcohol advertising. Some research indicates that the number of alcohol advertisements in a neighbourhood is positively associated with alcohol use in US adolescents (Tobler et al. 2009).

In conclusion, research indicates that the perceived availability at the individual and community levels and the actual density of alcohol outlets are important determinants of alcohol use at least among young people. A recent review also concludes that there is some indication for an association between higher outlet density as well as exposure to advertisement and alcohol use, especially among adolescents (Bryden et al. 2012).

With regard to other drugs, the quantification of availability and association with its use is less well researched as these drugs are illicit. Observations from the Netherlands where cannabis has been decriminalised and sold in coffee shops since the 1980s do not indicate a direct link between cannabis availability and use. Although the availability of cannabis is high in the Netherlands, the prevalence of cannabis use among Dutch adults is somewhat below the European average (Monshouwer et al. 2011). However, the availability of cannabis in the Netherlands certainly has an effect on tourists visiting the country. Thus, trends in cannabis use among Dutch people seem to develop rather independently from cannabis policies and availability (Korf 2002).

Implications for Prevention

Overall, one can conclude from research on neighbourhood structure and AOD use that several characteristics of neighbourhoods have an impact on AOD use. This influence, however, is modest in comparison to the more proximal predictors of AOD use such as individual factors and the immediate social environment of families and peers. Figure 15.1 summarises the different exolevel factors at neighbourhood level on AOD use and relates them to other relevant factors at macro-, meso- and microsystem level. The effects of neighbourhood characteristics on drug use also show conflicting results and suggest a complex interplay between contextual influences, intermediate factors and individual behaviour. The hypothesis that disadvantaged neighbourhoods are a general risk for drug use needs to be considered with caution. With regard to illicit drug use, there is some evidence that neighbourhood disadvantage and neighbourhood disorganisation increase the risk for substance availability and use, but most of this evidence is limited to urban settings in the United States. In relation to alcohol, one can conclude that neighbourhood effects exist, but the direction of the effects differs between countries, neighbourhood setting, population groups and outcomes studied. Research including path analysis indicates that several factors serve as buffers or amplifiers of neighbourhood influences on AOD use. Mediators include family norms and parenting practices as well as availability of alcohol and availability of services. Alcohol consumption is not linked straightforwardly to social class in many Western countries, and poor or disadvantaged neighbourhoods do not necessarily have a high concentration of alcohol outlets (Ellaway et al. 2010). In many countries, shops selling alcohol are more concentrated in poorer neighbourhoods, while bars and restaurants are more concentrated in more advantaged neighbourhoods. Based on this summary of the effects of neighbourhood context on AOD use, we suggest some implications for prevention on macro-, exo- and microsystem levels.

Macrosystem Approaches

It has long been established that interventions which address the 'upstream' determinants of health, such as poverty, unemployment, poor housing, income and education inequality, have the potential to influence population health more profoundly than individually oriented behavioural programmes (Galea et al. 2007a). Research on neighbourhood context as a risk factor for AOD use supports such an approach. Social policies to reduce poverty together with public investments into neighbourhood physical and social capacities and resources have the potential to reduce the harmful effects of neighbourhood contexts and to strengthen protective neighbourhood characteristics. Research indicates that the following neighbourhood characteristics pose a risk for AOD use: the presence of negative role models such as drunken people or visible substance consumption, and a high level of neighbourhood disorganisation indicated by abandoned buildings and other signs of neglect. Other neighbourhood characteristics are likely to protect against AOD use such as a high level of social capital, neighbourhood strength and social cohesion. Social policies at national, regional and local levels have the potential to create neighbourhoods with a more equal level of housing quality, as well as safety and social norms within a given country. In most European countries, particularly in the Scandinavian welfare states, such policies exist and result in less absolute inequalities between rich and poor, although relative differences still exist. As a consequence, European studies do not show the same impact of neighbourhood characteristics on AOD use as seen in most studies based on urban neighbourhoods in the USA.

Exosystem Approaches

Some research on neighbourhood contexts and AOD use inform intervention at the neighbourhood (exosystem) level directly. The positive association between outlet density and alcohol use suggests that reduction of the number of bars, pubs, discos and restaurants together with reducing underage sales of alcohol in these establishments could prove promising (Kuntsche et al. 2008). Law enforcement measures (Waagenar et al. 2005) and training programmes for staff serving alcohol have also been shown to lower adolescent alcohol use (Grube 1997).

Another approach at the neighbourhood level would be community interventions based on participatory and empowerment strategies to strengthen social cohesion and sense of community. Such programmes have been shown to increase social capital and other indictors of community strength (Minkler and Wallerstein 2007). However, evidence is still lacking that such programmes are also effective in reducing AOD use. A community intervention programme in the Netherlands has shown more promising results in increasing fruit consumption than in changing alcohol consumption (Kloek et al. 2006). However, in this programme, the intervention activities have been initiated by the communities in self-directed manners and community activities directed towards reducing alcohol use were not prioritised (Kloek et al. 2006). The lack of effects on alcohol consumption can therefore be explained by a lack of community activities addressing this issue.

Approaches Interacting with Microsystem Factors

While reducing availability acts on neighbourhood context directly, some evidence suggests that neighbourhood context also plays a role when intervening at other levels. For example, a recent cluster randomised controlled trial in nine European centres suggested that a school-based prevention programme had more favourable effects in schools in lower socio-economic neighbourhoods (Caria et al. 2011). While adolescents in schools of low socio-economic level were more likely to report problem drinking at baseline, participation in the programme was associated with lower levels of problem drinking. No significant programme effects were noted for adolescents from schools in more privileged social environments (Caria et al. 2011). Therefore, neighbourhood context can play a role in targeting setting-based interventions towards neighbourhoods with highest vulnerability.

Research on neighbourhood contexts and AOD use indicates that families play an important role in mediating between neighbourhood risks and AOD use among youth (Chuang et al. 2005; Tobler et al. 2009). Programmes to support parents in parenting and monitoring practices in order to strengthen their buffering and preventive effects especially in neighbourhoods with disorganisation characteristics may be beneficial.

References

Agrawal, A., Scherrer, J. F., Lynskey, M. T., Sartor, C. E., Grant, J. D., Haber, J. R., et al. (2011). Patterns of use, sequences of onsets and correlates of tobacco and cannabis. *Addictive Behaviors, 36*, 1141–1147.

Ali, M. M., & Dwyer, D. S. (2009). Estimating peer effects in adolescent smoking behaviour: A longitudinal analysis. *The Journal of Adolescent Health, 45*, 402–408.

Ali, M., & Dwyer, D. (2010). Social network effects in alcohol consumption among adolescents. *Addictive Behaviors, 35*, 337–342.

Andersen, A., Holstein, B. E., & Due, P. (2006). School-related factors for drunkenness among adolescents: Risk factors differ between socio-economic groups. *European Journal of Public Health, 17*(1), 27–32.

Babor, T., Caukins, J., Edwards, G., Fischer, B., Foxcroft, D., Humphreys, K., et al. (2010). *Drug policy and the public good*. Oxford: Oxford University Press.

Bachman, J. G., Wallace, J. M., O'Malley, P. M., Johnston, L. D., Kurth, C. L., & Neighbors, H. S. (1991). Racial/ethnic differences in smoking, drinking and illicit drug use among American high school seniors. *American Journal of Public Health, 81*, 372–377.

Bergmark, K. H., & Andersson, T. (1999). Development of advanced drinking habits in adolescence. *Substance Use & Misuse, 34*, 171–194.

Bjarnason, T., Andersson, B., Choquet, M., Elekes, Z., Morgan, M., & Rapinett, G. (2003). Alcohol cutlure, family structure and adolescent alcohol use: Multilevel modeling of frequency of heavy drinking among 15–16 year old students in 11 European countries. *Journal of Studies on Alcohol, 64*, 200–208.

Bjarnason, T., Davidaviciene, A. G., Miller, P., Nociar, A., Pavlakis, A., & Stergar, E. (2003). Family structure and adolescent cigarette smoking in eleven European countries. *Addiction, 98*, 815–824.

Boardman, J. D., Finch, B. K., Ellison, C. G., Williams, D. R., & Jackson, J. S. (2001). Neighborhood disadvantage, stress, and drug use among adults. *Journal of Health and Social Behavior, 42*(2), 151–165.

Brenner, A. B., Bauermeister, J. A., & Zimmermann, M. A. (2011). Neighbourhood variation in adolescent alcohol use: Examination of sociological and social disorganisation theories. *Journal of Studies on Alcohol and Drugs, 72*, 651–659.

Bryden, A., Roberts, B., McKee, M., & Petticrew, M. A. (2012). Systematic review of the influence on alcohol use of community level availability and marketing of alcohol. *Health & Place, 18*(2), 349–357.

Caria, M. P., Faggiano, F., Belloco, R., & Galanti, M. R. (2011). The influence of socioeconomic environment on the effectiveness of alcohol prevention among European students: A cluster randomized controlled trail. *BMC Public Health, 11*, 312.

Cerdá, M., Diez-Roux, A. V., Tchetgen, E. T., Gordon-Larsen, P., & Kiefe, C. (2010). The relationship between neighborhood poverty and alcohol use: Estimation by marginal structural models. *Epidemiology, 21*(4), 482–489.

Chen, M. J., Grube, J. W., & Gruenewald, P. J. (2010). Community alcohol outlet density and underage drinking. *Addiction, 105*(2), 270–278.

Christakis, N. A., & Fowler, J. H. (2008). The collective dynamics of smoking in a large network. *New England Journal of Medicine, 358*, 2249–2258.

Chuang, Y. C., Ennett, S. T., Bauman, K. E., & Foshee, V. A. (2005). Neighbourhood influences on adolescent cigarette and alcohol use: Mediating effects through parent and peer behaviours. *Journal of Health and Social Behavior, 46*, 187–204.

Chuang, Y. C., Li, Y. S., Wu, Y. H., & Chao, H. J. (2007). A multilevel analysis of neighborhood and individual effects on individual smoking and drinking in Taiwan. *BMC Public Health, 7*, 151.

Clark, A., & Loheac, Y. (2007). It wasn't me, it was them! Social influence in risky behaviour by adolescents. *Journal of Health Economics, 26*, 763–784.

Cornaz, S., Taffé, P., & Santos-Eggimann, B. (2009). Life-course socioeconomic environment and health risk behaviours. A multilevel small-area analysis of young-old persons in an urban neighbourhood in Lausanne, Switzerland. *Health & Place, 15*(1), 273–283.

Crum, R. M., Lillie-Blanton, M., & Anthony, J. C. (1996). Neighbourhood environment and opportunity to use cocaine and other drugs in late childhood and early adolescence. *Drug and Alcohol Dependence, 43*(3), 155–161.

Currie, C., Molcho, M., Boyce, W., Holstein, B., Torsheim, T., & Richter, M. (2008). Research health inequalities in adolescents: The development of the Health Behaviour in School-aged Children (HBSC) Family Affluence Scale. *Social Science & Medicine, 66*(6), 1429–1436.

Degenhart, L., Chiu, W. T., Conway, K., Dierker, L., Glantz, M., Kalaydjian, A., et al. (2009). Does the 'gateway' matter? Associations between the order of drug use initiation and the development of drug dependence in the National comorbidity study replication. *Psychological Medicine, 39*(1), 157–167.

Duncan, S. C., Duncan, T. E., & Stykler, L. A. (2002). A multilevel analysis of neighbourhood context and youth alcohol and drug problems. *Prevention Science, 3*, 125–133.

Ellaway, A., Macdonald, L., Forsyth, A., & Macintyre, S. (2010). The socio-spatial distribution of alcohol outlets in Glasgow city. *Health & Place, 16*(1), 167–172.

Ennett, S. T., Flewelling, R. L., Lindrooth, R. C., & Norton, E. C. (1997). School and neighbourhood characteristics associated with school rates of alcohol, cigarette, and marijuana use. *Journal of Health and Social Behavior, 38*(1), 55–71.

Ennett, S. T., Foshee, V. A., Bauman, K. E., Hussong, A., Cai, L., Reyes, H. L., et al. (2008). The social ecology of adolescent alcohol misuse. *Child Development, 79*(6), 1777–1791.

Fang, J., Madhavan, S., Bosworth, W., & Alderman, M. H. (1998). Residential segregation and mortality in New York City. *Social Science & Medicine, 47*, 469–476.

Furr-Holden, C. D., Campbell, K. D., Milam, A. J., Smart, M. J., Ialongo, N. A., & Leaf, P. J. (2010). Metric properties of the Neighbourhood Inventory for Environmental Typology (NIfETy): An environmental assessment tool for measuring indicators of violence, alcohol, tobacco, and other drug exposures. *Evaluation Review, 34*(3), 159–184.

Furr-Holden, C. D., Lee, M. H., Milam, A. J., Johnson, R. M., Lee, K. S., & Ialongo, N. S. (2011). The growth of neighborhood disorder and marijuana use among urban adolescents: A case for policy and environmental interventions. *Journal of Studies on Alcohol and Drugs, 72*(3), 371–379.

Galea, S., Ahem, J., Tracy, M., Rudenstine, S., & Vlahov, D. (2007a). Education inequality and use of cigarettes, alcohol, and marijuana. *Drug and Alcohol Dependence, 90*(Suppl 1), 4–15.

Galea, S., Ahem, J., Tracy, M., & Vlahov, D. (2007b). Neighbourhood income and income distribution and the use of cigarettes, alcohol, an marijuana. *American Journal of Public Health, 32*(6), 195–202.

Grube, J. W. (1997). Preventing sales of alcohol to minors: Results from a community trial. *Addiction, 92*, 251–260.

Gruenewald, P. J., Johnson, F. W., & Treno, A. J. (2002). Outlets, drinking and driving: A multilevel analysis of availability. *Journal of Studies on Alcohol, 63*(4), 460–468.

Gruenewald, P. J., Millar, A. B., & Treno, A. J. (1993). Alcohol availability and the ecology of drinking behaviour. *Alcohol Health and Research World, 17*, 39–45.
Hanson, M. D., & Chen, E. (2007). Socioeconomic status and health behaviours in adolescence: A review of the literature. *Journal of Behavioral Medicine, 30*, 263–285.
Hawkins, J. D., Catalano, R. F., & Miller, J. Y. (1992). Risk and protective factors for alcohol and other drug use in adolescence and early adulthood: Implications for substance abuse prevention. *Psychological Bulletin, 112*, 64–105.
Hawkins, J. D., Lishner, D. M., Catalano, R. F., & Howard, M. O. (1986). Childhood predictors of adolescent substance abuse: Toward an empirically grounded theory. *Journal of Children in Contemporary Society, 8*, 11–48.
Hibell, B., Guttmormsson, U., Ahlström, S., Balakireva, O., Bjarnason, T., Kokkevi, A., et al. (2009). *The 2007 ESPAD Report Substance use among students in 35 European countries*. Stockholm: The Swedish Council for Information on Alcohol and Other Drugs (CAN).
Kalesan, B., Stine, J., & Alberg, A. J. (2006). The joint influence of parental modeling and positive parental concern on cigarette smoking in middle and high school students. *Journal of School Health, 76*, 402–407.
Kandel, D. B. (1986). Processes of peer influence in adolescence. In R. Silberstein (Ed.), *Development as action in context: Problem behaviour and normal youth development* (pp. 203–228). New York: Springer.
Karvonen, S., & Rimpelä, A. (1996). Socio-regional context as a determinant of adolescents' health behaviour in Finland. *Social Science & Medicine, 43*(10), 1467–1474.
Kawachi, I., Kennedy, B. P., Lochner, K., & Prothrow-Stith, D. (1997). Social capital, income inequality and mortality. *American Journal of Public Health, 87*, 1491–1498.
Kloek, G. C., van Lenthe, F. J., van Nierop, P. W. M., Koelen, M. A., & Mackenbach, J. P. (2006). Impact evaluation of a Dutch community intervention to improve health-related behaviour in deprived neighbourhoods. *Health & Place, 12*, 665–677.
Kokkevi, A. E., Arapaki, A. A., Richardson, C., Florescu, S., Kuzman, M., & Stergar, E. (2007a). Further investigation of psychological and environmental correlates of substance use in adolescence in six European countries. *Drug and Alcohol Dependence, 88*, 308–312.
Kokkevi, A., Richardson, C., Florescu, S., Kuzman, M., & Stergar, E. (2007b). Psychosocial correlates of substance use in adolescence: A cross-national study in sex European countries. *Drug and Alcohol Dependence, 86*, 67–74.
Korf, D. J. (2002). Dutch coffee shops and trends in cannabis use. *Addictive Behaviors, 27*(6), 851–866.
Kuntsche, E., Kuendig, H., & Gmel, G. (2008). Alcohol outlet density, perceived availability and adolescent alcohol use: A multilevel structural equation model. *Journal of Epidemiology and Community Health, 62*, 811–816.
Latkin, C. A., & Curry, A. D. (2003). Stressful neighbourhoods and depression: A prospective study of the impact of neighbourhood disorder. *Journal of Health and Social Behavior, 44*(1), 34–44.
Leventhal, T., & Brooks-Gunn, J. (2000). The neighbourhoods they live in: The effects of neighbourhood residence on child and adolescent outcomes. *Psychological Bulletin, 126*, 309–337.
Leventhal, T., & Brooks-Gunn, J. (2003). Children and youth in neighbourhood contexts. *Current Directions in Psychological Science, 12*, 27–31.
Lundborg, P. (2006). Having the wrong friends? Peer effects in adolescent substance use. *Journal of Health Economics, 25*, 214–233.
Lynch, J., Kaplan, G. A., & Salonen, J. T. (1997). Why do poor people behave poorly? Variation in adult health behaviours and psychological characteristics by stages of the socioeconomic lifecourse. *Social Science & Medicine, 44*(6), 809–819.
Mair, J. S., & Mair, M. (2003). Violence prevention and control through environmental modifications. *Annual Review of Public Health, 24*, 209–225.
Mathers, M., Toumbourou, J. W., Catalano, R. F., Williams, J., & Patton, G. C. (2006). Consequences of youth tobacco use: A review of prospective behavioural studies. *Addiction, 101*, 948–958.

Merikangas, K. R., Mehta, R. L., Molnar, B. E., Walters, E. E., Swendsen, J. D., Aguilar-Gaziola, S., et al. (1998). Comorbidity of substance use disorders with mood and anxiety disorders: Results of the international consortium in psychiatric epidemiology. *Addictive Behaviors, 23*, 893–907.
Miller, P. (1997). Family structure, personality, drinking, smoking and illicit drug use: A study of UK teenagers. *Drug and Alcohol Dependence, 45*, 121–129.
Minkler, M., & Wallerstein, N. (2007). Improving health through community organisation and community building: A health education perspective. In M. Minkler (Ed.), *Community organizing and community building for health* (pp. 26–50). New Brunswick: Rutgers University Press.
Monden, C. W. S., van Lenthe, F. J., & Mackenbach, J. P. (2006). A simultaneous analysis of neighbourhood and childhood socio-economic environment with self-assessed health and health-related behaviours. *Health & Place, 12*, 394–403.
Monshouwer, K., Van Laar, M., & Vollebergh, W. A. (2011). Buying cannabis in "coffee shops". *Drug and Alcohol Review, 30*(2), 148–156.
Newcomb, M. D., Maddahian, E., & Bentler, P. (1986). Risk factors for drug use among adolescents: Concurrent and longitudinal analyses. *American Journal of Public Health, 76*, 525–530.
Poortinga, W. (2006). Do health behaviors mediate the association between social capital and health? *Preventive Medicine, 43*(6), 488–493.
Presley, C. A., Meilman, P. W., & Leichliter, J. S. (2002). College factors that influence drinking. *Journal of Studies on Alcohol, 14*(Suppl), 82–90.
Reifman, A., Barnes, G. M., Dintcheff, B. A., Farrell, M. P., & Uhteg, L. (1998). Parental and peer influences on the onset of heavier drinking among adolescents. *Journal of Studies on Alcohol, 59*, 311–317.
Rhodes, J. E., & Jason, L. A. (1990). A social stress model of substance use. *Journal of Consulting and Clinical Psychology, 58*, 395–401.
Richter, M., Leppin, A., & Gabhainn, S. N. (2006). The relationship between parental socio-economic status and episodes of drunkenness among adolescents: Findings from a cross-national survey. *BMC Public Health, 6*, 289. http://www.biomedcentral.com/1471-2458/6/289.
Rodgers, G. (1979). Income inequality as determinants of mortality: An international cross section analysis. *Population Studies, 31*, 182–191.
Rosenquist, J. N., Murabito, J., Fowler, J. H., & Christakis, N. A. (2010). The spread of alcohol consumption behaviour in a large social network. *Annals of Internal Medicine, 152*, 426–433.
Sampson, J. R., & Groves, W. B. (1989). Community structure and crime: Testing social-disorganisation theory. *The American Journal of Sociology, 94*, 774–802.
Scribner, R. A., Cohen, D. A., & Fisher, W. (2000). Evidence of a structural effect for outlet density: A multilevel analysis. *Alcoholism, Clinical and Experimental Research, 24*(2), 188–195.
Simons-Morton, B. G., Farhat, T., ter Bogt, T. F. M., Hublet, A., Kuntsche, E., Gabhainn, S. N., et al. (2009). Gender specific trends in alcohol use: Cross-cultural comparisons from 1998 to 2006 in 24 countries and regions. *International Journal of Public Health, 54*, 199–208.
Stock, C., Ejstrud, B., Vinther-Larsen, M., Schlattmann, P., Curtis, T., Grønbæk, M., et al. (2011). Effects of school district factors on alcohol consumption: Results of a multi-level analysis among Danish adolescents. *European Journal of Public Health, 21*(4), 449–455.
Stock, C., Mikolajzcyk, R., Bloomfield, K., Maxwell, A. E., Ozebe, H., Petkeviciene, J., et al. (2009). Alcohol consumption and attitudes towards banning alcohol sales on campus among European university students. *Public Health, 123*, 122–129.
Sunder, P. K., Grady, J. J., & Wu, Z. H. (2007). Neighbourhood and individual factors in marijuana and other illicit drug use in a sample of low-income women. *American Journal of Community Psychology, 40*, 167–180.
Tobler, A. L., Komro, K. A., & Maldonado-Molina, M. M. (2009). Relationship between neighbourhood context, family management practices and alcohol, use among urban, multi-ethnic, young adolescents. *Prevention Science, 10*(4), 313–324.

Waagenar, A. C., Toomey, T. L., & Erickson, D. J. (2005). Preventing youth access to alcohol: Outcomes from a multi-community time-series trial. *Addiction, 100*, 335–345.

Weitzman, E. R., Folkman, A., Folkman, M. P., & Wechsler, H. (2003). The relationship of alcohol outlet density to heavy and frequent drinking and drinking-related problems among college students at eight universities. *Health & Place, 9*(1), 1–6.

Wicki, M., Kuntsche, E., & Gmel, G. (2010). Drinking at European universities? A review of students' alcohol use. *Addictive Behaviours, 35*, 913–924.

Wilson, J. Q., & Kelling, G. L. (1982). Broken windows: The police and neighbourhood safety. *Atlantic Monthly, 211*, 29–38.

Winstanley, E. L., Steinwachs, D. M., Ensminger, M. E., Latkin, C. A., Stitzler, M. L. & Olsen, Y. (2008). The association of self-reported neighborhood disorganization and social capital with adolescent alcohol use and drug use, dependence, and access to treatment. *Drug and Alcohol Dependence, 92*, 173–182.

Chapter 16
Neighbourhoods and Healthy Nutrition

Fiona Crawford

Influences on Food Choices and Nutrition

Introduction

The contemporary Scottish diet is widely regarded as unhealthy and a risk factor for a number of chronic diseases including cancer, diabetes and cardiovascular disease. Poor diet in Scotland is also thought to be a contributor to the growing prevalence of obesity amongst all age groups. Levels of obesity in Scotland have been rising even faster than in comparable countries. The Scottish Public Health Observatory reported in 2007 that the prevalence of obesity in Scotland was now one of the highest in the developed world, second only to the USA and higher than Mexico, Canada, the UK and Australia (Scottish Public Health Observatory 2007). Obesity is also seen as a serious public health issue at a UK level. The Foresight report, produced by an expert working group in order 'to produce a long-term vision of how we can deliver a sustainable response to obesity in the UK over the next 40 years', estimated that, unless urgent action was taken, economic costs attributable to obesity at a UK level would rise from £15.8 billion in 2007 to £49.9 billion by 2050 (Foresight 2007).

There are a large and growing number of research studies using increasingly sophisticated methodologies to explore the relationship between neighbourhood environments and eating behaviour. The evidence presented in this section will focus primarily on UK and European evidence rather than that from the USA or Australia as there are distinct geographical, political, commercial, social and cultural differences between the two continents in relation to planning, distribution and usage of food retail outlets.

F. Crawford (✉)
Glasgow Centre for Population Health, House 6, 1st Floor, 94 Elmbank Street,
Glasgow G2 4DL, Scotland
e-mail: Fiona.Crawford@glasgow.gov.uk

C. Stock and A. Ellaway (eds.), *Neighbourhood Structure and Health Promotion*,
DOI 10.1007/978-1-4614-6672-7_16,

Equitable Access to Healthy Food

For over a century, access to healthy food at an affordable price has been recognised as important for good nutrition, particularly in disadvantaged communities, and there have been a number of studies exploring and assessing potential facilitators and barriers to healthy nutrition. The concept of 'food deserts' became prominent in the late twentieth century in the UK to describe deprived urban neighbourhoods where there were thought to be few retail food outlets and therefore poorer access to healthy, affordable foodstuffs than in more affluent neighbourhoods. The concept was widely disseminated and incorporated into various government policies on nutrition, inequalities in health and social exclusion. Although some UK research has supported the view that deprived areas provide less access to health-promoting amenities, including healthy, low-cost food (Swinburn et al. 2004; Taylor et al. 2006; Clark et al. 2002), an increasing number of other UK studies have found very little evidence that areas with large proportions of deprived residents have poor access to retail food outlets (Cummins and Macintyre 1999, 2002a, b; White et al. 2004). Researchers in the field have suggested that the concept of food deserts is a 'factoid', an assertion that is repeated so often that it becomes accepted as true (Cummins and Macintyre 2002a, b).

However, as well as considering concrete empirical evidence in exploring access to healthy, accessible foodstuffs, it has been proposed that it is important to include consideration of socio-economic and cultural contexts, rural/urban planning issues and the design of the built environment (Macintyre 2007). A study exploring people's food shopping practices in four socially contrasting neighbourhoods in Glasgow found that, despite the fact that most grocery shopping was done in supermarkets, poorer people and those living in poorer neighbourhoods were more likely than more affluent people to buy basic foods such as bread, milk, fruit and vegetables in local shops where prices were generally higher and quality of such items often poorer (Ellaway and Macintyre 2000). One proposed explanation was that families opted to shop little and often at local grocery stores because they did not have the financial resources to bulk-buy from large supermarkets (Dobson et al. 1994). Other questions have been posed as to whether locating supermarkets in deprived neighbourhoods meets demand in the locality as these supermarkets may be patronised by customers from richer areas not by local people who do not regard the facilities to be 'for them'. Research conducted in Glasgow exploring usage of a newly opened large chain supermarket in a poor neighbourhood in Glasgow found the main beneficiaries to be people from outside the area rather than local residents who continued to shop in smaller local shops (Cummins et al. 2005, 2008).

Other English research concluded that access to food, healthy or otherwise, was predicated on proximity of outlet, price, desirability and peer pressure/prevailing social norms so consideration of the built environment in exploring food intake was necessary but insufficient to understand eating behaviour (Hackett et al. 2008). Shaw has proposed that 'ability', 'asset' and 'attitude' problems present specific barriers to a healthy diet (Shaw 2006). 'Ability problems' are anything that physically prevents access to food which a consumer can afford and would like to purchase; 'asset problems' arise from a lack of financial means and storage/cooking facilities which she or he can otherwise physically access and would like to consume; and 'attitude' problems' are any state of mind that prevents an individual from accessing foods she or he is able to purchase and can otherwise bring into the home.

Takeaway Food

The amount of food and drinks purchased and consumed from takeaway food outlets is on the increase. Market value of the fast-food/takeaway and home-delivery sector in the UK reached £10.8 billion by 2005 and is predicted to continue rising (Keynote 2006). There is clear evidence that takeaway foods are less healthy than food prepared in the home (Astrup 2005). The UK National Consumer Council investigated the nutritional content of takeaway meals and associated nutrition information available to consumers in seven major chain takeaway restaurants (National Consumer Council 2008). Results showed that the nutrition content of meals was often high in salt, saturated fat and sugar and, although nutrition information was available in some outlets, it was often hard to find and difficult to understand. The Consumer Council recommended that takeaway outlets make clear, effective, understandable nutritional information more widely available to customers along with healthier options.

Evidence is mixed as to whether or not there are higher concentrations of takeaway food outlets in deprived or affluent neighbourhoods. One study which analysed data on population, deprivation and the location of McDonald's restaurants (fast-food outlets) in Scotland and England found that there were greater numbers of outlets in deprived than affluent areas (Cummins et al. 2005). An observational study conducted in Leeds found that children living in areas of higher deprivation had more fast-food outlets in their local area and lived closer to fast-food outlets than less deprived children (Fraser et al. 2010). In contrast, a study of out-of-home outlets and area deprivation in Glasgow, Scotland, found no evidence that out-of-home outlets, takeaways or fast-food chain restaurants were more likely to be found in more deprived areas of Glasgow (Macintyre et al. 2005). The research team concluded that 'Further critical evaluation of the role of access to foods eaten outside the home in the aetiology of obesity is warranted. This relationship may well be more complex than simple proximity to an outlet, and may vary with macro and more local cultural and socioeconomic factors' (Macintyre et al. 2005, p.6).

A semi-systematic review of the geography of fast-food outlets (Fraser et al. 2010) found a positive association between proximity and density of fast-food outlets and increasing deprivation. The research team speculated that this might be due to companies targeting more deprived areas as the land was cheaper or that demand from consumers in these areas was greater. Either way, they regarded this as an important issue to highlight to policymakers as it was pertinent to land use planning and licensing decisions.

Food Poverty

Food poverty has been defined as the inability to obtain healthy affordable food. This has obvious implications for healthy nutrition. Research conducted in 2002 documented the circumstances of low-income consumers that limited their access to an adequate diet. The researchers concluded that achieving a nutritious diet on a low income required extraordinary levels of persistence, flexibility and awareness (Hitchman et al. 2002). There is also evidence that low-income households in the UK may commonly experience 'food insecurity', which has previously been described as 'limited or uncertain availability of nutritionally adequate safe foods, or limited or uncertain ability to acquire foods in socially acceptable ways' (Life Sciences Research Office 1990, p.1560). Experiences of food insecurity that have been cited include running out of food, running out of money to buy food, skipping meals, experiencing hunger and being unable to buy food or buying cheaper foods because of financial constraints (Tingay et al. 2003).

Whilst many poor adults, especially women, adopt coping strategies such as strict budgeting, using local discount stores and not risking unfamiliar foods for fear of waste (Beardsworth and Keil 1997), a particular area of significance is around children's diets. Many parents/carers on low incomes find contemporary food culture in relation to children a challenge or constant source of anxiety (Dowler 2002). Many children are susceptible to marketing strategies that promote foods that are high in fat, sugar and salt. Food is the largest category of product advertised to children and accounts for about 40 % of advertising during children's programming. A systematic review on the effects of food promotion to children (Hastings et al. 2003) concluded that targeted advertising by the 'big five' of pre-sugared breakfast cereals, soft drinks, confectionery, savoury snacks and fast-food restaurants influenced what children claimed to like, what they bought and what they ate.

The Policy Context

Introduction

Public health/health improvement strategies, policies and programmes to promote healthy nutrition are regarded as having important potential in the successful promotion of healthy eating although the evidence of their effectiveness is uncertain unless robust evaluation of their impact accompanies delivery. Evaluation of impact in this arena is not straightforward as measures to promote healthy nutrition are multifaceted and complex. Some nutritional interventions, such as school meals legislation, have been described as 'natural experiments' (Medical Research Council 2011) which present methodological challenges in evaluation but which are regarded as having a great deal to offer.

In recognition of the importance of healthy eating, the World Health Organisation has published a *Global Strategy on Diet, Physical Activity and Health*, which has been adopted by all member states (World Health Organisation 2004). The overall aim of this strategy is to substantially reduce deaths and disease worldwide by improving diet and promoting physical activity. At its outset, the document outlines a number of relevant and important principles that it recommends strategies, policies and programmes should incorporate in the promotion of healthy diets and nutrition. These principles include adoption of:

- Comprehensive, multi-sectoral approaches based on the best available scientific research and evidence, which take a life-course perspective and which are part of broader, comprehensive and coordinated public health efforts.
- Involvement of all sectors of society in a multidisciplinary and participative way, recognising the complex interactions between personal choice, social norms and economic and environmental factors.
- Inequality sensitive practice, i.e. activities should be prioritised that have a positive impact on the poorest population groups and communities; also, programmes and initiatives should be sensitive to gender and cultural differences.

At a UK level, in recognition of the importance of a healthy diet for good cardiovascular health, the National Institute for Health and Clinical Excellence (NICE) has produced evidence-based guidelines for the prevention of cardiovascular disease (NICE 2010). Recommendations make direct reference to the need for food producers and caterers to reduce salt, saturated fats and trans fats in everyday foods. The guidance calls for much wider restrictions on marketing and promotions of unhealthy foods and drinks aimed at children and young people, clear product labelling of packaged foods using a simple traffic light system as proposed by the Food Standards Agency (Kelly et al. 2009) and use of local government licensing and planning powers to control numbers and density of food retail outlets in specific areas, such as near schools.

Scottish Nutrition Policy

During the 1990s, in response to growing evidence and widespread concern regarding poor nutrition and its impacts on population health in Scotland, a major national policy on diet was published by the Scottish Office—*The Scottish Diet Action Plan* (The Scottish Office 1996). The plan made a number of recommendations aiming to improve consumer understanding and behaviour in relation to healthy eating and to work with the food industry to encourage measures that would promote the accessibility and popularity of healthy foods and drinks on sale in commercial outlets. A ten-year timescale was set for a number of dietary targets. A subsequent review of this policy (Lang et al. 2006) concluded that dietary targets set for 2005 had not been met and that population trends in food consumption and nutrient intake over the previous ten years were largely moving in the wrong direction. The authors presented a number of plausible explanations including:

- An underestimation of the impact of inequalities and too thin a spread of resources and initiatives across a broad range of actions rather than a focus on achieving population level impact within a few priority areas (i.e. a scattergun approach)
- The use of a wholly consensual partnership approach to 'working with' the food industry, underplaying the powerful role of the food supply chain in shaping food content, access, availability and consumer demand
- Little use of regulation and legislation to control the food supply chain and help generate demand
- The need for more effective alignment of institutions and leadership across stakeholders involved in the food supply chain

The evaluation panel concluded that the direction of policy on food, diet and nutrition needed a serious rethink if Scotland's dietary trends were to improve, stating that:

> 'If Scotland's current dietary trends continue they will remain a contributing factor to its poor relative position on health within the UK and Western Europe, with a toll of unnecessary premature death, longstanding illness and dental ill-health' (Lang et al. 2006).

Following this lack of success in achieving better nutrition in Scotland, during the last decade, several further policies and plans have been published, driven by converging policy agendas in relation to poor nutrition in many population groups in Scotland, steadily increasing prevalence of obesity in children and adults and calls for greater sustainability and ecological responsibility in relation to food production and consumption. Policies and plans have included *Eating for Health—meeting the Challenge*, published in 2004, a strategic framework produced by the Scottish Executive intended to develop food and health policy and to guide national and local health action plans (Scottish Executive 2004); *Healthy Eating, Active Living (08–11)*, published in 2008, the Scottish Government's action plan to improve diet, increase physical activity and tackle obesity (Scottish Government 2008); and, most recently, *Preventing Overweight and Obesity in Scotland: A route map towards healthy weight* (Scottish Government 2010a), which sets out plans and actions to prevent obesity at a population level including priorities regarding energy consumption that include measures to control exposure to foods that are high in energy.

School Food Policy

School food policy has been recognised for over a century in the UK as being important for the promotion of healthy nutrition amongst children and young people. Legislation to provide a universal school meals service introduced in England and Wales in 1906 and in Scotland in 1908 was a direct response to concern around levels of malnourishment identified in many young recruits for the Boer War (Gillard 2003). School meals were provided by local authorities until the onset of the First World War when the service declined due to economic pressures. Following the Second World War, partly due to rationing and state-provided meals, people in Britain were reputedly better nourished than at any time in history. Legislation has continued to impact on school meals provision. The *1980 Education (Scotland) Act* (UK Government 1980) removed the obligation of local authorities to provide school meals and only required them to provide meals for children whose parents claimed supplementary benefit or family income supplement. The act also abolished the minimum nutritional standards that controlled the quality of school meals and the fixed price 'national charge for school meals' leading to an erosion of standards of quality of meals as well as unregulated costs.

Now, at the beginning of the twenty-first century, nutritional standards and subsidised, fixed price charges for school meals have been reintroduced, initially under *Hungry for Success* (Scottish Executive 2003) and subsequently through *The Schools (Nutrition and Health Promotion) (Scotland) Act* (Scottish Parliament 2007). *Hungry for Success*, the report of the Scottish Executive's expert panel on school meals, set out a vision for a revitalised school meals service in Scotland. It provided national guidelines and standards for school meals in primary and secondary schools across Scotland calling for a whole-child, whole-school approach to food, complementing the current government commitment to make all schools health-promoting institutions. It also recommended that nutrient standards for school meals be established, better links be made between the curriculum and food provision in schools, stigma for free-meal recipients be eliminated, partnership working in the planning and delivery of school meals be strengthened and improvements be made to the physical and social environment in schools. *The Schools (Nutrition and Health Promotion) (Scotland) Act* has built on *Hungry for Success* to embed school-based provision and promotion of healthy food and drinks into legislation introducing statutory nutritional standards and requirements with which all educational establishments must comply.

Evaluating the Impact of Healthy School Food Policy

Research conducted in Glasgow to evaluate the impact of policies and legislation aiming to improve the school lunchtime environment and raise school meal standards shows that they have had a positive impact on pupils' attitudes and behaviour in relation to healthy eating, particularly within the primary school sector; healthy eating initiatives and programmes have been well received by pupils, parents and school staff (GCPH 2007a). However, in contrast to the primary school sector, changes to school food policy and practice within secondary schools have been much more difficult. Increasing numbers of secondary school pupils across Scotland are leaving school premises at lunchtime to purchase food and drinks from high street outlets and mobile vans (Scottish Government 2010a, b). Further qualitative research, facilitated by the Glasgow Centre for Population Health, recommended that lunchtime ‘stay-on-site’ policies for junior secondary pupils be tested out in order to encourage pupils to stay within the school grounds at lunchtime (GCPH 2007b). An evaluation of the impact of these ‘stay-on-site’ policies concluded that they offer multiple benefits for junior secondary pupils which not only relate to healthy eating but also include increased safety, support with the transition from primary to secondary school and the establishment of good relationships between school staff and pupils and between pupils themselves (GCPH 2012). However, the research highlighted staff and parental/carers concerns about the presence of commercial outlets in the vicinity of schools utilising marketing/promotional strategies to encourage pupils to buy unhealthy, convenience food and drinks.

Recent analysis exploring numbers and density of food outlets near secondary schools in Glasgow by Ellaway and colleagues (Ellaway et al. 2012) has found that there is an average of 35 food outlets per secondary school where energy dense foods can be purchased at lunchtime. The research team concluded that the environment around Glasgow schools provides ample opportunities to purchase takeaway food options and ease of access appears to be similar between affluent and deprived areas. As has already been discussed, the nutritional quality of takeaway foods available to school pupils is also questionable. A pilot study conducted in 2011 assessed the quality of popular foods purchased by pupils from outlets near secondary schools against Scottish nutrient standards for school lunches (GCPH 2012). Approximately half of the samples exceeded recommended energy levels; over a half exceeded recommended fat and saturated fat levels and over a third exceeded recommended salt levels. Thirty-seven of the 45 savoury food items sampled did not comply with one or more of the nutrient standards for fat, saturated fat and salt. Given the fact that a number of pupils were observed augmenting savoury food items with sweetened carbonated drinks, crisps and confectionery, it is likely that their lunchtime energy, fat and salt consumption will be even greater than that revealed by the nutritional analysis. These two studies provide clear evidence that neighbourhoods around secondary schools provide and promote access to unhealthy food and drinks, effectively undermining efforts school-based healthy eating policies and programmes. Given the growing concerns about poor nutrition and rising levels of obesity amongst children and young people in Scotland, there is an urgent need for effective measures to tackle this issue.

Food Policies for Healthy Urban Neighbourhoods

There are a number of potential regulatory levers out with the school setting that could help restrict exposure to unhealthy foods and drinks and benefit children, young people and adults alike (Scottish Collaboration for Public Health Research and Policy 2011). Evidence is growing that health-related food taxes can improve population health, particularly if accompanied by subsidies on healthy foods (Mytton et al. 2012). Sales tax on sugared drinks, sweets and snacks has been introduced in the USA, Australia and in several European countries (Andreyeva et al. 2010). Politicians in the UK have called for the introduction of taxes on unhealthy food and drinks to be considered to help tackle growing obesity levels (Guardian Website 2012). Modelling studies predict that a 20 % tax on sugared drinks in the USA would reduce the overall prevalence of obesity by 3.5 % (Hall et al. 2011).

The challenge for governments in creating healthy food policy is that it cuts across departmental boundaries. The Foresight report on obesity pointed out that although health services pick up the costs of obesity, many of the policy levers for change lie outside its jurisdiction; the same applies for other diet-related diseases (Foresight 2007). Therefore, system-wide action is necessary.

Conclusions

The idea that what we eat affects our health is almost too obvious to state, but it is becoming very clear that twenty-first century food policies and eating habits are damaging our health. The food industry has been cited as a major contributor to this problem—global food markets are promoting overconsumption, in developed (and increasingly developing) countries, of food and drinks that are calorific and high in fat, sugar and salt. UK and European policies on diet have relied heavily on more and better education for consumers to make healthy choices, based on the notion that consumer behaviour will shape markets but as well as education and information, governance mechanisms are needed for pricing, marketing, promotion and more equitable availability of healthy foods. There is some evidence that deprived communities are more exposed to unhealthy food and drinks through a combination of economic, social and cultural influences. Many governments worldwide are beginning to realise the enormity of the challenge of addressing poor nutrition and growing prevalence of obesity. In 2011, the United Nations released a political declaration emphasising the need for the implementation of multi-sectoral, cost-effective, population-wide interventions in order to reduce the impact of unhealthy diets and other causes of non-communicable disease (United Nations 2011).

The message is clear—single issue solutions will not work. In their discussion of how to overcome policy cacophony on obesity (a consequence of an unhealthy diet), Lang and Rayner propose that change will only be achieved by ‘big thinking, many changes’ (Lang and Rayner 2007, page 178). They argue that coherence and optimism with firm political leadership across government, supply chains and civil society is essential.

To conclude, if healthy nutrition across our neighbourhoods is to become a reality, a range of factors and influences at local, regional, national and global level need to be considered and addressed. This will not happen overnight, but progress in this arena will yield enormous dividends in relation to future population health. In the words of Susan Jebb, an expert in the field: ‘Food policy is a matter for everyone and needs partnerships and alliances at all levels to drive change—individuals making choices for themselves and their families, communities and local government taking action, businesses acting responsibly, and government leading and coordinating action across departments and sectors' (Jebb 2012, p. 11).

References

Andreyeva, T., Long, M. W., & Brownell, K. D. (2010). The impact of food prices on consumption: A systematic review of research on the price elasticity of demand for food. *American Journal of Public Health, 100*, 216–222.

Astrup, A. (2005). Supersized and diabetic by frequent fast food consumption? *Lancet, 365*, 4–5.

Beardsworth, A., & Keil, T. (1997). *Sociology on the Menu*. London: Routledge.

Clark, G., Eyre, H., & Guy, C. (2002). Deriving indicators of access to food retail provision in British cities: Studies of Cardiff, Leeds and Bradford. *Urban Studies, 39*, 2041–2060.

Cummins, S., Findlay, A., Petticrew, M., & Sparks, L. (2008). Reducing inequalities in health and diet: The impact of food retail development. *Environment and Planning A, 40*(2), 402–422.

Cummins, S., & Macintyre, S. (1999). The location of food stores in urban areas: A case study in Glasgow. *British Food Journal, 101*(7), 545–553.

Cummins, S., & Macintyre, S. (2002a). A systematic study of an urban food-scape: The price and availability of food in greater Glasgow. *Urban Studies, 39*(11), 2115–2130.

Cummins, A., & Macintyre, S. (2002b). 'Food deserts'—evidence and assumption in health policy making. *BMJ, 325*, 436–438.

Cummins, S., Petticrew, M., Higgins, C., Findlay, A., & Sparks, L. (2005). Large scale food retailing as an intervention for diet and health: Quasi-experimental evaluation of a natural experiment. *Journal of Epidemiology and Community Health, 59*, 1035–1104.

Dobson, A., Beardsworth, T., Keil, T., & Walker, R. (1994). *Diet, choice and poverty: Social cultural and nutritional aspects of food consumption among low-income families*. Loughborough: Family Policy Studies Centre.

Dowler, E. (2002). Food and poverty in Britain: Rights and responsibilities. *Social Policy & Administration, 36*(6), 698–717.

Ellaway, A., Macdonald, L., Lamb, K., Day, P., Thornton, L., & Pearce, J. (2012). Do obesity-promoting food environments cluster around socially disadvantaged schools in Glasgow? *Health & Place, 18*(6), 1335–1340.

Ellaway, A., & Macintyre, S. (2000). Shopping for food in socially contrasting localities. *British Food Journal, 102*(1), 52–59.

Fraser, L. K., Edwards, K. L., Cade, J., & Clarke, P. C. (2010). The geography of fast food outlets: A review. *International Journal of Environmental Research and Public Health, 7*, 2290–2308.

GCPH. (2007a). *Healthy Food Provision and Promotion in Primary School: What impact is it having on food choices?* Glasgow: GCPH.

GCPH. (2007b). *Healthy food provision and promotion in primary and secondary school. Impacts in school and beyond.* Glasgow: GCPH.

GCPH. (2012). *Are school lunchtime stay-on-site policies sustainable? A follow-up study.* Glasgow: GCPH.

Gillard, D. (2003). Food for thought: Child nutrition, the school dinner and the food industry. http://www.educationengland.org.uk/articles/22food.html. Accessed May 2012.

Government Office for Science. Foresight. (2007). Tackling obesities: future choices. Project report. http://www.bis.gov.uk/foresight/our-work/projects/published-projects/tackling-obesities/reports-and-publications. Accessed June 2012.

Guardian Website. (2012). UK could introduce 'fat tax', says David Cameron. http://www.guardian.co.uk/politics/2011/oct/04/uk-obesity-tax-david-cameron. Accessed May 2012.

Hackett, L., BoddyL, B. J., Dummer, T. F. B., Johnson, B., & Stratton, G. (2008). Mapping dietary habits may provide clues about the factors that determine food choice. *Journal of Human Nutrition and Dietetics, 2008*(21), 428–437.

Hall, K. D., Sacks, G., Chandramohan, D., Chow, C. C., Wang, Y. C., Gortmaker, S. L., et al. (2011). Quantification of the effect of energy imbalance on bodyweight. *Lancet, 378*, 826–837.

Hastings, G., Stead, M., McDermott, L., Forsyth, A., MacKintosh, A., Raynor, M., et al. (2003). *Review of research on the effects of food promotion to children*. London: Food Standards Agency.

Hitchman, C., Christie, I., Harrison, M., & Lang, T. (2002). *Inconvenience food. The struggle to eat well on a low income*. London: Demos.

Jebb, S. (2012). A system-wide challenge for UK food policy. *BMJ, 344*, e3414.

Kelly, B., Hughes, C., Chapman, K., Louie, J. C.-Y., Dixon, H., Crawford, J., et al. (2009). Consumer testing of the acceptability and effectiveness of front-of-pack food labelling systems for the Australian grocery market. *Health Promotion International, 24*(2), 120–129.

Keynote. (2006). UK fast food and home delivery outlets. http://www.reportlinker.com/p040211-summary/UK-Fast-Food-Home-Delivery-Outlets.html. Accessed Dec 2011.

Lang, T., Barling, D., & Caraher, M. (2009). *Food policy*. Oxford: Oxford University Press.

Lang, T., Dowler, E., & Hunter, D. (2006). *Review of the Scottish Diet Action Plan: Progress and impacts 1996–2005*. Edinburgh: NHS Health Scotland.

Life Sciences Research Office, Federation of American Societies for Experimental Biology. (1990). Core indicators of nutritional state for difficult-to-sample populations. *Journal of Nutrition, 120*(suppl), 1559–1600.

Lang, T., & Rayner, G. (2007). Overcoming policy cacophony on obesity: an ecological public health framework for policy-makers. *Obesity reviews, 8*(1 Suppl) 165–181.

Macintyre, S. (2007). Deprivation amplification revisited; or, is it always true that poorer places have poorer access to resources for healthy diets and physical activity? *International Journal of Behavioral Nutrition and Physical Activity*. doi:10.1186/1479-5868-4-32.

Macintyre, S., McKay, L., Cummins, S., & Burns, C. (2005). Out-of-home food outlets and area deprivation: A case study in Glasgow, UK. *International Journal of Behavioral Nutrition and Physical Activity, 2*, 16. doi:10.1186/1479-5868-2-16.

Medical Research Council. (2011). Using natural experiments to evaluate population health interventions. http://www.mrc.ac.uk/naturalexperimentsguidance. Accessed June 2012.

Mytton, O., Clarke, D., & Rayner, M. (2012). Taxing unhealthy food and drinks to improve health. *BMJ, 344*, 1–7.

National Institute for Health and Clinical Excellence. (2010). Prevention of Cardiovascular Disease: quick reference guide. http://guidance.nice.org.uk/PH25/QuickRefGuide/pdf/English. Accessed November 2011.

National Consumer Council. (2008). *Takeaway Foods; how takeaway foods can affect your choice of a healthy diet*. London: National Consumer Council.

Scottish Collaboration for Public Health Research and Policy. (2011). *Policy interventions to tackle the obesogenic environment. Focusing on adults of working age in Scotland*. Edinburgh: Scottish Collaboration for Public Health Research and Policy.

Scottish Executive's Expert Panel on School Meals. (2003). Hungry for Success: A Whole School Approach to School Meals in Scotland. Edinburgh: HMSO.

Scottish Public Health Observatory. (2007). *Obesity in Scotland: An epidemiological briefing*. Edinburgh: ScotPHO.

Scottish Parliament. (2007). *Schools (Nutrition and Health Promotion) (Scotland) Act*. Edinburgh: HMSO.

Shaw, H. J. (2006). Food deserts: Towards the development of a classification. *Geografiska Annaler Series B-Human Geography, 88B*, 231–247.

Swinburn, B., Caterson, I., Seidall, J., & James, W. (2004). Diet, nutrition and prevention of excess weight gain and obesity. *Public Health Nutrition, 7*(1(A)), 123–146.

Taylor, W. C., Poston, C., Jones, L., & Kraft, M. K. (2006). Environmental justice: Obesity, physical activity and healthy eating. *Journal of Physical Activity and Health, 3*(I), S30–S54.

The Scottish Government. (2008). Healthy eating, active living: An action plan to improve diet, increase physical activity and tackle obesity (2008–2011). http://www.scotland.gov.uk/Publications/2008/06/20155902/0. Accessed July 2008.

The Scottish Executive. (2004). *Eating for health - meeting the challenge*. Edinburgh: Scottish Executive.

The Scottish Government. (2010a). Preventing overweight and obesity in Scotland: A route map towards healthy weight. http://www.scotland.gov.uk/Publications/2010/02/17140721/0. Accessed May 2010.

The Scottish Government. (2010b). *School meals in Scotland 2010*. Edinburgh: The Scottish Government.

The Scottish Office. (1996). *Scotland's health a challenge to us all. Eating for Health. A diet action plan for Scotland*. Edinburgh: The Scottish Office Department of Health.

Tingay, R. S., Tan, C. J., Tan, N. C.-W., Tang, S., Teoh, P. F., Wong, R., et al. (2003). Food insecurity and low income in an English inner city. *Journal of Public Health Medicine, 25*(2), 156–159.

UK Government. (1980). *1980 Education (Scotland) Act*. London: HMSO.

United Nations General Assembly. (2011). Political declaration of the high-level meeting of the general assembly on the prevention and control of non-communicable diseases. http://www.ncdalliance.org/sites/default/files/UN%20Political%20Declaration%20on%20NCDs.pdf. Accessed June 2012.

White, M., Williams, E., Raybould, S., Adamson, A., Bunting, J., & Mathers, J. (2004). *Do food deserts exist? A multi-level geographical analysis of the relationship between retail food access, socio-economic position and dietary intake. (Final report to Food Standards Agency)*. Newcastle: School of Population and Health Sciences, University of Newcastle upon Tyne.

World Health Organisation. (2004). Global strategy on diet, physical activity and health. http://www.who.int/dietphysicalactivity/strategy/eb11344/strategy_english_web.pdf. Accessed Dec 2011.

Chapter 17
School Neighbourhoods and Obesity Prevention in Youth

Chalida Svastisalee

Introduction

Schools are important environments for children and adolescents. In many parts of the world, children spend more than 6 h per day in school on average or approximately 195 days per year (Rahman et al. 2011; Euridice Network 2010, 2011). Not only do they spend a great deal of time in school, young people are more likely to be bound to the neighbourhood areas surrounding their schools, unlike adults who may travel further distances between the home and the workplace. The reasons for this include attendance in schools within catchment areas that are in close proximity to the home or participation in extracurricular activities at school (Feldman and Matjasko 2005, 2007). Another factor may be that parents restrict how far their child travels due to fears over traffic exposure (Cole et al. 2007; Villanueva et al. 2012) or personal safety (Cole et al. 2007; Jago et al. 2009; McDonald et al. 2010; Faulkner et al. 2010). Thus, schools and their underlying neighbourhoods serve as important living environments for youth.

Due to the substantial amount of time children spend in school, it has become natural for health specialists to use schools as platforms for the promotion of healthy lifestyle practices. While there are many scientific and professional investigations that have focused on health promotion programmes *within* schools, this chapter will focus on the physical and structural resources in neighbourhoods surrounding schools and how they may impact the health and health behaviours of the children and adolescents who attend them. Evidence addressing the relationship between social characteristics (either at the individual or neighbourhood levels) and built environment exposure is still emerging (Boone-Heinonen et al. 2010b; Charreire

C. Svastisalee (✉)
National Institute of Public Health, University of Southern Denmark,
Øster Farimagsgade 5A 2, DK-1353 Copenhagen, Denmark

Metropolitan University College, Pustervig 8, 1126 Copenhagen K, Denmark
e-mail: chsv@si-folkesundhed.dk; cams@phmetropol.dk

C. Stock and A. Ellaway (eds.), *Neighbourhood Structure and Health Promotion*,
DOI 10.1007/978-1-4614-6672-7_17,

et al. 2010) and will also not be addressed in this chapter. However, in the future, examinations of these interactions may help us further our understanding of how place contributes to health inequalities among youth.

Another reason why emphasis is based on schools and surrounding environments is that there is a broad policy and scientific interest in examining to what extent schools contribute to child health. This chapter is not meant to be an exhaustive summary, but will highlight some of the primary research study areas aimed at examining built environments of school communities and child health, such as dietary behaviour, active transport, physical activity and obesity. While scholarly and policy-oriented work regarding alcohol and tobacco outlet exposure surrounding schools is also a relevant area of study for child and adolescent health (Pasch et al. 2009; Ogneva-Himmelberger et al. 2011; Stock et al. 2011), this chapter will focus on predictors of obesity due to the urgency placed within both public policy and urban planning (Popkin et al. 2005; Sallis and Glanz 2006; Slater et al. 2007; Yancey et al. 2007; Maziak et al. 2008; Stanley and Daube 2009) to optimize school settings for obesity prevention (Ashe et al. 2007; Jaime and Lock 2009; Story et al. 2009; Sallis and Glanz 2009). In closing, this chapter will also highlight potential contributions of school environments within obesity prevention policy.

Measures of Built Environments

Although the school may be one frame of reference within health-based research that defines a specific place-based context, there are still many ways to delineate where school boundaries should be placed. The identification of neighbourhood size is important because it may determine the strength of associations between levels of neighbourhood exposure and the health outcome of interest (Boone-Heinonen et al. 2010c; Ding et al. 2011). Another struggle in examining the relationship between place and health is in developing standards for GIS-based measures, which, as they are currently in constant development, still makes it difficult to make cross-comparisons between countries. In the body of literature reviewed in this chapter, scholars have defined the size of school neighbourhoods in many ways. Due to the ease and availability of information aggregated for census purposes, initial studies classically defined school neighbourhoods within administrative units, such as school districts (Sallis et al. 1996), school postal codes (Kipke et al. 2007; Powell et al. 2007a, b) or other census boundaries (Powell and Bao 2009). School neighbourhoods have also been defined by locational measures such as circular radii (buffer zones) where the school or the home serves as the central measure of focus (Pate et al. 2008; Sturm 2008; van der Horst et al. 2008; Charreire et al. 2010). Presentation of neighbourhoods in this manner has typically approached exposure to resources such as food outlets by expressions of density (Charreire et al. 2010).

Another way that school surroundings have been conceptualized is by distance measure, which may be expressed by travel time, by straight-line distances or by travel network (Charreire et al. 2010). With the increased use of locational positioning via Global Positioning Systems (GPS), especially for physical activity studies, the school is represented as one destination or one of many along a particular street network. The advantage of this method may be a more realistic reflection of typical travel from one place to another (Wiehe et al. 2008a, b; Jones et al. 2009; Cooper et al. 2010; Troped et al. 2010; Rodriguez et al. 2011) and indicates to what extent study participants use their community surroundings.

Given the differences in defining neighbourhoods and measures of exposure, comparability of studies is difficult, prompting requests for more detailed methodology (Ding et al. 2011) and until standardization of measures is reached (Feng et al. 2010), then expression of neighbourhood measures using multiple distances (Boone-Heinonen et al. 2010c) should be considered to allow for placement of relevant policy or intervention within an appropriate setting or neighbourhood scale (Handy et al. 2002; Giles-Corti et al. 2005; Ding et al. 2011).

Food Outlets Surrounding Schools

Over the last recent decades, the number of fast food outlets worldwide has increased (Datamonitor 2006; Sipahi 2010), while small individually owned grocers have been displaced by large chain supermarkets (Myers 2004; Reardon and Hopkins 2006; Danish National Consumer Agency 2007). This shift in the food shopping landscape may impact access to healthy food and result in altered eating behaviour. Initial examinations of the spatial distribution of food outlets surrounding schools indicate that in North America, schools are generally within 400–800-m walking distances to places where calorie-dense, nutrient poor foods are usually sold, such as fast food restaurants or convenience stores (Austin et al. 2005; Simon et al. 2008; Sturm 2008; Zenk and Powell 2008; Davis and Carpenter 2009; Kipke et al. 2007; Kestens and Daniel 2010; Kwate and Loh 2010; Neckerman et al. 2010). Many of these food outlets are often placed around schools in lower income neighbourhoods (Simon et al. 2008; Sturm 2008; Zenk and Powell 2008; Kestens and Daniel 2010; Kwate and Loh 2010; Neckerman et al. 2010). There is little but emerging evidence regarding the patterning of food outlets surrounding schools outside of North America, although similar findings have been shown in New Zealand (Day and Pearce 2011). Nevertheless, these initial findings are troubling given the relatively easy access young people may have to calorie-dense foods as students pass these shops during their travel to and from school. Such exposures may prime children into not making healthy food choices (Hackett et al. 2008).

Whether the exposure to food outlets around schools has an impact on dietary behaviour among youth is still unclear. Potential differences in study results may be due to variations in size of the study, urban design, distances measured or the types of food outlets available. For example, a US study (Davis and Carpenter 2009) investigating pooled information from over 500,000 students in California reported a decrease in fruit and vegetable consumption as well as increased soda intake with the presence of fast food outlets within 0.5 mile (800 m) from the school. While in the city of Norfolk (UK), Skidmore et al. (2009) found that although 9–10-year-old children ($n = 1{,}721$) increased vegetable intake with increasing density of supermarkets in the school neighbourhood (at a distance of 800 m), they also increased their intake of other foods such as potato crisps and white bread. By contrast, a study conducted in the city of Rotterdam in the Netherlands (van der Horst et al. 2008) found little association between soft drink and snack consumption and food outlets within 500 m from the school in approximately 1,300 adolescents (12–15 years). Likewise, a US study (Laska et al. 2010) in the city of Minneapolis/St. Paul found little association between the exposure of any food outlets in surrounding school areas and dietary intake of 349 adolescents (11–18 years) when using distance measures of 800, 1,600 and 3,000 m from the school. Based on the evidence so far, the relationship between food environments surrounding schools and eating behaviour prompts further investigation despite potential neighbourhood exposure to food outlets within close proximity to schools.

Active Transport to Schools

While examinations of food environments external to the school prompt more attention, other scholars examine whether schools may provide opportunities for physical activity, with active transportation to school as one possibility. In many Western countries, the prevalence of children and adolescents who either cycle or walk to school has fallen steadily, with proportions declining with age. In the USA, transport by either cycling or walking to school declined from 40.7 % in 1969 to 12 % in 2001 (McDonald 2007). In Canada, the proportion of adolescents walking to school between 1986 and 2001 was reduced by 11 % among 11–13-year-olds and by 8 % among 14–15-year-olds (Buliung et al. 2009). Similar but less drastic reductions are shown in the UK between the periods of 1975 and 2009 among 11–16-year-old adolescents for walking (53–38 %) and for cycling (7–3 %) (Department of Transport 2009). Lastly, in Australia, trips to school by either walking or cycling declined by 50 % in 1985 and by 80 % in 2001 (Salmon et al. 2005).

Despite the overall decline in many countries, active transport to schools (ATS) is emerging to be an important source of physical activity (Carver et al. 2011; Mendoza et al. 2010a) and may be especially important for adolescent health, as indicated so far by a longitudinal study in Australia (Carver et al. 2011). Additionally, children and adolescents who travel to school have higher levels of aerobic fitness (Andersen et al. 2009) and decreased weight (Rosenberg et al. 2006). Because school transport is a potentially easy way to ensure children and adolescents achieve recommended levels of daily physical activity, emphasis has been made on investigating the features of the built environmental associated with ATS. These features have been identified by either self-reported or GIS measures. Recent reviews of the scientific literature identified perceived characteristics such as short distances between home and school (Pont et al. 2009), the presence of cycling or walking paths (Ewing et al. 2004; Fulton et al. 2005; Kerr et al. 2006) and direct routes (Panter et al. 2008) to be positive predictors of active transport. In addition, land use characteristics may provide a backdrop for why certain transportation features exist. For example, a newly published Danish study found school districts with higher proportions of single homes may have more positive characteristics such as interconnected streets or aesthetic and safety features more conducive towards ATS compared to rural areas (Stock et al. 2012). On the other hand, concerns about safety (Evenson et al. 2006; Kerr et al. 2006) tended to be negative predictors. Among characteristics identified through GIS measures, Pont (Pont et al. 2009) and Wong (Wong et al. 2011) both concluded that only distance between the home and school was consistently negatively associated with ATS, with commuting to school more likely if residing within a range of 0.5 miles (800 m) (Timperio et al. 2006) to 2.5 miles (4 km) (Schlossberg et al. 2006). However, criterion studies from Belgium note that these distances may differ according to age groups. D'Haese et al. (2011) determined distances for walking at 1.5 km for walking and 3.0 km for cycling for younger Belgian adolescents (11–12 years of age). On the other hand, van Dyck found distances for walking (2 km) and cycling (8.0 km) to be relevant for older Belgian adolescents between 17 and 18 years of age (Van Dyck et al. 2010). The results of these studies suggest that ATS strategies should tailor according to age and distance from home, as well as by mode of transport.

Sports or Recreational Facilities Around Schools

In comparison to literature available on active modes of transport to school, studies examining the contribution of objectively measured parks and recreation centres to physical activity are relatively fewer and understudied (Moody et al. 2004; Limstrand 2008; Ding et al. 2011) with the majority of these findings based on perceived information. A recent review of 103 studies with a majority coming from North America ($n = 68$) concluded objectively measured sport or recreation centres to be positively associated with reported physical activity levels among children but inconsistent evidence for access to parks (Ding et al. 2011). For adolescents, the accumulated evidence is inconsistent for reported levels of physical activity and objectively measured access to parks and sports or recreation facilities (Ding et al. 2011).

Exposure to sports or recreational facilities based on schools as the central reference point is not readily available as most studies use the home as a point of reference. Exceptions to these studies using the school as the central point of measure include two national studies conducted in the USA, which examined whether there were positive relationships between frequent levels of physical activity and access to commercial physical activity facilities within school zipcodes. In the first study by Powell et al. (2007b), these associations were primarily found for adolescent girls and older children. The second study by Isgor and Powell (2011) also showed significant and positive associations for adolescent girls, with greater associations among those from higher income. These results show on a national level in the USA that an increase in the availability of commercial physical activity facilities may help increase physical activity levels in adolescent girls and especially those from low-income backgrounds. In addition, a study in Norway of 662 participants indicated that girls, older adolescents (14–16 years) and those reporting low levels of physical activity outside of school tended to use sports facilities (within a 5.2 km^2 study area) less than boys, younger children (6–13 years) and those reporting higher levels of physical activity (Limstrand and Rehrer 2008). Furthermore, non-specialized multifunction sports centres were used more widely than specialized sports facilities, such as ice skating rinks. Lastly, perceived proximity to the facility, especially those considered to be plentiful within the local area, was a significant predictor of physical activity. Given the results of these studies, it may be likely that an increase in sports centres that cater to a variety of sports and are widely accessible may be one solution to create environments supportive of physical activity in young people.

Because perceived access to sports or recreational opportunities may be influenced by lifestyle or travel route (Scott et al. 2007), it is also worth noting several studies using both perceived and objective measures, even though these studies use the home as a centre of reference. These studies compared which type of information would best predict physical activity in a young population. A study conducted in Baltimore, United States, found adolescents (14–16 years) who perceived public recreational facilities within 10-min walk from their home were more likely to use them for physical activity than private ones, while significant associations were not observed with objectively measured facilities (Ries et al. 2011). These associations were also significant for objectively measured moderate-to-vigorous physical activity (MVPA). Using the US Trial of Activity for Adolescent Girls (TAAG), Scott et al. (2007) reported that among sixth grade girls ($n=1,367$), both perception that a facility was nearby and the total number of perceived facilities near the home were associated with accelerometer-measured MVPA. There were no apparent associations with facilities objectively measured from the home, which included specialized and commercial sports facilities and parks within a 1-mile radius. Other studies examining both perceived and objective measures of both parks and sports facilities include two analyses from the Netherlands (Prins et al. 2009, 2011). The study by Prins et al. (2009) examined objective and perceived measures of available parks and sports facilities 1,500 m from the homes of 13–15-year-old adolescents and found no direct association with engagement in sports activities or cycling or walking in leisure time. However, perceived availability of parks and sports facilities was significantly associated with sports and leisure time cycling and walking. Likewise, no significant associations were found between parks and sports facilities objectively measured within 400, 800 and 2,000 m buffers from participant homes and objectively assessed MVPA, even when mediating variables such as self-efficacy, attitude and perceived availability of parks and sporting facilities were introduced in the analytical models. However, the authors did observe an association between objectively measured availability of sports facilities and perceived availability of parks and sports grounds at 800 and 2,000 m (Prins et al. 2011). The results of these studies highlight the value of incorporating both perceived and objective assessments in examinations of the built environment and physical activity behaviour and that both measures offer varying associations. It may be useful to enhance perception of the availability of parks and sports facilities by using objective information to increase local knowledge of sports and recreation facilities in the area.

Green Space, Parks and Schools

Scholars examining the association between objectively measured park exposure and physical activity have been inconclusive (Ding et al. 2011) due to lack of detailed objective measures (Kaczynski and Henderson 2008), especially with regard to the provision and quality of park amenities (Brownson et al. 2009). In addition, most studies examining park exposure and physical activity in children use the home as a central measure of reference, not the school. Where schools are concerned, studies generally highlight school playgrounds as potential sites of physical activity. For instance, a study by Willenberg et al. (2010) found using a mixed methods approach among 23 schools in Australia that habitual upkeep of playground equipment, play boundary markings, and teacher presence would likely enhance opportunities for increased physical activity in 9–11-year-old children. These findings are also supported in an observational study with schoolyard assessment in the USA (Colabianchi et al. 2011). Overall, renovated schoolyards with a significant number of attributes and shading were associated with greater utilization. Likewise, a study in Norway among 130 schools (Haug et al. 2010) showed a greater likelihood of physical activity among boys and girls attending schools with a greater number of outdoor facilities (e.g. hopscotch/rope skipping areas or sledding hills) than those with fewer outdoor facilities. Thus, improvement of playground equipment may be essential in promoting play through physical activity in children.

Other studies examining the relationship between objectively measured park exposure and physical activity tend to highlight home-based rather than school-based access. Some of these studies showing a positive relationship are outlined here and suggest that various provisions and park upkeep may be important to enhance physical activity in children. For example, a study conducted in six US cities (Cohen et al. 2006) indicated that adolescent girls who live near parks within 1 mile (1.60 km) from their home engage in more physical activity than those who live near fewer parks. This association was particularly noted for girls who lived near parks with amenities conducive to walking. Findings are also similar in a study of 12th grade girls in South Carolina, USA, by Pate et al. (2008), in which significant associations were reported between physical activity facilities within 0.75-mile street-network home buffer and reported vigorous physical activity; likewise, the number of parks within home buffers was associated with total METs in white girls. A national US study of over 10,000 adolescents (grades 7–12) showed availability of major or neighbourhood parks from the home was associated with higher participation in active sports (Boone-Heinonen et al. 2010a). In females, park availability was also associated with wheel-based activity and reporting five or more MVPA bouts/week. Greater green space coverage was also associated with reporting five or more MVPA bouts/week in males and females as well as exercise participation in females. A study reported by Rodriguez et al. (2011) using both GPS positioning and accelerometry in 293 adolescent females (age 15–18 years) in the US cities of Minneapolis and San Diego showed an increase in the likelihood of physical activity was greater among girls living near parks and schools but lower in areas with more roads and food outlets. Finally, a study in Ontario, Canada (Potwarka et al. 2008), showed children (2–17 years) living near a park playground within 1 km from the home were more likely to be classified as healthy weight compared to those at risk for overweight. These results also suggest that park amenities or design may be important characteristics associated with park usage among youth, and the result of park renovations can enhance physical activity in children and adolescents (Barrett et al. 2011).

Similar to studies regarding sports and recreational facilities, perceived exposure to parks may be as essential to physical activity engagement as objectively measured information, but the literature also suggests that relations between physical activity behaviours and perceived park access are complex. Often park perception is intricately woven with other socially related ones, such as perceptions of safety or neighbourhood cohesion (McCormack et al. 2010). A study by Ries et al. (2009) involving 369 adolescents in Baltimore, MD (USA), found that perceived measures of park availability, quality and use by friends were more likely predictors of park usage perceptions of greater park than objective measures. Perceptions of park availability were also associated with higher levels of physical activity, although marginally significant. On the other hand, a study by Perry et al. (2011) concluded among a study of middle school Latinos in a rural community in Washington State (USA) that park use was positively associated with younger age, participation in an after-school activity and team sport identification. The odds of being active in the parks were greater for boys and Latinos, while older age and alcohol use were correlated with sedentary park behaviour.

Schools and Obesogenic Environments

So far, this chapter has examined the built environment correlates of food and physical activity behaviours among children and adolescents in school and residential neighbourhoods. As both diet and physical activity are involved in energy input and utilization, it is important to describe whether food or physical activity environments (i.e. obesogenic environments) may contribute to adiposity or sedentary behaviour. Yet few studies examine the combined impact of both objectively measured nutrition and physical activity environments on child or adolescent obesity (Sallis and Glanz 2006). Furthermore, the environmental findings are generally inconsistent with adiposity due to limitations in methodology and conceptualization (Dunton et al. 2009).

One of the few studies examining both school and residential exposure to food outlets and environmental supports for physical activity and the association with adiposity is a study by Harrison et al. (2011) in 9–10-year-old children in Norfolk, UK. Results of this study indicate gender- and place-based differences in the association with fat mass index (FMI), such that among girls, exposure to supermarkets and greengrocers in the home neighbourhood was associated with lower FMI but higher FMI with greater exposure to takeaways and convenience stores surrounding homes and schools. In addition, a higher proportion of open land and lower land use mix was related to higher FMI among girls. On the other hand, boys who did not actively travel to school had higher FMI in the presence of major roads in the home neighbourhood, while lower FMI were detected among those who actively travel to schools with major roads. There were no associations between the food environment and FMI among boys. Study findings further suggest future studies should consider travel mode as part of the interaction between the built environment and adiposity and that additional investigation is needed to examine gender-based associations with the built environment.

Other studies examine the relationship between weight status and either the food or physical activity built environment in school neighbourhoods as separate entities. Among school-based studies examining obesogenic food environments, a study by Chiang et al. (2011) demonstrated in 2,283 Taiwanese schoolchildren (6–13 years) a significant relationship between BMI among boys and fast food outlet density within 500 m from the school, while fast food outlet density was positively associated with height in girls. Similarly, Davis and Carpenter (2009) reported a greater likelihood of overweight among students attending schools with fast food restaurants within 0.5 mile (800 m) vicinity from schools in California, USA. Lastly, Jennings et al. (2011), in examining school and home environments, found significant associations between lowered indicators of adiposity (i.e. body weight, BMI, BMI z-score, waist circumference and percentage body fat) and obesity preventing food outlets, such as supermarkets and fruit and vegetable stores. An association was also observed between neighbourhood exposure to obesity promoting food outlets (fast food outlets and convenience stores) and higher indicators of adiposity. Increased intake in unhealthy food was also observed in association with the presence of obesity promoting food outlets.

Studies examining the relationship between supports for physical activity and adiposity are also limited, with several highlighted studies including a wide age range of children. A national US study by Slater et al. (2010) reported an association between self-reported neighbourhood physical disorder (e.g. people loitering in the streets or dilapidated housing) and higher BMI and obesity prevalence among 33,000 eighth and tenth grade students. On the other hand, an objective measure of neighbourhood compactness, which is characterized by higher walkability, was associated with lower prevalence of BMI and obesity. These findings are also supported by Grafova (2008), who observed in 2,482 children and adolescents in the USA positive associations between likelihood of being overweight and neighbourhood physical disorder, the presence of neighbourhood convenience stores and living in a newer neighbourhood (developments built after 1969). A lack of physical disorder was associated with likelihood of not being overweight. Neighbourhood supports for walking and access to public transportation may also be important environmental supports for the prevention of obesity. In another large US study of 21,008 children (2–18 years) in Massachusetts, Oreskovic et al. (2009) observed when socio-demographic factors were controlled, only subway station density within 400 m home radius was associated with the odds of being overweight. Lastly, proximity to recreational facilities may also be important characteristics to consider.

A study by Potwarka et al. (2008) and others found the likelihood of being overweight was decreased with the presence of parks within 1 km from the home in 108 Canadian children (2–17 years). This finding is supported by Nelson and Woods (2009), who showed adolescents in the USA were 2 % less likely to be overweight when reporting physical activity facilities within 5–10-min walk along frequent routes to and from school or home. Overall, the results of these studies suggest the potential importance of mobility and recreational supports for obesity prevention in children and adolescents, but other characteristics, such as neighbourhood disorder and safety, should also be considered.

Policies Based on School Neighbourhood Environments

There is no doubt that the application of GIS methods to health research has allowed scholars new insight in identifying and conceptualizing how context shapes health. Furthermore, health experts have been able to use study findings to engage in dialogue with urban and transportation planners as well as decision-makers about how to best improve or build physical resources that support health. Scholars who engage in policy discourse aimed at obesity prevention in children and adolescents stress the need for integrated and community-wide action (Wakefield 2004) and that schools provide key opportunities to elicit change and that these sentiments are echoed on a global scale (Katzmarzyk et al. 2008; Pate et al. 2011). Of special note was the recent United Nations NCD summit held in September of 2011, which included both physical activity and an unhealthy diet as two of the four key risk factors (http://www.who.int/nmh/events/un_ncd_summit2011/en/) and addressed special concerns of young populations.

In terms of policies directly addressing food environments surrounding schools, it is still unclear whether there is an impact on eating behaviour, even though ecological studies (mainly from North America) show schools in close proximity to food outlets selling calorie-dense but nutrient poor foods, especially in low-income communities. Despite the little evidence on altered individual dietary behaviour due to these nearby food outlets, well-intentioned regulations such as the 2008 building ban of fast food outlets in Los Angeles, CA (Sturm and Cohen 2009), may not address health problems of target populations (Creighton 2009) because it does not provide or offer opportunities to educate about healthy eating (Sturm and Cohen 2009), questions autonomy (Creighton 2009) and perhaps lacks an awareness of interactions between user and facility location. Nevertheless, the subject of zoning of fast food outlets is broadly maintained as a potential policy-based strategy to curb obesity (Mair et al. 2005) and perhaps prompts one to realize broader boundaries that shape the food environment (Gittelsohn and Kumar 2007). Another potential area for community-based policy involving schools could be targeted towards placement advertising of unhealthy foods to diminish potential food-based cues that prompt eating (Maher et al. 2005). However, this is a very new area of research, and associations with eating behaviour are difficult to demonstrate. School-based food policies, however, that primarily focus on the availability or sale of energy dense food or beverages within school campuses worldwide are numerous (Jaime and Lock 2009; Masse et al. 2007). While some changes have been effective in positively changing dietary intake (Jaime and Lock 2009; Story et al. 2009; Haroun et al. 2011; Mendoza et al. 2010b), they have yet to demonstrate long-lasting effects on obesity reduction. Added to the complexity of the problem, especially in the USA (Wakefield 2004; Johnston et al. 2007), is the contractual relationship schools have with food vendors to raise revenue through daily food and beverage sales or fund-raising events in exchange for sports or club sponsorships.

In a recent review of policies aimed at increasing physical activity among youth in Europe, the Americas, Asia and Oceania, Pate et al. (2011) summarized six common arenas for enhanced physical activity (1) physical education curriculum in school, (2) physical activity promotion in health education, (3) community environmental supports, (4) school environmental supports, (5) active transport and (6) mass media/advertising. Of these themes mentioned, at least four (themes 1, 2, 4 and 5) use schools as potential backdrops to initiate policy, and three (themes 3, 4 and 5) have implications for the improvement or building of structural supports within school neighbourhoods.

Given the trend among schools to either reduce recess time or physical education curricula in favour of raising academic standards (Eyler et al. 2008) or reduced funding (Wakefield 2004), active transport to school initiatives seems to be one practical solution to incorporate daily physical activity into the lives of youth. Shared characteristics of active transport to school policies include built environment characteristics, such as physical infrastructure (e.g. presence of cycle lanes or sidewalks) devoted to bicycle travel or to walking, as well as traffic and personal safety concerns (Eyler et al. 2008). Not only is the physical infrastructure important to encourage active travel to school, but these environmental supports cannot occur without understanding how economic investment, travel destinations and travel choice play a role in prioritizing travel infrastructure (Frank 2004). If priorities shift to more active forms of travel, such goals cannot be realized in the absence of trans-disciplinary collaboration, which involves key stakeholders in transportation and urban planning, community leaders, school districts, the media, legislation and the children and parents of the schools themselves (Eyler et al. 2008). Finally, even if active transport infrastructure is enhanced, there may still be cultural aspects to overcome, as car-dependent societies need to consider walking and cycling as legitimate means of transport (Buliung et al. 2009; Franco et al. 2010).

Another area of policy where schools and communities may play a role is to address community-based supports of physical activity and create integrated strategies to devise where physical activity may occur, either through physical activity programming at public sports venues or via after-school activities (Feldman and Matjasko 2007). Equity of access to sports and recreational facilities is a potential concern, especially in underserved communities in the USA (Spengler et al. 2010). Thus, schools also present as potential venues for hosting physical activity events or other athletic opportunities that may be open to the community outside of school hours. In addition to ensuring community and political support, liability is another important barrier to consider in allowing public use of school property (Spengler et al. 2010).

There is a keen policy interest to include schools as health promoting sites for the prevention of obesity in children, but there is also increasing recognition that change cannot occur only within school boundaries. There is some evidence that aspects of the built environment surrounding schools may have an impact on dietary behaviour (Davis and Carpenter 2009) and growing evidence in support of the need to encourage active transport to school, especially in enhancing environmental supports for those who live longer distances from school (Pont et al. 2009; Wong et al. 2011). Exposure to other physical activity supports such as sports centres and levels of physical activity is inconsistent in adolescents but positively associated in children. Relationships are inconsistent for park exposure and physical activity in both children and adolescents (Ding et al. 2011). While there is progress in the scientific literature supporting the relationship between environmental characteristics and child adiposity, further study is needed to improve understanding of how neighbourhood factors work, especially in concert with each other and in relationship to psychosocial and social factors. Improvements in methodology and conceptualization should be made to ensure comparability of results (Dunton et al. 2009; Galvez et al. 2010; Feng et al. 2010). In tandem, academics need to continue and engage in policy dialogue aimed at obesity prevention in children and adolescents, which not only stress integrated and community supports but also strengthen partnerships and shared vision (Wakefield 2004; Uyeda et al. 2009).

References

Andersen, L. B., Lawlor, D. A., Cooper, A. R., Froberg, K., & Anderssen, S. A. (2009). Physical fitness in relation to transport to school in adolescents: The Danish youth and sports study. *Scandinavian Journal of Medicine & Science in Sports, 19*(3), 406–411.

Ashe, M., Feldstein, L. M., Graff, S., Kline, R., Pinkas, D., & Zellers, L. (2007). Local venues for change: Legal strategies for healthy environments. *The Journal of Law, Medicine & Ethics, 35*(1), 138–147.

Austin, S. B., Melly, S. J., Sanchez, B. N., Patel, A., Buka, S., & Gortmaker, S. L. (2005). Clustering of fast-food restaurants around schools: A novel application of spatial statistics to the study of food environments. *American Journal of Public Health, 95*(9), 1575–1581.

Barrett, J. L., Hannon, C., Keefe, L., Gortmaker, S. L., & Cradock, A. L. (2011). Playground renovations and quality at public parks in Boston, Massachusetts, 1996–2007. *Preventing Chronic Disease, 8*(4), A72.

Boone-Heinonen, J., Casanova, K., Richardson, A. S., & Gordon-Larsen, P. (2010a). Where can they play? Outdoor spaces and physical activity among adolescents in U.S. urbanized areas. *Preventive Medicine, 51*(3–4), 295–298.

Boone-Heinonen, J., Evenson, K. R., Song, Y., & Gordon-Larsen, P. (2010b). Built and socioeconomic environments: Patterning and associations with physical activity in U.S. adolescents. *International Journal of Behavioral Nutrition and Physical Activity, 20*(7), 45.

Boone-Heinonen, J., Popkin, B. M., Song, Y., & Gordon-Larsen, P. (2010c). What neighborhood area captures built environment features related to adolescent physical activity? *Health & Place, 16*(6), 1280–1286.

Brownson, R. C., Hoehner, C. M., Day, K., Forsyth, A., & Sallis, J. F. (2009). Measuring the built environment for physical activity: State of the science. *American Journal of Preventive Medicine, 36*(4 Suppl), S99–123.e12.

Buliung, R. N., Mitra, R., & Faulkner, G. (2009). Active school transportation in the Greater Toronto Area, Canada: An exploration of trends in space and time (1986–2006). *Preventive Medicine, 48*(6), 507–512.

Carver, A., Timperio, A., Hesketh, K., & Crawford, D. (2011). Are safety-related features of the road environment associated with smaller declines in physical activity among youth? *Journal of Urban Health, 8*(1), 29–43.

Charreire, H., Casey, R., Salze, P., Simon, C., Chaix, B., Banos, A., Badariotti, D., Weber, C., & Oppert, J. M. (2010). Measuring the food environment using geographical information systems: A methodological review. *Public Health Nutrition, 13*(11), 1773–1785.

Chiang, P. H., Wahlqvist, M. L., Lee, M. S., Huang, L. Y., Chen, H. H., & Huang, S. T. (2011). Fast-food outlets and walkability in school neighbourhoods predict fatness in boys and height in girls: A Taiwanese population study. *Public Health Nutrition, 14*(9), 1601–1609.

Cohen, D. A., Ashwood, J. S., Scott, M. M., Overton, A., Evenson, K. R., Staten, L. K., Porter, D., McKenzie, T. L., & Catellier, D. (2006). Public parks and physical activity among adolescent girls. *Pediatrics, 118*(5), e1381–1389.

Colabianchi, N., Maslow, A. L., & Swayampakala, K. (2011). Features and amenities of school playgrounds: A direct observation study of utilization and physical activity levels outside of school time. *International Journal of Behavioral Nutrition and Physical Activity, 14*(8), 32.

Cole, R., Leslie, E., Donald, M., Cerin, E., & Owen, N. (2007). Residential proximity to school and the active travel choices of parents. *Health Promotion Journal of Australia, 18*(2), 127–134.

Cooper, A. R., Page, A. S., Wheeler, B. W., Griew, P., Davis, L., Hillsdon, M., & Jago, R. (2010). Mapping the walk to school using accelerometry combined with a global positioning system. *American Journal of Preventive Medicine, 38*(2), 178–183.

Creighton, R. (2009). Cheeseburgers, race, and paternalism Los Angeles' ban on fast food restaurants. *The Journal of Legal Medicine, 30*(2), 249–267.

D'Haese, S., De Meester, F., De Bourdeaudhuij, I., Deforche, B., & Cardon, G. (2011). Criterion distances and environmental correlates of active commuting to school in children. *International Journal of Behavioral Nutrition and Physical Activity, 10*(8), 88.

Danish National Consumer Agency (2007). Chapter 3. Danskernes adfærd og vaner på fødevaremarkedet [Danish food habits and purchasing behavior]. In Danish. *Consumer Report 2007*. Danish National Consumer Agency, Copenhagen.

Datamonitor (2006). Fast food in Europe. Datamonitor Europe. doi:0201–2230.

Davis, B., & Carpenter, C. (2009). Proximity of fast-food restaurants to schools and adolescent obesity. *American Journal of Public Health, 99*(3), 505–510.

Day, P. L., & Pearce, J. (2011). Obesity-promoting food environments and the spatial clustering of food outlets around schools. *American Journal of Preventive Medicine, 40*(2), 113–121.

Department of Transport. (2009). Local government and the regions. In *National Travel Survey: 2009*. London: National Statistics.

Ding, D., Sallis, J. F., Kerr, J., Lee, S., & Rosenberg, D. E. (2011). Neighborhood environment and physical activity among youth a review. *American Journal of Preventive Medicine, 41*(4), 442–455.

Dunton, G. F., Kaplan, J., Wolch, J., Jerrett, M., & Reynolds, K. D. (2009). Physical environmental correlates of childhood obesity: A systematic review. *Obesity Reviews, 10*(4), 393–402.

Euridice Network (2010). Recommended annual taught time in full-time compulsory education. (ed): Arlette Delhaxhe. Brussels: European Commission. Education, Audiovisual and Culture Executive Agency. http://eacea.ec.europa.eu/education/eurydice/documents/tools/taught_time_11-12.pdf. Accessed Dec 2011.

Euridice Network (2011). Organisation of school time in Europe: Primary and general secondary education 2011/12 school year. Brussels: European Commission. Education, Audiovisual and Culture Executive Agency. http://eacea.ec.europa.eu/education/eurydice/documents/calendars/school_calendar_EN.pdf.pdf. Accessed Dec 2011

Evenson, K. R., Birnbaum, A. S., Bedimo-Rung, A. L., Sallis, J. F., Voorhees, C. C., Ring, K., & Elder, J. P. (2006). Girls' perception of physical environmental factors and transportation:

Reliability and association with physical activity and active transport to school. *International Journal of Behavioral Nutrition and Physical Activity, 14*(3), 28.

Ewing, R., Schroeer, W., & Greene, W. (2004). School locations and student travel. *Transportation Research Record, 1895*, 55–63.

Eyler, A. A., Brownson, R. C., Doescher, M. P., Evenson, K. R., Fesperman, C. E., Litt, J. S., Pluto, D., Steinman, L. E., Terpstra, J. L., Troped, P. J., & Schmid, T. L. (2008). Policies related to active transport to and from school: A multisite case study. *Health Education Research, 23*(6), 963–975.

Faulkner, G. E., Richichi, V., Buliung, R. N., Fusco, C., & Moola, F. (2010). What's "quickest and easiest?": Parental decision making about school trip mode. *International Journal of Behavioral Nutrition and Physical Activity, 6*(7), 62.

Feldman, A. F., & Matjasko, J. L. (2005). The role of school-based extracurricular activities in adolescent development: A comprehensive review and future directions. *Review Educational Research, 75*(2), 159–210.

Feldman, A. F., & Matjasko, J. L. (2007). Profiles and portfolios of adolescent school-based extracurricular activity participation. *Journal of Adolescence, 30*(2), 313–332.

Feng, J., Glass, T., Curriero, F. C., Stewart, W. F., & Schwartz, B. S. (2010). The built environment and obesity: A systematic review of the epidemiologic evidence. *Health & Place, 16*, 175–190.

Franco, M., Sanz, B., Otero, L., Dominguez-Vila, A., & Caballero, B. (2010). Prevention of childhood obesity in Spain: A focus on policies outside the health sector. SESPAS report 2010. *Gaceta Sanitaria, 24*(Suppl 1), 49–55.

Frank, L. D. (2004). Economic determinants of urban form: Resulting trade-offs between active and sedentary forms of travel. *American Journal of Preventive Medicine, 27*(3 Suppl), 146–153.

Fulton, J. E., Shisler, J. L., Yore, M. M., & Caspersen, C. J. (2005). Active transportation to school: Findings from a national survey. *Research Quarterly for Exercise and Sport, 76*(3), 352–357.

Galvez, M. P., Pearl, M., & Yen, I. H. (2010). Childhood obesity and the built environment. *Current Opinion in Pediatrics, 22*(2), 202–207.

Giles-Corti, B., Timperio, A., Bull, F., & Pikora, T. (2005). Understanding physical activity environmental correlates: Increased specificity for ecological models. *Exercise and Sport Sciences Reviews, 33*(4), 175–181.

Gittelsohn, J., & Kumar, M. B. (2007). Preventing childhood obesity and diabetes: Is it time to move out of the school? *Pediatric Diabetes, 8*(Suppl 9), 55–69.

Grafova, I. B. (2008). Overweight children: Assessing the contribution of the built environment. *Preventive Medicine, 47*(3), 304–308.

Hackett, A., Boddy, L., Boothby, J., Dummer, T. J., Johnson, B., & Stratton, G. (2008). Mapping dietary habits may provide clues about the factors that determine food choice. *Journal of Human Nutrition and Dietetics, 21*(5), 428–437.

Handy, S. L., Boarnet, M. G., Ewing, R., & Killingsworth, R. E. (2002). How the built environment affects physical activity: Views from urban planning. *American Journal of Preventive Medicine, 23*(2 Suppl), 64–73.

Haroun, D., Wood, L., Harper, C., & Nelson, M. (2011). Nutrient-based standards for school lunches complement food-based standards and improve pupils' nutrient intake profile. *British Journal of Nutrition, 106*(4), 472–474.

Harrison, F., Jones, A. P., van Sluijs, E. M., Cassidy, A., Bentham, G., & Griffin, S. J. (2011). Environmental correlates of adiposity in 9–10 year old children: Considering home and school neighbourhoods and routes to school. *Social Science & Medicine, 72*(9), 1411–1419.

Haug, E., Torsheim, T., Sallis, J. F., & Samdal, O. (2010). The characteristics of the outdoor school environment associated with physical activity. *Health Education Research, 25*(2), 248–256. http://eacea.ec.europa.eu/education/eurydice/documents/calendars/school_calendar_EN.pdf. pdf. Accessed Dec 2011.

Isgor, Z., & Powell, L. M. (2011). Availability of commercial physical activity facilities and physical activity outside of school among high school students. *Journal of Physical Activity & Health, 8*(5), 707–715.

Jago, R., Thompson, J. L., Page, A. S., Brockman, R., Cartwright, K., & Fox, K. R. (2009). Licence to be active: Parental concerns and 10–11-year-old children's ability to be independently physically active. *Journal of Public Health (Oxford, England), 31*(4), 472–477.

Jaime, P. C., & Lock, K. (2009). Do school based food and nutrition policies improve diet and reduce obesity? *Preventive Medicine, 48*(1), 45–53.

Jennings, A., Welch, A., Jones, A. P., Harrison, F., Bentham, G., van Sluijs, E. M., Griffin, S. J., & Cassidy, A. (2011). Local food outlets, weight status, and dietary intake: Associations in children aged 9–10 years. *American Journal of Preventive Medicine, 40*(4), 405–410.

Johnston, L. D., Delva, J., & O'Malley, P. M. (2007). Soft drink availability, contracts, and revenues in American secondary schools. *American Journal of Preventive Medicine, 33*(4 Suppl), S209–225.

Jones, A. P., Coombes, E. G., Griffin, S. J., & van Sluijs, E. M. (2009). Environmental supportiveness for physical activity in English schoolchildren: A study using global positioning systems. *International Journal of Behavioral Nutrition and Physical Activity, 17*(6), 42.

Kaczynski, A. T., & Henderson, K. A. (2008). Parks and recreation settings and active living: A review of associations with physical activity function and intensity. *Journal of Physical Activity & Health, 5*(4), 619–632.

Katzmarzyk, P. T., Baur, L. A., Blair, S. N., Lambert, E. V., Oppert, J. M., Riddoch, C., Force, F. T., & Panel, T. C. (2008). International conference on physical activity and obesity in children: Summary statement and recommendations. *International Journal of Pediatric Obesity, 3*(1), 3–21.

Kerr, J., Rosenberg, D., Sallis, J. F., Saelens, B. E., Frank, L. D., & Conway, T. L. (2006). Active commuting to school: Associations with environment and parental concerns. *Medicine & Science in Sports & Exercise, 38*(4), 787–794.

Kestens, Y., & Daniel, M. (2010). Social inequalities in food exposure around schools in an urban area. *American Journal of Preventive Medicine, 39*(1), 33–40.

Kipke, M. D., Iverson, E., Moore, D., Booker, C., Ruelas, V., Peters, A. L., & Kaufman, F. (2007). Food and park environments: Neighborhood-level risks for childhood obesity in east Los Angeles. *The Journal of Adolescent Health, 40*(4), 325–333.

Kwate, N. O., & Loh, J. M. (2010). Separate and unequal: The influence of neighborhood and school characteristics on spatial proximity between fast food and schools. *Preventive Medicine, 51*(2), 153–156.

Laska, M. N., Hearst, M. O., Forsyth, A., Pasch, K. E., & Lytle, L. (2010). Neighbourhood food environments: Are they associated with adolescent dietary intake, food purchases and weight status? *Public Health Nutrition, 13*(11), 1757–1763.

Limstrand, T. (2008). Environmental characteristics relevant to young people's use of sports facilities: A review. *Scandinavian Journal of Medicine & Science in Sports, 18*(3), 275–287.

Limstrand, T., & Rehrer, N. J. (2008). Young people's use of sports facilities: A Norwegian study on physical activity. *Scandinavian Journal of Public Health, 36*(5), 452–459.

Maher, A., Wilson, N., & Signal, L. (2005). Advertising and availability of 'obesogenic' foods around New Zealand secondary schools: A pilot study. *The New Zealand Medical Journal, 118*(1218), U1556.

Mair, J. S., Pierce, M. W., Teret, S. P. (2005). The use of zoning to restrict fast food outlets: A potential strategy to combat obesity. The Center for Law and the Public's Health at Johns Hopkins & Georgetown Universities. http://www.publichealthlaw.net/Zoning %20Fast %20 Food %20Outlets.pdf. Accessed Dec 2011.

Masse, L. C., Frosh, M. M., Chriqui, J. F., Yaroch, A. L., Agurs-Collins, T., Blanck, H. M., Atienza, A. A., McKenna, M. L., & Igoe, J. F. (2007). Development of a school nutrition-environment state policy classification system (SNESPCS). *American Journal of Preventive Medicine, 33* (4 Suppl), S277–291.

Maziak, W., Ward, K. D., & Stockton, M. B. (2008). Childhood obesity: Are we missing the big picture? *Obesity Reviews, 9*(1), 35–42.

McCormack, G. R., Rock, M., Toohey, A. M., & Hignell, D. (2010). Characteristics of urban parks associated with park use and physical activity: A review of qualitative research. *Health & Place, 16*(4), 712–726.

McDonald, N. C. (2007). Active transportation to school: Trends among U.S. schoolchildren, 1969–2001. *American Journal of Preventive Medicine, 32*(6), 509–516.

McDonald, N. C., Deakin, E., & Aalborg, A. E. (2010). Influence of the social environment on children's school travel. *Preventive Medicine, 50*(Suppl 1), S65–68.

Mendoza, J. A., Watson, K., Baranowski, T., Nicklas, T. A., Uscanga, D. K., & Hanfling, M. J. (2010a). Validity of instruments to assess students' travel and pedestrian safety. *BMC Public Health, 18*(10), 257.

Mendoza, J. A., Watson, K., & Cullen, K. W. (2010b). Change in dietary energy density after implementation of the Texas Public School Nutrition Policy. *Journal of the American Dietetic Association, 110*(3), 434–440.

Moody, J. S., Prochaska, J. J., Sallis, J. F., McKenzie, T. L., Brown, M., & Conway, T. L. (2004). Viability of parks and recreation centers as sites for youth physical activity promotion. *Health Promotion Practice, 5*(4), 438–443.

Myers, H. (2004). Trends in the food retail sector across Europe. *European Retail Digest, 41*, 1–3.

Neckerman, K. M., Bader, M. D., Richards, C. A., Purciel, M., Quinn, J. W., Thomas, J. S., Warbelow, C., Weiss, C. C., Lovasi, G. S., & Rundle, A. (2010). Disparities in the food environments of New York City public schools. *American Journal of Preventive Medicine, 39*(3), 195–202.

Nelson, N. M., & Woods, C. B. (2009). Obesogenic environments: Are neighbourhood environments that limit physical activity obesogenic? *Health & Place, 15*(4), 917–924.

Ogneva-Himmelberger, Y., Ross, L., Burdick, W., & Simpson, S. A. (2011). Using geographic information systems to compare the density of stores selling tobacco and alcohol: Youth making an argument for increased regulation of the tobacco permitting process in Worcester, Massachusetts, USA. *Tobacco Control, 19*(6), 475–480.

Oreskovic, N. M., Winickoff, J. P., Kuhlthau, K. A., Romm, D., & Perrin, J. M. (2009). Obesity and the built environment among Massachusetts children. *Clinical Pediatrics (Philadelphia), 48*(9), 904–912.

Panter, J. R., Jones, A. P., & van Sluijs, E. M. (2008). Environmental determinants of active travel in youth: A review and framework for future research. *International Journal of Behavioral Nutrition and Physical Activity, 23*(5), 34.

Pasch, K. E., Hearst, M. O., Nelson, M. C., Forsyth, A., & Lytle, L. A. (2009). Alcohol outlets and youth alcohol use: Exposure in suburban areas. *Health & Place, 15*(2), 642–646.

Pate, R. R., Colabianchi, N., Porter, D., Almeida, M. J., Lobelo, F., & Dowda, M. (2008). Physical activity and neighborhood resources in high school girls. *American Journal of Preventive Medicine, 34*(5), 413–419.

Pate, R., Trilk, J. L., Byun, W., & Wang, J. (2011). Policies to increase physical activity in children and youth. *Journal of Exercise Science & Fitness, 9*(1), 1–14.

Perry, C. K., Saelens, B. E., & Thompson, B. (2011). Rural Latino youth park use: Characteristics, park amenities, and physical activity. *Journal of Community Health, 36*(3), 389–397.

Pont, K., Ziviani, J., Wadley, D., Bennett, S., & Abbott, R. (2009). Environmental correlates of children's active transportation: A systematic literature review. *Health & Place, 15*(3), 827–840.

Popkin, B. M., Duffey, K., & Gordon-Larsen, P. (2005). Environmental influences on food choice, physical activity and energy balance. *Physiology & Behavior, 86*(5), 603–613.

Potwarka, L. R., Kaczynski, A. T., & Flack, A. L. (2008). Places to play: Association of park space and facilities with healthy weight status among children. *Journal of Community Health, 33*(5), 344–350.

Powell, L. M., Auld, M. C., Chaloupka, F. J., O'Malley, P. M., & Johnston, L. D. (2007a). Associations between access to food stores and adolescent body mass index. *American Journal of Preventive Medicine, 33*(4Suppl), S301–307.

Powell, L. M., & Bao, Y. (2009). Food prices, access to food outlets and child weight. *Economics and Human Biology, 7*(1), 64–72.

Powell, L. M., Chaloupka, F. J., Slater, S. J., Johnston, L. D., & O'Malley, P. M. (2007b). The availability of local-area commercial physical activity-related facilities and physical activity among adolescents. *American Journal of Preventive Medicine, 33*(4 Suppl), 292–300.

Prins, R. R., Ball, K., Timperio, A., Salmon, J., Oenema, A., Brug, J., & Crawford, D. (2011). Associations between availability of facilities within three different neighbourhood buffer sizes and objectively assessed physical activity in adolescents. *Health & Place, 17*(6), 1228–1234.

Prins, R. G., Oenema, A., van der Horst, K., & Brug, J. (2009). Objective and perceived availability of physical activity opportunities: Differences in associations with physical activity behavior among urban adolescents. *International Journal of Behavioral Nutrition and Physical Activity, 15*(6), 70.

Rahman, T., Cushing, R. A., & Jackson, R. J. (2011). Contributions of built environment to childhood obesity. *The Mount Sinai Journal of Medicine, 78*(1), 49–57.

Reardon, T., & Hopkins, R. (2006). The supermarket revolution in developing countries: Policies to address emerging tensions among supermarkets, suppliers and traditional retailers. *European Journal of Development Research, 18*(4), 522–545.

Ries, A. V., Voorhees, C. C., Roche, K. M., Gittelsohn, J., Yan, A. F., & Astone, N. M. (2009). A quantitative examination of park characteristics related to park use and physical activity among urban youth. *The Journal of Adolescent Health, 45*(3 Suppl), S64–70.

Ries, A. V., Yan, A. F., & Voorhees, C. C. (2011). The neighborhood recreational environment and physical activity among urban youth: An examination of public and private recreational facilities. *Journal of Community Health, 36*(4), 640–649.

Rodriguez, D. A., Cho, G. H., Evenson, K. R., Conway, T. L., Cohen, D., Ghosh-Dastidar, B., Pickrel, J. L., Veblen-Mortenson, S., & Lytle, L. A. (2011). Out and about: Association of the built environment with physical activity behaviors of adolescent females. *Health & Place, 18*(1), 55–62.

Rosenberg, D. E., Sallis, J. F., Conway, T. L., Cain, K. L., & McKenzie, T. L. (2006). Active transportation to school over 2 years in relation to weight status and physical activity. *Obesity (Silver Spring), 14*(10), 1771–1776.

Sallis, J. F., & Glanz, K. (2006). The role of built environments in physical activity, eating, and obesity in childhood. *The Future of Children, 16*(1), 89–108.

Sallis, J. F., & Glanz, K. (2009). Physical activity and food environments: Solutions to the obesity epidemic. *The Milbank Quarterly, 87*(1), 123–154.

Sallis, J. F., Zakarian, J. M., Hovell, M. F., & Hofstetter, C. R. (1996). Ethnic, socioeconomic, and sex differences in physical activity among adolescents. *Journal of Clinical Epidemiology, 49*(2), 125–134.

Salmon, J., Timperio, A., Cleland, V., & Venn, A. (2005). Trends in children's physical activity and weight status in high and low socio-economic status areas of Melbourne, Victoria, 1985–2001. *Australian and New Zealand Journal of Public Health, 29*(4), 337–342.

Schlossberg, M., Greene, J., Phillips, P., Johnson, B., & Parker, B. (2006). School trips: Effects of urban form and distance on travel mode. *Journal of American Planning Association, 72*(3), 337–346.

Scott, M. M., Evenson, K. R., Cohen, D. A., & Cox, C. E. (2007). Comparing perceived and objectively measured access to recreational facilities as predictors of physical activity in adolescent girls. *Journal of Urban Health, 84*(3), 346–359.

Simon, P. A., Kwan, D., Angelescu, A., Shih, M., & Fielding, J. E. (2008). Proximity of fast food restaurants to schools: Do neighborhood income and type of school matter? *Preventive Medicine, 47*(3), 284–288.

Sipahi, S. (2010). Expanding operations in fast-food industry under uncertain market conditions. *International Journal of Trade, Economics, and Finance, 1*(1), 74–79.

Skidmore, P., Welch, A., van Sluijs, E., Jones, A., Harvey, I., Harrison, F., Griffin, S., & Cassidy, A. (2009). Impact of neighbourhood food environment on food consumption in children aged 9–10 years in the UK SPEEDY (Sport, Physical Activity and Eating behaviour: Environmental Determinants in Young people) study. *Public Health Nutrition, 13*(7), 1022–1030.

Slater, S. J., Ewing, R., Powell, L. M., Chaloupka, F. J., Johnston, L. D., & O'Malley, P. M. (2010). The association between community physical activity settings and youth physical activity, obesity, and body mass index. *The Journal of Adolescent Health, 47*(5), 496–503.

Slater, S. J., Powell, L. M., & Chaloupka, F. J. (2007). Missed opportunities: Local health departments as providers of obesity prevention programs for adolescents. *American Journal of Preventive Medicine, 33*(4 Suppl), S246–250.

Spengler, J. O., Carroll, M. S., Connaughton, D. P., & Evenson, K. R. (2010). Policies to promote the community use of schools: A review of state recreational user statutes. *American Journal of Preventive Medicine, 39*(1), 81–88.
Stanley, F., & Daube, M. (2009). Should industry care for children? Public health advocacy and law in Australia. *Public Health, 123*(3), 283–286.
Stock, C., Bloomfield, K., Ejstrud, B., Vinther-Larsen, M., Meijer, M., Grønbæk, M., & Grittner, U. (2012). Are characteristics of the school district associated with active transportation to school in Danish adolescents? *European Journal of Public Health, 22*(3), 398–404.
Stock, C., Ejstrud, B., Vinther-Larsen, M., Schlattmann, P., Curtis, T., Grønbaek, M., & Bloomfield, K. (2011). Effects of school district factors on alcohol consumption: Results of a multi-level analysis among Danish adolescents. *European Journal of Public Health, 21*(4), 449–455.
Story, M., Nanney, M. S., & Schwartz, M. B. (2009). Schools and obesity prevention: Creating school environments and policies to promote healthy eating and physical activity. *The Milbank Quarterly, 87*(1), 71–100.
Sturm, R. (2008). Disparities in the food environment surrounding US middle and high schools. *Public Health, 122*(7), 681–690.
Sturm, R., & Cohen, D. A. (2009). Zoning for health? The year-old ban on new fast-food restaurants in South LA. *Health Affairs (Millwood), 28*(6), w1088–1097.
Timperio, A., Ball, K., Salmon, J., Roberts, R., Giles-Corti, B., Simmons, D., Baur, L. A., & Crawford, D. (2006). Personal, family, social, and environmental correlates of active commuting to school. *American Journal of Preventive Medicine, 30*(1), 45–51.
Troped, P. J., Wilson, J. S., Matthews, C. E., Cromley, E. K., & Melly, S. J. (2010). The built environment and location-based physical activity. *American Journal of Preventive Medicine, 38*(4), 429–438.
Uyeda, K., Bogart, L. M., Hawes-Dawson, J., & Schuster, M. A. (2009). Development and implementation of a school-based obesity prevention intervention: Lessons learned from community-based participatory research. *Progress in Community Health Partnerships, 3*(3), 249–255.
van der Horst, K., Timperio, A., Crawford, D., Roberts, R., Brug, J., & Oenema, A. (2008). The school food environment associations with adolescent soft drink and snack consumption. *American Journal of Preventive Medicine, 35*(3), 217–223.
Van Dyck, D., De Bourdeaudhuij, I., Cardon, G., & Deforche, B. (2010). Criterion distances and correlates of active transportation to school in Belgian older adolescents. *International Journal of Behavioral Nutrition and Physical Activity, 7*(87), 1–9.
Villanueva, K., Giles-Corti, B., Bulsara, M., McCormack, G. R., Timperio, A., Middleton, N., Beesley, B., & Trapp, G. (2012). How far do children travel from their homes? Exploring children's activity spaces in their neighborhood. *Health & Place, 18*(2), 263–273.
Wakefield, J. (2004). Fighting obesity through the built environment. *Environmental Health Perspectives, 112*(11), A616–618.
Wiehe, S. E., Carroll, A. E., Liu, G. C., Haberkorn, K. L., Hoch, S. C., Wilson, J. S., & Fortenberry, J. D. (2008a). Using GPS-enabled cell phones to track the travel patterns of adolescents. *International Journal of Health Geographics, 21*(7), 22.
Wiehe, S. E., Hoch, S. C., Liu, G. C., Carroll, A. E., Wilson, J. S., & Fortenberry, J. D. (2008b). Adolescent travel patterns: Pilot data indicating distance from home varies by time of day and day of week. *The Journal of Adolescent Health, 42*(4), 418–420.
Willenberg, L. J., Ashbolt, R., Holland, D., Gibbs, L., MacDougall, C., Garrard, J., Green, J. B., & Waters, E. (2010). Increasing school playground physical activity: A mixed methods study combining environmental measures and children's perspectives. *Journal of Science and Medicine in Sport, 13*(2), 210–216.
Wong, B. Y., Faulkner, G., & Buliung, R. (2011). GIS measured environmental correlates of active school transport: A systematic review of 14 studies. *International Journal of Behavioral Nutrition and Physical Activity, 6*(8), 39.
Yancey, A. K., Fielding, J. E., Flores, G. R., Sallis, J. F., McCarthy, W. J., & Breslow, L. (2007). Creating a robust public health infrastructure for physical activity promotion. *American Journal of Preventive Medicine, 32*(1), 68–78.
Zenk, S. N., & Powell, L. M. (2008). US secondary schools and food outlets. *Health & Place, 14*(2), 336–346.

Chapter 18
Connecting Gender, Space and Place: Are There Gender Differences in the Relationships Between the Social Environment and Health-Related Behaviours?

Anne Ellaway and Carol Emslie

Introduction

Neighbourhood of residence may influence the health of men and women in different ways. For example, stronger associations among men than among women in life expectancy and area deprivation have been noted in England (Raleigh and Kiri 1997), the United States (Singh and Siahpush 2006) and Canada (Auger et al. 2010). Wider area differences in self-rated health over time have been observed among men compared to women (Ellaway et al. 2012). Neighbourhood social fragmentation appears to be more strongly related to women's mental health than that of men (Ivory et al. 2011). Findings such as these suggest that there may be gender differences in the social meanings and experience of place; in differential exposure, vulnerability or sensitivity to social and physical environments (Ellaway et al. 2001; Stafford et al. 2005b) and in the health-related responses of men and women (van Praag et al. 2009). In this chapter we will briefly review the literature on gender differences in perceptions of the neighbourhood. We will then focus on two health behaviours (smoking cigarettes and drinking alcohol) in order to explore how relationships between gender, space and smoking and drinking vary across contexts and by scale.

A. Ellaway (✉)
MRC Social and Public Health Sciences Unit, University of Glasgow, 4 Lilybank Gardens, Glasgow, G12 8RZ, UK
e-mail: anne@sphsu.mrc.ac.uk

C. Emslie
Institute for Applied Health Research, School of Health & Life Sciences, Buchanan House, Glasgow Caledonian University, Cowcaddens Road, Glasgow, G4 0BA, United Kingdom
e-mail: carol.emslie@gcu.ac.uk

C. Stock and A. Ellaway (eds.), *Neighbourhood Structure and Health Promotion*,
DOI 10.1007/978-1-4614-6672-7_18,

Gender Differences in Neighbourhood Perception

A substantial body of work shows that women tend to view the world as a more risky place than do men (Gustafson 1996). Women express greater concern about environmental hazards in their neighbourhoods, at home and in their workplaces (Emslie et al. 1999; Flynn et al. 1994; Karpowicz-Lazreg and Mullet 1993; Savage 1993). Explanations to account for gender differences in risk perception include women feeling more personally threatened by environmental problems than men, women tending to be more involved in loc.l activities than men and therefore being more knowledgeable about environmental issues and women being more concerned than men with nurturing and maintaining life and less concerned than men with jobs and economic growth (Blocker and Eckberg 1989; Stern and Kalof 1993). Others have argued that the observed relationship between gender and risk perception is still under-theorised (Henwood et al. 2008).

A number of studies have shown that how residents perceive their local neighbourhood varies by gender and is related to health and health behaviours in different ways for men and for women. For example, a study in the United States found that for women, it was their perceptions of the *social* quality of their local community (including problems such as unemployment, access to health care, youth violence and the quality of public education) that were associated with their self-assessed health, whereas for men, it was their perceptions of the *physical* quality of their local community (such as the quality of indoor and outdoor air, drinking water and waste disposal) that were associated with their self-assessed health (Molinari 1998). In a study in the West of Scotland, we explored gender differences in people's perceptions of their neighbourhood and in the links between these perceptions and self-rated health (Ellaway and Macintyre 2001). We found that there were no gender differences in perceived neighbourhood cohesion, but women had significantly more negative assessments than men of problems in the local area. Gender differences seem to be related to domestic circumstances, the most negative perceptions being in women with children who were not employed outside the home. This lends some support to the idea that women at home with children may be more exposed, or more sensitive, to features of their local neighbourhood than men or women in employment. Poor opinions of the neighbourhood were more strongly associated with mental health among men and more strongly associated with physical symptoms among women (Ellaway and Macintyre 2001). A study in Wales, UK, also found little difference between men and women in the reporting of the levels of social cohesion in their neighbourhood. However, there were gender differences in the associations between perceptions of social cohesion and health as it was linked with self-rated health among women, but not among men (Poortinga et al. 2007).

Other studies have explored the influence of social and material context, as measured by routine data sources rather than residents' perceptions. For example, Stafford et al. measured sociopolitical and physical environment, amenities and indicators of economic deprivation and affluence in neighbourhoods in the UK and investigated their relationship with self-rated health using multilevel regression models (Stafford et al. 2005a). Each of these contextual domains was associated with self-rated health over and above individual socioeconomic characteristics. The magnitude of the association was larger for women in each case. Statistically significant interactions between gender and residential environment were found for trust, integration into wider society, left-wing political climate, physical quality of the residential environment and unemployment rate.

A number of studies, therefore, have shown that men and women may experience place differently with subsequently differential impacts upon health. In the following we will focus on two health behaviours (smoking cigarettes and drinking alcohol) in order to explore how relationships between gender, space and smoking and drinking vary across contexts and by scale.

Neighbourhood, Gender and Smoking

Increasingly, researchers have examined neighbourhood effects on health behaviours such as smoking. As also shown in Chap. 14, a number of studies across the world have shown that where people live is associated with the likelihood of smoking even after controlling for individual socioeconomic factors (Chaix et al. 2004; Davey Smith et al. 1998; Duncan et al. 1999; Reijneveld 1998; Ross 2000; Shohaimi et al. 2003; Sundquist et al. 1999).

Gender differences in perceptions of the local neighbourhood have been noted in relation to smoking. In a Scottish study, we found that for both men and women, perceived neighbourhood problems were associated with the likelihood of smoking but mainly among those with the most negative view of the local neighbourhood (Ellaway and Macintyre 2009). However, there were gender differences in these relationships. For example, perceptions of the provision of neighbourhood amenities seem to be more strongly associated with women's compared to men's smoking status, whereas the perceived quality of the local neighbourhood appears to be a better predictor of men's smoking. Further to this, we examined whether smoking behaviour was associated with neighbourhood crime and whether there were gender differences in any relationships found (Shareck and Ellaway 2011a). Crime and safety measures represent sociocultural features of neighbourhoods which may act as chronic stressors (Nielsen et al. 2008) and as such, may influence smoking through pathways such as stress or psychological well-being (Pearce et al. 2012; Weden et al. 2008). Most studies of crime-related exposures and smoking have investigated subjective measures of safety as perceived by respondents or municipal authorities, while few have relied on more objective measures of crime such as rates recorded by police authorities. We investigated the association between smoking behaviour and neighbourhood crime using both 'objective' (as recorded by police) and 'subjective' measures (as perceived by participants). We found that residents living in areas characterised by high and medium police-recorded crime rates were more likely to be current smokers than residents of low crime areas. Similarly, individuals perceiving high crime in their neighbourhood were more likely to be smokers than those perceiving low crime levels. These associations remained statistically significant even after adjusting for individual characteristics. The association between both crime measures and smoking was more pronounced among women than men lending some support to the notion that women may be more aware of, or sensitive to, what happens in their neighbourhood; alternatively, women might be more exposed to their local area than men due to their spending more time there, on a daily basis (Shareck and Ellaway 2011b).

Using data from a qualitative study which explored possible pathways between area of residence and smoking, Stead et al. found gender differences in the relationship between smoking behaviour and features of the local social and physical environment. A poorly resourced local environment, strong community norms, isolation from wider social norms and limited opportunities for recreation seemed to not only foster smoking but also appeared to discourage or undermine smoking cessation (Stead et al. 2001). This study also found that there were considerable gender differences in the ways in which the respondents used and experienced their neighbourhood. For example, there were differences between men and women in sources to alleviate the influence of a stressful neighbourhood; women tended to socialise with friends and family in their homes, whereas men tended to visit the pub. However, both forms of recreation were 'bound up' with drinking, drug taking and, in particular, smoking (Stead et al. 2001). After the advent of the introduction of the smoking ban in public places in Scotland in 2006, a study of the impact among residents of deprived neighbourhoods found that women's smoking rates remained relatively stable after the ban as their preferred place to smoke was already within their own home (Robinson et al. 2010). Whereas for men, the ban had more of an impact as their opportunity for smoking was more restricted (Robinson et al. 2010).

Gender, Place and Drinking Alcohol

Gender differences in alcohol consumption and alcohol-related harm are found consistently across cultures (Rehm et al. 2006; Makela et al. 2006); indeed, alcohol-related deaths account for around 20 % of the overall gender gap in mortality across Europe (McCartney et al. 2011). Men are more likely to drink alcohol than women, to drink excessively and to experience or cause problems related to alcohol (Plant 2008). Little research on women and alcohol existed until the 1970s and, as frequently reported with regard to other conditions (O'Donnell et al. 2004), men's experiences were taken as the 'norm'. For example, Makela et al. (2006) have challenged the common division of European countries according to wine, beer or spirit consumption, as they argue that these distinctions only apply to male drinking patterns. There have also been rapid transformations in the social context of drinking. In the UK, for example, recent changes include an increase in alcohol consumption among women, the feminisation of the 'night time economy' with a proliferation of different types of style bars at the expense of traditional working men's pubs, alcohol being more affordable and easily available (e.g. in supermarkets) and the marketing of brands of alcohol which explicitly draw on different gendered identities.

There is a complex relationship between neighbourhood and alcohol consumption (see also Chap. 15). In the UK as a whole, the total amount of alcohol consumed varies little by social class or neighbourhood; however, the *way* people drink and the effects of alcohol *do* vary by both social class and area of residence. A greater proportion of both men and women in the least deprived areas reported exceeding 21 and 14 units, respectively, in the last week than those in the most deprived areas of Scotland. However, for men only, those living in the most deprived areas were more likely to drink 'harmfully' (exceed 50 units in a week) (ISD Scotland 2011).

Alcohol problems occur in all social groups, but there is a marked socioeconomic gradient in alcohol-related morbidity. People from the most deprived areas in Scotland have rates of alcohol-related discharge from general acute hospitals which are more than seven times greater than from those in the least deprived areas. They are also six times more likely to die from an alcohol-related condition than those living in the least deprived areas (ISD Scotland 2011).

In this section, we begin with an overview of quantitative studies which consider gender, place and alcohol and then take a micro-level approach to explore how masculinities and femininities are (re)constructed through drinking in different ways in different places.

Quantitative Approaches: Associations Between Area, Alcohol and Gender

Much of the work on alcohol and place merely controls for sex or reports findings for men and women separately without discussing what these results may mean. Wilsnack et al. (2000) have commented on this lack of satisfactory explanations for gender differences in drinking behaviour: 'Despite a growing reservoir of data on drinking practices around the world, few studies go beyond analyses showing that men use and abuse alcohol more than women do. Remarkably little is known about how gender differences in alcohol use and abuse vary or form patterns, across cultures and over time. Even less is known about how women and men may differ in the causes, context, and consequences of their drinking behaviour' (p. 253). Similarly, Jayne et al. (2008) have noted how drinking and drunkenness takes place in specific spaces and places but that geography (and – we would add – gender) is considered a peripheral issue; for example, we cannot explore 'moral panics' around binge drinking without investigating how they are centred on specific groups, at specific times, in particular places (often when there are structural changes taking place in society).

However, some researchers have attempted to take both gender and geography into account when exploring drinking patterns. For example, we used a spatial approach to explore whether the kinds of social environments which are associated with alcohol-related death were the same for men and women in Scotland (Emslie and Mitchell 2009). One hypothesis was that, on one hand, localities which produce hazardous drinking men (and high rates of alcohol-related death) might be the same as those which produce hazardous drinking women. On the other hand, area variation in gendered drinking cultures, or in the norms which influence whether men and women seek help for problem drinking, might lead to different relationships between the alcohol-related mortality rate of men and women. The first hypothesis was confirmed; in most places in Scotland, similar processes were important in determining the risk of mortality from alcohol for both men and women. Thus, while area of residence was strongly associated with alcohol-related death, it appeared only rarely to influence the 'gender gap' in alcohol-related death in this research (Emslie and Mitchell 2009).

A number of other studies have also found that the relationship between neighbourhood characteristics and drinking is similar for men and women. For example, Kavanagh et al. (2011) found an association between the density of alcohol outlets and harmful drinking for both men and women in Melbourne, Australia. Chuang et al. (2007) found that living in areas with 'high social disorganisation' (high percentage of unemployment, divorced and separated and single-parent families) intensified the effects of individual socioeconomic status (SES) for both men and women in Taiwan; high social disorganisation was associated with increased drinking only for low SES men and women. In contrast, Matheson et al. (2011) found that while neighbourhood material deprivation was associated with weekly drinking for men in Canada, this was not the case for women. They suggest that men in poor neighbourhoods may use alcohol to relieve stress, while women in similar situations may be more likely to develop symptoms of depression.

Working at a larger scale, McCartney et al. (2011) highlighted the variability in the gender gap in alcohol-related deaths across Europe. The smallest gender gap was found in Iceland (men: 59 deaths per 100,000 population per year; women: 30), while the largest gap was found in Ukraine (Men: 317; women: 77). This variability – as well as rapid changes over time – reminds us of the importance of cultural and geographical factors when attempting to explain gender differences in drinking and alcohol-related harm. Alcohol-related deaths were particularly high in Eastern Europe. Other researchers have commented on the increase in alcohol-related mortality in this region, given the huge political and socioeconomic changes after the fall of communism. For example, Rehm et al. (2007) calculated that 25 % of premature male and 14 % of premature female adult deaths in Hungary were attributable to alcohol, while Wojtyniak et al. (2005) found a sharp rise in alcohol poisoning among both men and women – although men's mortality was roughly 10 times that of women's – after the transition to a market economy in Poland. There has also been interest in the very high rates of alcohol-related death among men in Russia, attributed to heavy episodic drinking combined with a preference for spirits and the consumption of ethanol-based liquids not intended to be drunk, as well as broader social change (Leon et al. 2007). Jukkala et al. (2008) found that while men with economic problems were more likely to drink than those not experiencing problems, this was not the case for women; this may help to explain the large gender gap in alcohol-related deaths in Russia. In addition, being married or cohabiting was a protective factor for women, but not for men. They concluded that increased unemployment and wage reductions had demoralised Russian men who hold traditional views about their roles as breadwinners. Thus, heavy drinking – which is linked to traditional forms of masculinity and viewed as a gender-appropriate and culturally acceptable form of self-medication – may be one response to stressful economic situations for men in Russia (Pietila and Rytkonen 2008).

A comparative study of alcohol consumption in Denmark and the UK (Measham and Ostergaard 2009) found that young women's consumption of alcohol in these two countries was the highest, and had the narrowest gender gap, in Europe (using data from the European School Survey Project on Alcohol and Other Drugs, ESPAD, http://www.espad.org). Concerns over levels of female drinking and public drunkenness and media portrayals of 'ladettes' highlight the social anxieties around young women's alcohol consumption (Jackson and Tinkler 2007). However, as Measham and Ostergaard note, there is evidence of stability and decline in alcohol consumption among young women aged 16–24 in recent years (Hibell et al. 2009). In comparison, the consumption of alcohol by women in professional and managerial occupations in the UK in terms of frequency and excessive drinking is steadily increasing and has received much less attention as it is more likely to take place within the home rather than in public spheres (Holloway et al. 2008).

Qualitative Approaches: Masculinities, Femininities, Alcohol and the Pub

Qualitative work allows us to understand how alcohol is used as a tool to help people 'perform' gendered identities in different contexts (Lyons 2009). For example, 'drinking like a man' has historically involved public displays of excessive drinking while still appearing to remain in control (Lemle and Mishkind 1989). More recently, alcohol marketing and cultural portrayals of drinking have changed to encompass women's increased access to, and consumption of, alcohol while still constructing men's drinking as 'different' to women's (Lyons et al. 2006). In this section, we explore how gendered relationships are played out in public drinking houses.

Campbell's (2000) classic study highlights the importance of the pub as a site of male power. His ethnography of a rural community in New Zealand revealed how hegemonic (culturally dominant) masculinity was constructed and reproduced in public bars during after-work drinking, where the most influential men in the community occupied the bar stools, lower status men sat elsewhere and women and tourists were excluded. Campbell described an extremely competitive, hierarchical social context where 'conversational cockfighting' (e.g. verbal abuse and one-upmanship) and maintaining bodily control while consuming large amounts of alcohol were central to the performance of pub(lic) masculinity. Displaying detailed local knowledge and an intimate familiarity of the history of people and places was also important, as was longtime residence (over generations) in the locality. Work on rural pubs in the UK had similar findings; although women were present, they tended to 'dress down' and position themselves unobtrusively in the side spaces of pubs in order to avoid sexist comments (Leyshon 2008), and there was much less tolerance of women's excessive drinking compared to men (Burns 2002). Like Campbell (2000), Leyshon concluded that 'the rural pub.. is constructed, through embodied drinking practices and talk, as a masculine heterosexual space the effects of which extend beyond the closed space of the bar' (p. 277).

In contrast, recent research on men's drinking in midlife (Emslie et al. 2013) took place in an urban setting in Scotland. Here, many traditional working men's pubs have been replaced by cosmopolitan café and bars creating 'feminised public arenas' (Lyons and Willott 2008), and men and women are equally likely to agree that getting drunk is acceptable (Ormston and Webster 2008), although women's public drunkenness is still viewed more negatively than men's (Day et al. 2004). The most common location for drinking in Scotland is people's own homes (ISD Scotland 2011), so it was notable that men's accounts focused on the pub as a key location for forming and maintaining male friendships. Pubs were seen as male meeting places; the suggestion that men would routinely go out to restaurants or coffee shops together was perceived as laughable, as these locations were symbolically associated with women or gay men. Respondents described the 'abuse' and banter they traded with each, which often depended on narratives which denigrated women and lower status men (Gough and Edwards 1998). Thus, despite huge changes in drinking environments, the reciprocal purchase and consumption of pints of beer in the pub was constructed as an 'act of friendship' and functioned as a social lubricant and a gender-appropriate way for men to communicate with each other. In contrast, women were constructed as 'naturally' sociable and able to form friendships in other spaces (e.g. in cafes, at home) without the need of 'social lubricants' such as alcohol.

Research on women and alcohol has also provided important insights into gender and place. Women are currently heavily targeted by alcohol companies as consumers (Plant 2008), but in the past female patrons were dissuaded from entering public drinking spaces. For example, a study of Liverpool, England, between 1860 and 1914 demonstrated how women were discouraged through social and legal norms from participating in the social world of the pub (Beckingham 2012). However, given that drinking still took place in the home, it was unclear whether it was the alcohol consumption per se or the space where it took place (i.e. public houses) which was the most important factor (Beckingham 2012). Efforts to prevent women from frequenting public houses risked encouraging women to consume alcohol in the home – where they were beyond the reach of the police or licensing laws (Kneale 1999).

Lyons and Willott (2008) argue that urban-dwelling women in New Zealand are currently redefining their gendered identities through their drinking behaviours in relation to the traditional male practice of consuming alcohol in public. The young women in their study discussed their heavy drinking and perceived drunkenness as part of enjoying a night out with friends, thus 'appropriating hegemonic masculine behaviours and legitimising alterative forms of femininity which functions to gain her some of the power of the dominant position' (p. 700). However, drinking beer remained linked to masculinity, and the few women who did drink beer had to work hard discursively to make this claim. While male and female respondents were broadly positive about women in their own friendship groups drinking excessively, the same behaviour among 'outsiders' – particularly older women and women who were very drunk in public – was positioned as deviant, embarrassing and possibly promiscuous by both men and women, reinforcing the traditional sexual double standard. Public drunkenness by women was still perceived as unacceptable, and the consensus was that these women should be removed from the public sphere: 'drunk women are aligned with domestic/private spaces ("take her home") whereas drunk men are aligned with public spaces ("ha ha skull another beer")' (Lyons and Willott 2008, p.705).

This brief overview of the qualitative literature confirms that 'drinking and drunkenness unfold in specific spaces and places' (Jayne et al. 2008) and suggests that the meanings attached to pub(lic) drinking vary for men and women. Thus, while quantitative research about gender, neighbourhood and alcohol consumption is valuable, it is important to complement this knowledge with qualitative research about how alcohol is used to (re)construct different masculinities and femininities and how this changes over time and across settings.

Conclusion

In this chapter we have highlighted some of the literature exploring the gendered nature of place on smoking and alcohol consumption. However, this is still a nascent area and more research needs to be done on how gender and place impact upon these two health behaviours in different contexts and across the life course as well as other health conditions related to major causes of death. For example, hypertension is a well-known risk factor for CVD, and there is increasing interest in the ways in which an individual's neighbourhood of residence influences their blood pressure (see, e.g. Mujahid et al. 2008); however, gender is not yet strongly featured in this work.

Therefore, it is important to examine statistical associations between area (at national, regional and local scales), gender and alcohol as well as to explore how 'alcohol, drinking and drunkenness unfold in specific spaces and places' (Jayne et al. 2008) and the ways that these 'performances' are gendered. The same might also be applied to smoking, as shown earlier women's smoking may be more confined to the home than that of men and is thus currently outside the scope of public health policy measures.

References

Auger, N., Alix, C., Zang, G., & Daniel, M. (2010). Sex, age deprivation and patterns in life expectancy in Quebec, Canada: A population-based study. *BMC Public Health, 10*, 161–169.

Beckingham, D. (2012). Gender, space and drunkenness: Liverpool's licensed premises, 1860–1914. *Annals of the Association of American Geographers, 102*(3), 647–666.

Blocker, T., & Eckberg, D. (1989). Environmental issues as women's issues: General concerns and local hazards. *Social Science Quarterly, 70*, 586–593.

Burns, N. H. (2002). Alcohol and Mental Health. Findings Paper no. 12. Glasgow, Scotland: Department of Geography and Topographic Science, University of Glasgow.

Campbell, H. (2000). The Glass Phallus: Pub(lic) Masculinity and drinking in rural New Zealand. *Rural Sociology, 65*(4), 562–581.

Chaix, B., Guilbert, P., & Chauvin, P. (2004). A multilevel analysis of tobacco use and tobacco consumption levels in France—Are there any combination risk groups? *European Journal of Public Health, 14*(2), 186–190.

Chuang, Y.-C., Li, Y.-S., Wu, Y.-H., & Chao, H. (2007). A multilevel analysis of neighborhood and individual effects on individual smoking and drinking in Taiwan. *BMC Public Health, 7*(1), 151.

Davey Smith, G., Hart, C., Watt, G., Hole, D., & Hawthorne, V. (1998). Individual social class, area-based deprivation, cardiovascular disease risk-factors and mortality: The Renfrew and Paisley study. *Journal of Epidemiology and Community Health, 52*(6), 399–405.

Day, K., Gough, B., & McFadden, M. (2004). Warning! Alcohol can seriously damage your feminine health. A discourse analysis of recent British newspaper coverage of women and drinking. *Feminist Media Studies, 4*(2), 165–183.

Duncan, C., Jones, K., & Moon, G. (1999). Smoking and deprivation: Are there neighbourhood effects? *Social Science & Medicine, 48*(4), 497–505.

Ellaway, A., & Macintyre, S. (2001). Women in their place: Gender and perceptions of neighbourhoods in the West of Scotland. In I. Dyck, N. Davis Lewis, & S. McLafferty (Eds.), *Geographies of women's health*. London, New York: Routledge.

Ellaway, A., & Macintyre, S. (2009). Are perceived neighbourhood problems associated with the likelihood of smoking? *Journal of Epidemiology and Community Health, 63*, 78–90.

Ellaway, A, Benzeval, M, Green, M., Leyland, A., & Macintyre, S. (2012). Getting sicker quicker: does living in a more deprived neighbourhood mean your health deteriorates faster? *Health & Place, 18*(2), 132–137.

Ellaway, A., Macintyre, S., & Kearns, A. (2001). Perceptions of place and health in socially contrasting neighbourhoods. *Urban Studies, 38*(12), 2299–2316.

Emslie, C., Hunt, K., & Lyons, A. (2013). The role of alcohol in (re)constructing masculinities and maintaining friendships between men in early mid-life. Health Psychology special issue on men's health. *Health Psychology, 32*(1), 33–41.

Emslie, C., Hunt, K., & Macintyre, S. (1999). 'Gender' or 'job' differences? Reported working conditions amongst men and women in similar white-collar occupations. *Work, Employment and Society, 13*(4), 711–729.

Emslie, C., & Mitchell, R. (2009). Are there gender differences in the geography of alcohol-related mortality in Scotland? An ecological study. *BMC Public Health, 9*, 58.

Flynn, J., Slovic, P., & Mertz, C. (1994). Gender, race, and perception of environmental health risks. *Risk Analysis, 14*(6), 1101–1108.

Gough, B., & Edwards, G. (1998). The beer talking: Four lads, a carry out and the reproduction of masculinities. *The Sociological Review, 46*(3), 409–455.

Gustafson, P. E. (1996). Gender differences in risk perception: Theoretical and methodological perspectives. *Risk Analysis, 18*(6), 805–811.

Henwood, K., Parkhill, K., & Pidgeon, N. (2008). Science, technology and risk perception: From gender differences to the effects made by gender. *Equal Opportunities International, 27*(8), 662–676.

Hibell, B., Guttorrmsson, U., Ahlstrom, S., Balakireva, O., Bjarnason, T., Kokkevi, A., et al. (2009). *The 2007 ESPAD report: Substance use among students in 35 European countries. The Swedish council for information on alcohol and other*. Stockholm: Drugs.

Holloway, S., Jayne, M., & Valentine, G. (2008). 'Sainsbury's is my local': English alcohol policy, domestic drinking practices and the meaning of home. *Transactions of the Institute of British Geographers, 33*, 532–547.

Ivory, V. C., Collings, S. C., Blakely, T., & Dew, K. (2011). When does neighbourhood matter? Multilevel relationships between neighbourhood social fragmentation and mental health. *Social Science & Medicine, 72*(12), 1993–2002. doi: 10.1016/j.socscimed.2011.04.015.

Jackson, C., & Tinkler, P. (2007). "Ladettes" and "modern girls": "Troublesome" young femininities. *The Sociological Review, 55*(2), 251–272.

Jayne, M., Valentine, G., & Holloway, S. L. (2008). The place of drink: Geographical contributions to alcohol studies. *Drugs education prevention and policy, 15*(3), 219–232.

Jukkala, T., Makinen, I. H., Kislitsyna, O., Ferlander, S., & Vagero, D. (2008). Economic strain, social relations, gender, and binge drinking in Moscow. *Social Science & Medicine, 66*(3), 663–674.

Karpowicz-Lazreg, C., & Mullet, E. (1993). Societal risk as perceived by the French public. *Risk Analysis, 13*, 253–258.

Kavanagh, A. M., Kelly, M. T., Krnjacki, L., Thornton, L., Jolley, D., Subramanian, S. V., et al. (2011). Access to alcohol outlets and harmful alcohol consumption: a multi-level study in Melbourne, Australia. *Addiction, 106*(10), 1772–1779.

Kneale, J. (1999). "A problem of supervision": Moral geographies of the nineteenth-century British public house. *Journal of Historical Geography, 25*(3), 333–348.

Lemle, R., & Mishkind, M. (1989). Alcohol and masculinity. *J Subst Abuse Treat, 6*(4), 213–222.

Leon, D. A., Saburova, L., Tomkins, S., Andreev, E., Kiryanov, N., McKee, M., et al. (2007). Hazardous alcohol drinking and premature mortality in Russia: A population based case-control study. *Lancet, 369*(9578), 2001–2009.

Leyshon, M. (2008). "We're stuck in the corner" Young women, embodiment and drinking in the countryside. *Drugs Education Prevention and Policy, 15*(3), 267–289.

Lyons, A. C. (2009). Masculinities, femininities, behaviour and health. *Social and Personality Psychology Compass, 3*(4), 394–412.

Lyons, A. C., Dalton, S. I., & Hoy, A. (2006). Hardcore drinking. Portrayal of alcohol consumption in young women's and men's magazines. *Journal of Health Psychology, 11*(2), 223–232.

Lyons, A. C., & Willott, S. A. (2008). Alcohol consumption, gender identities and women's changing social positions. *Sex Roles, 59*(9–10), 694–712.

Makela, P., Gmel, G., Grittner, U., Kuendig, H., Kuntsche, S., Bloomfield, K. I. M., et al. (2006). Drinking patterns and their gender differences in Europe. *Alcohol and Alcoholism, 41*(suppl 1), i8–i18.

Matheson, F. I., White, H. L., Moineddin, R., Dunn, J. R., & Glazier, R. H. (2011). Drinking in context: The influence of gender and neighbourhood deprivation on alcohol consumption. *Journal of Epidemiology and Community Health*. doi:10.1136/jech.2010.112441.

McCartney, G., Mahmood, L., Leyland, A. H., Batty, G. D., & Hunt, K. (2011). Contribution of smoking-related and alcohol-related deaths to the gender gap in mortality: Evidence from 30 European countries. *Tobacco Control, 20*(2), 166–168.

Measham, F., & Ostergaard, J. (2009). The public face of binge drinking: British and Danish young women, recent trends in alcohol consumption and the European binge drinking debate. *Probation Journal, 56*(4), 415–434.

Molinari, C. (1998). The relationship of community quality to the health of women and men. *Social Science & Medicine, 47*(8), 1113–1120.

Mujahid, M. S., Diez Roux, A. V., Morenoff, J. D., Raghunathan, T. E., Cooper, R. S., Ni, H., et al. (2008). Neighborhood characteristics and hypertension. *Epidemiology, 19*(4), 590–598.

Nielsen, L., Curtis, T., Kristensen, T. S., & Rod Nielsen, N. (2008). What characterizes persons with high levels of perceived stress in Denmark? A national representative study. *Scandinavian Journal of Public Health, 36*(4), 369–379.

O'Donnell, S., Condell, S., & Begley, C. M. (2004). 'Add women & stir'—the biomedical approach to cardiac research! *European Journal of Cardiovascular Nursing, 3*, 119–127.

Ormston, R., Webster, C. (2008). Scottish social attitudes survey 2007: Something to be ashamed of or part of our way of life? Attitudes towards alcohol in Scotland. Edinburgh: Scottish Centre for Social Research. http://www.scotland.gov.uk/Publications/2008/08/01112431/11.

Pearce, J., Barnett, R., & Moon, G. (2012). Socio-spatial inequalities in health-related behaviours: pathways linking place and smoking. *Progress in Human Geography, 36*, 3–21.

Pietila, I., & Rytkonen, M. (2008). Coping with stress and by stress: Russian men and women talking about transition, stress and health. *Social Science & Medicine, 66*(2), 327–338.

Plant, M. L. (2008). The role of alcohol in women's lives: a review of issues and responses. *Journal of Substance Use, 13*(3), 155–191.

Poortinga, W., Dunstan, F. D., & Fone, D. L. (2007). Perceptions of the neighbourhood environment and self rated health: a multilevel analysis of the Caerphilly Health and Social Needs Study. *BMC Public Health, 7*, 285.

Raleigh, V., & Kiri, V. (1997). Life expectancy in England: Variations and trends by gender, health authority, and level of deprivation. *Journal of Epidemiology and Community Health, 51*, 649–658.

Rehm, J., Sulkowska, U., Manczuk, M., Boffetta, P., Powles, J., Popova, S., et al. (2007). Alcohol accounts for a high proportion of premature mortality in central and Eastern Europe. *International Journal of Epidemiology, 36*(2), 458–467.

Rehm, J., Taylor, B., & Patra, J. (2006). Volume of alcohol consumption, patterns of drinking and burden of disease in the European region 2002. *Addiction, 101*(8), 1086–1095.

Reijneveld, S. A. (1998). The impact of individual and area characteristics on urban socioeconomic differences in health and smoking. *International Journal of Epidemiology, 27*(1), 33–40.

Robinson, J., Deborah, R., Amos, A., Cunningham-Burley, S., Ritchie, D., Greaves, L., et al. (2010). Waiting until they got home: Gender, smoking and tobacco exposure in households in Scotland. *Social Science & Medicine*, 71(5), 884–890.

Ross, C. E. (2000). Walking, exercising, and smoking: Does neighborhood matter? *Social Science & Medicine, 51*(2), 265–274.

Savage, I. (1993). Demographic influences on risk perceptions. *Risk Analysis, 13*, 413–420.

Scotland, I. S. D. (2011). *Alcohol statistics Scotland*. Edinburgh: NHS National Services Scotland.

Shareck, M., & Ellaway, A. (2011). Neighbourhood crime and smoking: The role of objective and perceived crime measures. *BMC Public Health, 11*, 930.

Shohaimi, S., Luben, R., Wareham, N., Day, N., Bingham, S., Welch, A., et al. (2003). Residential area deprivation predicts smoking habit independently of individual educational level and occupational social class. A cross sectional study in the Norfolk cohort of the European Investigation into Cancer (EPIC-Norfolk). *Journal of Epidemiology and Community Health, 57*(4), 270–276.

Singh, G., & Siahpush, M. (2006). Widening socioeconomic inequalities in US life expectancy, 1980–2000. *International Journal of Epidemiology, 35*, 969–979.

Stafford, M., Cummins, S., Macintyre, S., Ellaway, A., & Marmot, M. (2005). Gender differences in the associations between health and neighbourhood environment. *Social Science & Medicine, 60*(8), 1681–1692.

Stead, M., MacAskill, S., MacKintosh, A., Reece, J., & Eadie, D. (2001). It's as if you're locked in: Qualitative explanations for area effects on smoking in disadvantaged communities. *Health & Place, 7*(4), 333–343.

Stern, P., & Kalof, L. (1993). Value orientations, gender and environmental concerns. *Environment and Behavior, 25*, 322–348.

Sundquist, J., Malmstrom, M., & Johansson, S. (1999). Cardiovascular risk factors and the neighbourhood environment: A multilevel analysis. *International Journal of Epidemiology, 28*, 841–845.

van Praag, L., Bracke, P., Christiaens, W., Levecque, K., & Pattyn, E. (2009). Mental health in a gendered context: Gendered community effect on depression and problem drinking. *Health & Place, 15*(4), 990–998.

Weden, M., Carpiano, R., & Robert, S. (2008). Subjective and objective neighbourhood characteristics and adult health. *Social Science & Medicine, 66*, 1256–1270.

Wilsnack, R. W., Vogeltanz, N. D., Wilsnack, S. C., & Harris, T. R. (2000). Gender differences in alcohol consumption and adverse drinking consequences: Cross-cultural patterns. *Addiction, 95*(2), 251–265.

Wojtyniak, B., Moskalewicz, J., Stokwiszewski, J., & Rabczenko, D. (2005). Gender-specific mortality associated with alcohol consumption in Poland in transition. *Addiction, 100*(12), 1779–1789.

Chapter 19
From Neighbourhood and Health Research to Health Promotion Practice

Christiane Stock

Introduction

Health promotion differs from prevention or risk reduction approaches by being broader and not limited on targeting a single risk factor or disease (Naidoo and Wills 2000). In contrast, health promotion tries to enhance each person's ability to improve their own health. A central goal in this respect is to create environments that support health, well-being and healthy lifestyles. This means health promotion also seeks to create a context in which health can evolve spontaneously. In contrast to putting an emphasis on care, health promotion aims to prevent disease by modifying the social determinants of health or sometimes called 'causes of the causes'.

The Ottawa Charter for Health Promotion (Ottawa Charter 1986) has given a well-known discussion of health promotion approaches and has outlined five strategies. (1) *Building healthy public policy:* This strategy is related to the decisions made at all levels of government and by organisations that work towards health improvement. It includes legislation, policies, taxation and organisational change in areas such as recreation, welfare, transport, education and housing. This puts health on the agenda for all policymakers, directing them to be aware of the health consequences of their decisions. (2) *Creating supportive environments:* This strategy recognises the importance of environment for health and proposed a socio-ecological approach to health. The protection of the natural and built environments and the conservation of natural resources are central elements here in order to maintain a healthy physical environment. The strategy focuses on the places people live, work and play and on increasing people's ability, within these, to make health-promoting choices. (3) *Strengthening community action:* Health promotion requires

C. Stock (✉)
Unit for Health Promotion Research, Institute of Public Health,
University of Southern Denmark, Niels Bohrs Vej 9-10, 6700 Esbjerg, Denmark
e-mail: cstock@health.sdu.dk

C. Stock and A. Ellaway (eds.), *Neighbourhood Structure and Health Promotion*,
DOI 10.1007/978-1-4614-6672-7_19, © Springer Science+Business Media New York 2013

community empowerment and involvement in setting priorities, planning and implementing strategies to achieve better health. The focus is here to give communities the chance to identify and implement actions that address their health concerns. (4) *Developing personal skills:* Health promotion supports personal and social development through providing information and enhancing life skills. The aim is to empower the individual, increasing the option available to people and allowing them to exercise more control over their own health and their environments. (5) *Reorienting health services:* Health promotion argues for shifting health resources towards a more equal distribution between health care and preventing disease. Essentially, health services should be expanded to include the four strategies above in addition to conventional medical care. Responsibility for health promotion services should be shared amongst individuals, community groups, health professionals, health services and governments.

This chapter will explore the ways in which neighbourhood and health research can inform health promotion practice with respect to the five strategy areas outlined by the Ottawa Charter.

Building Healthy Public Policy with Impact on Neighbourhood Structure

Social and Housing Policy

Several factors identified as relevant in neighbourhood and health research, such as neighbourhood deprivation and disorganisation, call for intervening at policy level and thus to address the 'causes of the causes'. Interventions to address the 'upstream' determinants of health, such as poverty, unemployment, poor housing and income and education inequality, have the potential to influence population health more profoundly than individually oriented behavioural programmes (Galea et al. 2007). Governments can influence social inequality and its consequences such as neighbourhood deprivation in many ways through social policies. A World Health Organisation (WHO) report on the social determinants of health suggests that governments shall impact the distribution of income towards reducing inequality through policies on taxes, benefits, employment, education or economic management (Wilkinson and Marmot 2003). In particular, absolute poverty should be eliminated and material inequality reduced through minimum income guarantees and minimum wages legislation. Further, legislative measures should be put in place to protect minority and vulnerable groups from social exclusion as well as policies to reduce barriers to affordable housing. Social stratification as an underlying pattern of neighbourhood deprivation and disorganisation should be reduced through labour market, education and family welfare policies (Wilkinson and Marmot 2003).

Social policies at national, regional and local levels have the potential to create neighbourhoods with a more equal level of housing quality, as well as improved neighbourhood safety. In addition, residential segregation would be reduced leading to lower differences between neighbourhoods in the composition of residents in neighbourhoods regarding characteristics such as income, education or employment status. In most European countries and especially in the Scandinavian welfare states such policies exist and result in less absolute inequalities between rich and poor, although relative differences still exist (Eikemo et al. 2008). Consequently, European studies do not show the same impact of neighbourhood characteristics on, i.e. alcohol and other drug use as seen in most studies from urban neighbourhoods in the USA (see Chap. 15). This is also supported by the work of Wilkinson and Pickett (2009) claiming that for each of eleven different health and social problems, including trust and community life, outcomes are significantly worse in more unequal rich countries.

Urban Planning Policies

Although city planning originated out of concerns about health problems caused by poor housing and industries around the turn of the last century, the fields of public health and planning became uncoupled. Whilst public health took a more biomedical focus on individual determinants of health and epidemiology, the planning of built environments was often driven by a focus on car mobility. The WHO's Healthy Cities movement, initiated in 1988, encouraged attention again on urban planning as one of the important factors to improve health in the urban environment. Neighbourhood and health research contributes to the attention on urban planning to improve health conditions in cities. Several factors have been identified as relevant. Improving the walkability of neighbourhoods as well as access to green spaces has the potential to increase physical activity and reduce air pollution level (e.g. Ding et al. 2011, see also Chaps. 11 and 12). Other aspects of urban planning improving aesthetics and safety of neighbourhoods have also positive impact on well-being and mental health of residents but also encourage outdoor activity and mobility. Urban planning has also the potential to have an impact on availability of alcohol and on the food offered in neighbourhoods (see sections below).

A positive impact on walkability and use of public transport can, e.g. be reached through mixed density building. Mixed density refers to urban development taking a mix of housing types and a variety of development forms such as size and height into account. It is suggested that mixed density developments should be integrated with surrounding development, with public transport and with supporting infrastructure including walkways, public areas and cycle paths (http://www.healthyplaces.org.au). Land use mix is another component of the built environment that has been associated with positive health outcomes (LEED for Neighbourhood Development 2006). This is because mixing land uses leads to shorter trips and motivates residents to move from automobiles to pedestrian, bicycle and transit travel. It also makes it possible for people to combine trips, such as shopping and commuting, when retail and employment uses are close together. As a consequence, the total number of trips taken by automobile decreases and thus emissions are reduced.

The national health policy in the UK *Healthy Weight, Healthy Lives, 2008*, suggests that cycle pathways and walking should take priority when developing or maintaining roads, that new workplaces are linked to walking and cycling networks and to invest in training for planners (urban, rural and transport), architects and designers on the health implications of local plans, for example, spatial plans and planning applications (Department of Health 2008). The Swedish national public health policy is also supporting local partnerships in the development of urban planning strategies through structured mapping protocols regarding contextual social determinants of health (Wamela 2010). These are examples that neighbourhood and health research can result in national policies for urban planning. However, the effects of these policy approaches on urban and neighbourhood structures and moreover on reducing the equity in health gap still need to be studied in long-term monitoring and evaluation.

Transport Policy

Transport policy is closely intertwined with urban planning and serves partly the same purposes. A transport policy with potential to promote health should encourage active transport in order to increase daily physical activity level and reduce greenhouse gas emissions. Active transport encompasses non-motorised forms of transport involving physical activity, such as cycling and walking. Public transport can also be included, if longer distance trips are done, which usually include walking or cycling components as part of the journey. If the urban structure will be designed so that walking and cycling trips are convenient, pleasant and safe, active transport will be more attractive for many people. High levels of amenity, especially to key destinations such as workplaces, schools and shops, as well as mixed land uses and densities, and choices of destinations are key factors to encourage modes of active transport.

Beyond encouraging active transport through urban planning and public transport policies, other regulations and incentive systems can also support active transport. These measures can range from 'job tickets' subsidised by employers to fiscal measures discouraging car use as a mode of transport to work.

School-Based Policies with Impact on Area Around Schools

As Shalida Svatisalee describes in Chap. 17, schools have also a potential to influence surrounding neighbourhoods through school-based policies. As schools and also other educational institutions like universities are settings embedded in a wider community, they have a potential to reach out and have an impact on the residential area around them (Doherty et al. 2011). One option how school or other organisations' policy could potentially reach out and influence the neighbouring environment would be through local partnerships and co-operations. For example, school-based food policies could be accompanied by partnerships with shop owners to improve the availability and price promotion of healthy foods and snacks as suggested by Gabauer and Laska (2011).

Creating Supportive Environments in Residential Areas

Renewal Programmes

In some countries, neighbourhood renewal programmes have been launched in order to narrow the gap between deprived and non-deprived neighbourhoods (see also Chap. 14). One example exists in Northern Ireland, where in 2003, the government launched *People and Place—A strategy for Neighbourhood Renewal* (Department for Social Development 2011). This strategy was planned long term (7–10 years) and was targeted towards those communities throughout Northern Ireland suffering the highest levels of deprivation. Neighbourhood renewal understands itself as a cross government strategy and aims to bring together the work of all government departments in partnership with local people to tackle disadvantage and deprivation in all aspects of everyday life.

Neighbourhoods in the most deprived 10 % of wards across Northern Ireland were identified, and this resulted in a total of 36 areas, and a population of approximately 280,000 (one person in six in Northern Ireland), being targeted for intervention. In each neighbourhood renewal area partnerships have been established in order to lead local planning and implementation. Each neighbourhood partnership includes representatives of key political, statutory, voluntary, community and private sector stakeholders. Together, they have developed long-term visions and action plans designed to improve the quality of life for those living in the area. A midterm review has summarised some positive outcomes regarding unemployment, education and crime, whilst the health indicators remained unchanged (Department for Social Development 2011). It is stated in the report that there has been some narrowing of the gap between the neighbourhood renewal areas and the rest of Northern Ireland on a range of the outcome indicators. However, place-related outcomes have been shown to be easier to achieve than people-related outcomes. In addition, partnership formation has suffered from several problems in the intervention areas.

The *New Deal for Communities* programme was a key part of the UK government's strategy to tackle multiple deprivation in some of the most deprived neighbourhoods in the country, but the programme did not demonstrate a positive effect on health inequalities in the targeted areas in a two-year follow-up study (Stafford et al. 2008).

However, a more long-term evaluation showed more promising results on the national strategy for neighbourhood renewal that has been launched by the Labour government in the UK in 2001. After 10 years, the strategy has been evaluated and the summary report concluded: 'Whilst no case neighbourhood was able to consistently narrow the gap across all domains, individual examples of success amongst each domain have demonstrated the important role of local spatial interventions in helping to alleviate or contain neighbourhood deprivation' (Department for Communities and Local Government 2010, p. 9).

Availability of Alcohol and Tobacco

As summarised in Chap. 15, the density of alcohol outlets is associated with its use in several population groups (Grunewald et al. 1993; Scribner et al. 2000; Chen et al. 2010). It has therefore been suggested that regulation of outlet density may be a useful tool for the reduction of excessive alcohol consumption and related harm in neighbourhoods (Campbell et al. 2009). When reviewing the effectiveness of such an approach, Campbell et al. and the Task Force for Community Preventive Services concluded: 'Using a variety of different study methods, study populations, and alcohol measures, most of the studies included in this review reported that greater outlet density is associated with increased alcohol consumption and related harms, including medical harms, injuries, crime, and violence. This convergent evidence comes both from studies that directly evaluated outlet density (or changes in outlet density) and those that evaluated the effects of policy changes that had a substantial impact on outlet density, including studies of privatization, remonopolization, bans on alcohol sales and the removal of bans, and changes in density from known policy interventions and from unknown causes' (Campbell et al. 2009, p. 565–566). Alcohol outlet density may be controlled through licensing and zoning regulations. In addition, as mentioned above in the section on urban planning, restrictions on the use and development of land can also have an impact on the availability of alcohol in neighbourhoods (Ashe et al. 2003).

Similarly have policies and regulations limiting tobacco sale also the potential to reduce tobacco availability in neighbourhoods or in specific areas, such as areas around schools with demonstrated effects on smoking (Forster et al. 2007, see also Chap. 14).

From Obesogenic to Health-Promoting Neighbourhoods

Environmental factors play a crucial role in promoting poor diet and obesity, and disadvantaged neighbourhoods are often so-called obesogenic environments (Black and Macinko 2008; Harrison et al. 2011; see also Chap. 17). Some factors of neighbourhoods such as provision of safe green spaces in which to exercise contribute to physical activity, whilst the offer of healthy food options contribute to better diet choices. Both aspects of neighbourhoods need to be promoted in order to avoid obesogenic environments and to stimulate residents to take healthier choices. The following two sections will explore options in these two areas of neighbourhood-level intervention.

Influencing the Availability of Healthy Food Options

Not only in the USA where neighbourhoods are relatively homogenous with respect to socioeconomic characteristics but also in the UK, take-away food is more often found in deprived areas (see Chap. 16) and the density of fast-food outlets was found to correlate closely with levels of obesity amongst children (Fraser and Edwards 2010). Therefore, it has been recommended to provide local authorities with powers to prevent fast-food outlets opening near parks and schools (Aylott et al. 2008) as a governmental policy to reduce obesogenic environments. A *Local Government Act 2000* allows local authorities in England and Wales to intervene in order to promote the economic, social and environmental well-being of areas unless prohibited by law (Department for Communities and Local Government 2008). This option for regulatory approaches is increasingly used (Department for Communities and Local Government 2008). The idea is taken up at local level by public health practitioners to work with retailers to encourage them to offer healthy food choices (Hanratty et al. 2012). A qualitative study using interviews with directors, managers and public service staff concluded though that encouraging food outlets to contribute to tackling the obesogenic environment is a major challenge for local public health teams and that supportive national policies are needed (Hanratty et al. 2012). From these UK experiences, it can be concluded that at policy and local level, at least in some countries, awareness has increased that neighbourhood environments can promote poor nutrition and that local co-operations with retailers are important in order to change obesogenic environments. However, the existing approaches at local level do not seem to be adequately backed up by regulatory and legislative support, are still sparse and have had limited success (Hanratty et al. 2012). In another study with 45 senior representatives and policy decision makers in Australia, over one third of participants suggested planning regulations to limit the density of fast-food outlets and/or improve access to healthy fresh fruits, but these were still amongst the least supported interventions to promote healthy food environments, whilst food marketing and service interventions were more supported (Shill et al. 2012).

When Neighbourhoods Move Their Residents

Research evidence regarding the impact of the physical and built environment of neighbourhoods on the level of physical activity of residents (see Chaps. 11 and 12) has informed several intervention projects. Many city councils mainly in the United Kingdom, Germany and the Netherlands have set up *home zones* which are environments designed to support physical activity. Home zones work through the physical alteration of streets and roads in an area forcing motorists to drive with greater care and at lower speeds. The benches, flower beds, play areas, lamp posts, fences and trees used to alter the streets and roads offer many additional community benefits.

The *SPACE* project is an example from Denmark which aims at investigating the impact of structural interventions to promote physical activity amongst children and adolescents. The project includes 6–8 municipalities in which an intervention and a control neighbourhood will be established. The intervention is aimed at (1) promoting active transport, (2) improving the school's outdoor areas, (3) establishing *play-spots* which are places to attract young people to be physically active in the leisure time, and (4) organised physical fitness. Several physical improvements will be made in each of the four intervention areas to either modify existing structures or establish new ones. Such physical structural enhancement of the neighbourhoods will be followed up by organisational interventions that support the options for physical activity by, e.g. changed access conditions or traffic action plans (http://cirhp.rup.mico.dk/side.asp?side=8&id=17&ver=uk).

A similar project in Denmark is the *When Cities Move Children* project, which aims at studying the impact of a district revitalisation on 11–15-year-old children's level of physical activity and movement patterns in a disadvantaged neighbourhood in Copenhagen. The intervention is defined by the changes that will be made to the physical environment in the neighbourhood, including the improvement of buildings and open spaces, two urban renewal initiatives, four initiatives directed towards improving the cityscape and traffic schemes and a number of small building projects (http://cirhp.rup.mico.dk/side.asp?side=8&id=18&ver=uk).

Both projects will be scientifically evaluated partly with the use of GPS, accelerometers and GIS (for a description of these techniques, see Chap. 10).

Strengthening Community Action

Another approach at the neighbourhood level would be community interventions based on participatory and empowerment strategies to strengthen social cohesion and sense of community. Such programmes have been shown to increase social capital and other indictors of community strength (Minkler and Wallerstein 2007). However, evidence is still sparse on whether such programmes lead to health or health behaviour improvements. A community intervention programme in the Netherlands has shown some promising results in increasing fruit consumption but failed to find a decrease in alcohol consumption or other health improvements (Kloek et al. 2006). Community empowerment or participation approaches have the potential to reduce social isolation, increase self-efficacy to change health behaviours and increase access to care and other intermediate outcomes that may affect health indirectly (Minkler and Wallerstein 2007).

Even if community development programmes are leading to more social capital and community capacity, some authors have raised the concern of a potential victim-blaming attitude, that communities would be healthier if they would overcome their social deficit and just better work together to solve their problems (Warren et al. 2001). Therefore, such community development programmes are not an alternative to providing greater financial resources and public services to disadvantaged neighbourhoods.

Developing Personal Skills

Theories on area impact on health imply that both the physical and the social environments contribute to health inequalities (Diez Roux and Mair 2010). Consequently, interventions aiming at reducing health inequalities should intervene both on the level of the physical environment but also on the level of strengthening the personal skills and capabilities of residents living in disadvantaged areas. Macintyre et al. (2002) have pointed out that an exclusive focus on either the material or the psychosocial features of place is counterproductive for urban regeneration. Therefore, investment in places should best be accompanied by investment in people living in these areas.

An approach offering low-barrier and equal access options for the health improvement of residents living in disadvantaged neighbourhoods is the establishing of *Healthy Living Centres*. As one example, the *East End Healthy Living Centre* in Glasgow provides facilities and services which help improve the health of the community through offering opportunities for learning, for social interaction and for leisure activities (EastEnd Healthy Living Centre 2006).

The research finding of higher rates of adolescent smoking, poorer diet and lower level of physical activity in disadvantaged areas has also resulted in several projects allocating educational activities and prevention projects towards such neighbourhoods. As Sharek and Frohlich have argued in Chap. 14, such interventions are unlikely to be successful in reducing health inequalities if they are targeted on the individual only, such as offering smoking cessation in disadvantaged neighbourhoods. Even, if such community interventions involve community participation and coalition building, such as the *Wijkgezondheidswerk* project in the Netherlands (already cited in the section above), only a small impact on health behaviour could be demonstrated (Kloek et al. 2006). Limited effectiveness of the educational activities implemented was one explanation for the lack of positive health outcomes. Other research has shown that participation of residents in neighbourhood development initiatives depends on prior participation experience and ethnicity, which suggests that not all residents will be activated by such programmes in the same way (Fröding et al. 2012). Such research suggests that improving basic, in particular school education and skills training that enable people to actively participate in community programmes, is important.

Research on neighbourhood contexts and alcohol and drug use indicates that families play an important role in mediating between neighbourhood risks and consumption of alcohol and other drugs amongst youth (Chuang et al. 2005; Tobler et al. 2009). For example, it has been shown that mothers who perceive greater problems in their neighbourhoods use less effective monitoring strategies of their children (Byrnes et al. 2011). Byrnes et al. (2011) suggest that prevention programmes should address parental monitoring needs based upon neighbourhood differences. A study looking at parenting interventions within the *Sure Start* programme in Wales examined 153 parents from socially deprived areas and showed that a course teaching improved parenting skills had great benefits in reducing problem behaviour in young children (Hutchings et al. 2007), which may result in reduced drug-taking behaviour later in life.

Reorienting Health Services

One pathway through which disadvantaged areas may affect health is through services provided, which would contribute to the material or infrastructural resources of a residential area (Macintyre et al. 2002). Amongst the services with relevance to health, the health service is likely to be of special importance. Even in countries with universal access to medical care, unequal access to and quality of primary and secondary healthcare services, discrimination in the access or delivery of care, and/or other healthcare-related factors may contribute to lower primary and secondary healthcare provision in deprived neighbourhoods (Winkleby et al. 2007). The actual number of health professionals working in primary healthcare clinics can also vary considerably by neighbourhood type due to difficulties in recruiting and retaining healthcare personnel in high-deprivation neighbourhoods.

Indeed does empirical research from the UK suggest a mismatch between the number of general practitioners in areas and population served with a tendency for deprived areas being under-served and affluent areas being over-served (e.g. Benzeval and Judge 1996; Hippisley-Cox and Pringle 2000). Inequity in the supply of GPs between deprived and less deprived areas has been addressed in *The White Paper on Primary Care* (Department of Health 2006) giving a commitment to improving access to primary care services in a number of ways, but the main focus was on increasing supply in deprived areas.

However, even if more services are provided, the success of such policy is depending on the ability of people from vulnerable groups to use the services adequately. Although consultation rates amongst disadvantaged groups are usually high, some other barriers may exist that limited the effects of service provision amongst socially disadvantaged groups. For example, the *Sure Start* programme had some limited success in the socially deprived areas, which the programme targeted. The *Sure Start* programme was a major national initiative to enhance the health and development of children under 4 years and their families living in socially deprived areas by improving access to services and creating new ones, with services targeted at local needs (Department for Children, Schools and Families 2009). When *Sure Start* areas were compared with comparison areas (Belsky et al. 2006), the results showed that the differences between intervention areas and comparison areas were limited and varied by degree of social deprivation. Interestingly, the programme had beneficial effects on non-teenage mothers (better parenting, better social functioning in children) and adverse effects on children of teenage mothers (poorer social functioning) and children of single parents or parents who did not work (lower verbal ability). In conclusion, the policy was found to benefit the relatively less socially deprived parents and children but actually had an adverse effect on the most disadvantaged children.

Since the authors suggest that socially deprived families with greater personal resources were better able to take advantage of the services and resources provided in the *Sure Start* (Belsky et al. 2006), one can conclude that providing services alone has limited potential to reduce health inequalities in disadvantaged neighbourhoods and populations.

Conclusions

Research on neighbourhood structure and health can inform policy and health promotion practice in many ways and at different levels. This chapter does not claim to be comprehensive in summarising all relevant approaches but rather gives some examples and sheds light on how this area of research can add to the five strategies of health promotion outlined by the Ottawa Charter. When the ultimate aim of health promotion efforts at neighbourhood would bring about the *healthy neighbourhood,* the organising framework becomes complex and involves (1) the physical features of the environment, (2) the availability of healthy environments at home, work and play (3) services provided to support people in their daily lives (4) the sociocultural features of a neighbourhood and (5) the reputation of an area (Macintyre et al. 2002). The strategies of the Ottawa Charter address all these areas. Programmes that involve most of the strategies and are long term have the best chances to achieve sustainable effects but require organised intersectoral collaboration between policy makers, urban planners, health and welfare service providers, educational institutions, private businesses and retailers, public health experts and community organisations.

References

Ashe, M., Jernigan, D., Kline, R., & Galaz, R. (2003). Land use planning and the control of alcohol, tobacco, firearms, and fast food restaurants. *American Journal of Public Health, 93*(9), 1404–1408.

Aylott, J., Brown, I., Copeland, R., & Johnson, D. (2008). *Tackling obesities: The foresight report and recommendations for local authorities*. Sheffield: Sheffield Hallam University. http://www.idea.gov.uk/idk/aio/8268011.

Belsky, J., Melhuish, E., Barnes, J., Leyland, A. H., Romaniuk, H., & National Evaluation of Sure Start Research Team. (2006). Effects of Sure Start local programmes on children and families: Early findings from a quasi-experimental, cross sectional study. *BMJ, 332*(7556), 1476.

Benzeval, M., & Judge, K. (1996). Access to health care in England: Continuing inequalities in the distribution of GPs. *Journal of Public Health Medicine, 18*(1), 33–40.

Black, J. L., & Macinko, J. (2008). Neighborhoods and obesity. *Nutrition Reviews, 66*(1), 2–20.

Byrnes, H. F., Miller, B. A., Chen, M. J., & Grube, J. W. (2011). The roles of mothers' neighborhood perceptions and specific monitoring strategies in youths' problem behavior. *Journal of Youth and Adolescence, 40*(3), 347–360.

Campbell, C. A., Hahn, R. A., Elder, R., Brewer, R., Chattopadhyay, S., Fielding, J., et al. (2009). The effectiveness of limiting alcohol outlet density as a means of reducing excessive alcohol consumption and alcohol-related harms. *American Journal of Preventive Medicine, 37*(6), 556–569.

Chen, M. J., Grube, J. W., & Gruenewald, P. J. (2010). Community alcohol outlet density and underage drinking. *Addiction, 105*(2), 270–278.

Chuang, Y. C., Ennett, S. T., Bauman, K. E., & Foshee, V. A. (2005). Neighbourhood influences on adolescent cigarette and alcohol use: Mediating effects through parent and peer behaviours. *Journal of Health and Social Behavior, 46*, 187–204.

Department for Children, Schools and Families. (2009). *The 1998 Green Paper*. London: Department for Children, Schools and Families.

Department for Communities and Local Government. (2008). *Practical use of well-being power*. London: Department for Communities and Local Government. http://communities.gov.uk.

Department for Communities and Local Government. (2010). *Evaluation of the national strategy for neighbourhood renewal: Local research project*. London: Department for Communities and Local Government.

Department for Social Development. (2011). *People and place: A strategy for neighbourhood renewal—Midterm review*. Belfast: Department for Social Development.

Department of Health. (2006). *Our health, our care, our say: A new direction for community services*. London: Department of Health.

Department of Health. (2008). *Healthy weight, healthy lives*. London: Department of Health.

Diez Roux, A. V., & Mair, C. (2010). Neighbourhoods and health. *Annals of the New York Academy of Sciences, 1186*, 125–145.

Ding, D., Sallis, J. F., Kerr, J., Lee, S., & Rosenberg, D. E. (2011). Neighborhood environment and physical activity among youth: A review. *American Journal of Preventive Medicine, 41*(4), 442–455.

Doherty, S., Cawood, J., & Dooris, M. (2011). Applying the whole-settings approach to food within universities. *Perspectives in Public Health, 131*, 217–224.

EastEnd Healthy Living Centre. (2006). *Annual report 2006*. Glasgow: EastEnd Healthy Living Centre. http://www.eehlc.org.uk/Uploads/1260175548_annual_report_final_version.pdf.

Eikemo, T. A., Bambra, C., Joyce, K., & Dahl, E. (2008). Welfare state regimes and income-related health inequalities: A comparison of 23 European countries. *European Journal of Public Health, 18*(6), 593–599.

Forster, J. L., Widome, R., & Bernat, D. H. (2007). Policy interventions and surveillance as strategies to prevent tobacco use in adolescents and young adults. *American Journal of Preventive Medicine, 33*(6), 335–339.

Fraser, L. K., & Edwards, K. (2010). The association between the geography of fast food outlets and childhood obesity rates in Leeds, UK. *Health & Place, 16*(6), 1124–1128.

Fröding, K., Elander, I., & Eriksson, C. (2012). Neighbourhood development and public health initiatives: Who participates? *Health Promotion International, 27*(1), 102–116.

Galea, S., Ahem, J., Tracy, M., & Vlahov, D. (2007). Neighbourhood income and income distribution and the use of cigarettes, alcohol, and marijuana. *American Journal of Public Health, 32*(6), 195–202.

Gebauer, H., & Laska, M. N. (2011). Convenience stores surrounding urban schools: An assessment of health food availability, advertising, and product placement. *Journal of Urban Health, 88*(4), 616–622.

Grunewald, P. J., Millar, A. B., & Treno, A. J. (1993). Alcohol availability and the ecology of drinking behaviour. *Alcohol Health and Research World, 17*, 39–45.

Hanratty, B., Milton, B., Ashton, M., & Whitehead, M. (2012). "McDonalds and KFC, it's never going to happen": The challenges of working with food outlets to tackle the obesogenic environment. *Journal of Public Health, 34*(4), 548–554. doi:10.1093/pubmed/fds036.

Harrison, F., Jones, A. P., van Sluijs, E. M., Cassidy, A., Bentham, G., & Griffin, S. J. (2011). Environmental correlates of adiposity in 9–10 year old children: Considering home and school neighbourhoods and routes to school. *Social Science & Medicine, 72*(9), 1411–1419.

Hippisley-Cox, J., & Pringle, M. (2000). Inequalities in access to coronary angiography and re-vascularisation: The association of deprivation and location of primary care services. *British Journal of General Practice, 50*(455), 449–454.

Hutchings, J., Bywater, T., Daley, D., Gardner, F., Whitaker, C., Jones, K., et al. (2007). Parenting intervention in Sure Start services for children at risk of developing conduct disorder: Pragmatic randomised controlled trial. *BMJ, 334*(7595), 678. doi:10.1136/bmj.39126.620799.55.

Kloek, G. C., van Lenthe, F. J., van Nierop, P. W. M., Koelen, M. A., & Mackenback, J. P. (2006). Impact evaluation of a Dutch community intervention to improve health-related behaviour in deprived neighbourhoods. *Health & Place, 12*, 665–677.

LEED for Neighbourhood Development. (2006). Understanding the relationship between physical activity and obesity. Sydney, NSW Health Department and NSW Centre for public health and the built environment. LEED-ND Core Committee, USA.

Macintyre, S., Ellaway, A., & Cummings, S. (2002). Place effects on health: How can we conceptualise, operationalise and measure them? *Social Science & Medicine, 55*, 125–139.

Minkler, M., & Wallerstein, N. (2007). Improving health through community organization and community building: A health education perspective. In M. Minkler (Ed.), *Community organizing and community building for health* (pp. 26–50). New Brunswick, New Jersey, London: Rutgers University Press.

Naidoo, J., & Wills, J. (2000). *Health promotion: Foundations for practice*. Edinburgh: Elsevier Science.

Ottawa Charter. (1986). Ottawa Charter for Health Promotion. Health Promotion International 1:ii–v.

Scribner, R. A., Cohen, D. A., & Fisher, W. (2000). Evidence of a structural effect for outlet density: A multilevel analysis. *Alcoholism, Clinical and Experimental Research, 24*(2), 188–195.

Shill, J., Mavoa, H., Allender, S., Lawrence, M., Sacks, G., Peeters, A., et al. (2012). Government regulation to promote healthy food environments—A view from inside state governments. *Obesity Reviews, 13*(2), 162–173.

Stafford, M., Nazroo, J., Popay, J. M., & Whitehead, M. (2008). Tackling inequalities in health: Evaluating the new deal for communities initiative. *Journal of Epidemiology and Community Health, 62*(4), 298–304.

Tobler, A. L., Komro, K. A., & Maldonado-Molina, M. M. (2009). Relationship between neighbourhood context, family management practices and alcohol, use among urban, multi-ethnic, young adolescents. *Prevention Science, 10*(4), 313–324.

Wamela, S. (2010). *Is the Swedish national public health policy closing the gap? Lessons learned from the WHO Commission on the Social Determinants of Health.* Paper presented at the Expert conference, Moving forward equity in health, Madrid 21st April 2010. http://www.fhi.se/Documents/Aktuellt/Nyheter/Wamala-paper.pdf.

Warren, M. R., Thompson, J. P., & Saegert, S. (2001). The role of social capital in combating poverty. In S. Saegert, J. P. Thompson, & M. R. Warren (Eds.), *Social capital and poor communities* (pp. 1–28). New York: Sage Foundation.

Wilkinson, R., & Marmot, M. (2003). *Social determinants of health: The solid facts*. Copenhagen: World Health Organization.

Wilkinson, R., & Pickett, K. (2009). *The spirit level: Why more equal societies almost always do better*. London: Allan Lane.

Winkleby, M., Sundquist, K., & Cubbin, C. (2007). Inequities in CHD incidence and case fatality by neighborhood deprivation. *American Journal of Preventive Medicine, 32*(2), 97–106.

Index

C. Stock and A. Ellaway (eds.), *Neighbourhood Structure and Health Promotion*,
DOI 10.1007/978-1-4614-6672-7, © Springer Science+Business Media New York 2013

N

O

P

R

MIX
Papier aus verantwortungsvollen Quellen
Paper from responsible sources
FSC® C105338

If you have any concerns about our products,
you can contact us on
ProductSafety@springernature.com

In case Publisher is established outside the EU,
the EU authorized representative is:
Springer Nature Customer Service Center GmbH
Europaplatz 3, 69115 Heidelberg, Germany

Printed by Libri Plureos GmbH
in Hamburg, Germany